PRAISE FOR *APHRODISIAC*

"Kimberly Gallagher's life-changing, life-enhancing, and life-expanding book *Aphrodisiac* is quite simply delicious. She takes the reader on a spine-tingling, heart-opening, and pulse-quickening awakening of all of our senses, leading each of us to experience the expansive wonder of all the sensual delights that life can offer."
— Regena Thomashauer, *New York Times* best-selling author of *Pussy: A Reclamation* and Creatrix of Mama Gena's School of Womanly Arts

"*Aphrodisiac* is a sensuous delight and a love letter to life itself. It invites and entices us to engage in the everyday aspects of life as sensuous acts of pleasure, and then goes on to explain in lovely detail exactly how to do so. This is Eros as its finest. Kimberly will help you create new levels of rapture and ecstasy as well as deeper heart connections."
— Rosemary Gladstar, herbalist and author

"*Aphrodisiac* is the book that I've always wanted! It encompasses a truly holistic understanding of sexuality that includes our relationship with the natural world and its healing, life-enhancing, Eros-encouraging plants. Just reading the recipes alone is a huge turn-on! Let Kimberly be your brilliant, wise, and empowering guide to the luscious world of wondrous plants (along with rituals, meditations, and more) that have the power to enhance our erotic connections with ourselves, with others, and with nature."
— Sheri Winston, wholistic sexuality teacher, author of the award-winning *Women's Anatomy of Arousal* and *Succulent SexCraft*, founder of the Intimate Arts Center

"In an age characterized by stress and uncertainty, *Aphrodisiac* invites us to remember pleasure and how good life can feel. Imagine all the good things you know you should be doing for yourself and your relationships—connecting with nature, pampering yourself, improving communication, having mind-blowing orgasms . . . the things we aspire to do and rarely find the time for. *Aphrodisiac* is a guide to discovering self-care, joy, love, and beauty."
— Thomas Easley, author of *The Modern Herbal Dispensatory*

"Fifty years after the Sexual Revolution, when we were tossed into the mix with no information, guidelines, or help, Kimberly Gallagher brings us a book to finally fully accept ourselves and enjoy the vital, erotic side of our existence. The world has been waiting for such gentle, pure guidance."
— Tina Sams, Editor, *Essential Herbal Magazine*

"While plants have been used to enliven our sensuality since time immemorial, the idea of 'aphrodisiacs' is too often presented as something spurious, or something coercive. In reality, a person's sexuality is as important to their wellness as their digestion. Kimberly Gallagher offers us a guidebook to the use of herbs known to connect us to the fullness of our lives' and bodies' sensual health."
— jim mcdonald, herbalist

"Within just a few pages of *Aphrodisiac*, your center of gravity changes in relation to your concepts around sensuality, sexuality, and pleasure. This veritable feast of the senses will rock your world, leading you on a journey of sensory revelry unlike what you have experienced before. Kimberly Gallagher is your artful guide in discovering greater sexual fulfillment and harnessing sexual creativity to fuel all aspects of your life."

— Kami McBride, author of *The Herbal Kitchen*

"Kimberly Gallagher elevates the path of herbal aphrodisiacs to a higher plane, so that every reader may find steps to liberating deep desire and expressing joy. Plants on the physical plane provide sweet adventures for each of our paths to erotic bliss. *Aphrodisiac* should be given to every person who has loved and wants to love."

— Amanda McQuade Crawford, MA, MFT, MCPP, RH(AHG), Consulting Medical Herbalist

"Kimberly Gallagher has created a sumptuous feast for the senses, as she not only explores the use of herbal aphrodisiacs, but gently guides the reader towards a resplendent state of self-love and nurturance within relationship. Drawing upon a thorough review of the scientific and sexual literature, she explores aphrodisiac and vitality-enhancing herbs. *Aphrodisiac* is a well-rounded exploration of the sexual potency of herbal medicine."

— Todd Caldecott, author of *Food as Medicine*

"*Aphrodisiac* is a must-have for all lovers seeking healthy and fun ways to enhance intimacy. The book itself is as beautiful as its content, making reading as pleasurable as implementing its teachings. Whether you're looking for a little warmup or ready to crank the fire to high, this book will help you get there!"

— Emily Ruff, Director of Sage Mountain Botanical Sanctuary

"*Aphrodisiac* is a beautiful ode to love and healing where healthy sexuality, as a personal exploration, lies at the core of vibrant living. Kimberly offers us an opportunity to slow down and savor this enchanting journey, full of nurturing lifestyle support and herbal treasures to help us fall in love with life, ourselves, and our lovers—if we so choose."

— Dina Falconi, author of *Earthly Bodies & Heavenly Hair*

"Are you primed and poised to spice up your love life and fully explore your sensuality? Kimberly Gallagher has artfully strewn the botanical path to sexual fulfillment throughout the lush pages of Aphrodisiac. You'll find a refreshing blend of inspiration and guidance for living a richer life, filled with earthly pleasures."

— Juliet Blankespoor, Director of the Chestnut School of Herbal Medicine

"*Aphrodisiac* is a guide for living with heightened senses, so we can enjoy life. Kimberly Gallagher's guide blends practical herbal and life strategies with inspiration and beauty. This book is for anyone who is ready to walk a path of erotic fulfillment."

— Bevin Clare, M.S., R.H., CNS, author of *Spice Apothecary*

"*Aphrodisiac* redefines the word to encompass not just herbal remedies for sexual stimulation, but also using plants to help us heal. Part herbal, part relationship guide, and part cookbook to steam up life in the bedroom, Aphrodisiac is an incredible resource to open up an often neglected, but important, aspect of herbal medicine."

— Sajah Popham, author of *Evolutionary Herbalism*

APHRODISIAC

APHRODISIAC

THE HERBAL PATH TO HEALTHY
SEXUAL FULFILLMENT AND VITAL LIVING

KIMBERLY GALLAGHER

HAY HOUSE, INC.
Carlsbad, California • New York City
London • Sydney • New Delhi

CONTENTS

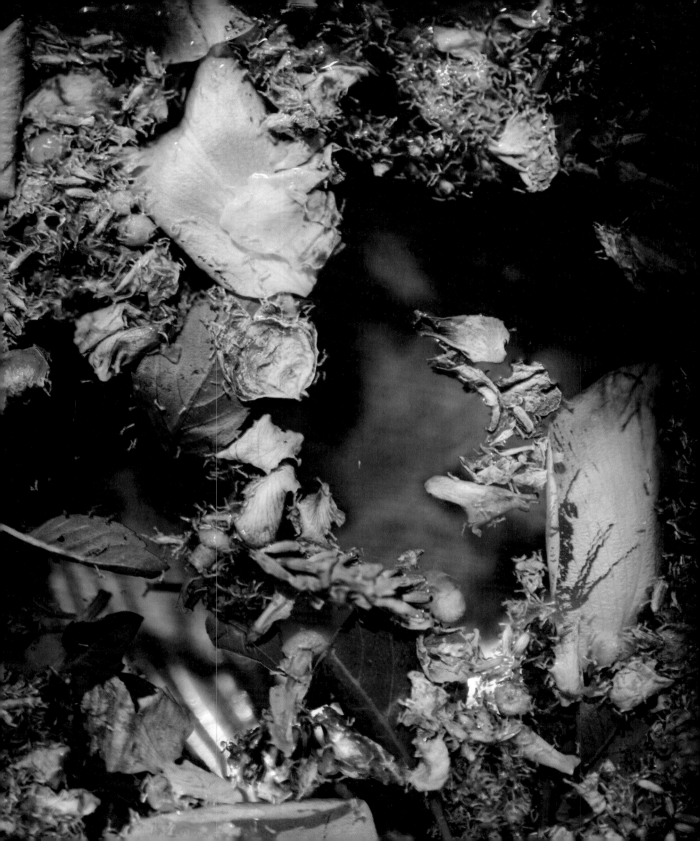

Introduction

Take a moment right now to lightly and slowly brush one finger across your lips. Feel the shape of them. Tune in to the exquisite sensation of your own touch. Sink into the joy of sensuality.

Sensual pleasure and healthy sexuality are our birthright. They are sources of deep satisfaction, joy, creativity, self-confidence, and success. They are fundamentally about connection—connection to our bodies, each other, and the world around us.

This book is a journey of exploration into the world of connection and sensation. The path we are stepping onto together is one of curiosity and discovery about our full capacity for pleasure and the deliciousness of living a sensually alive, vital, and even ecstatic life. I am your guide on this journey and the plants are our allies.

I have been working with herbs for the past 20 years. My husband, John, and I began as herbalists just as we were starting our family.

He was apprenticing at RavenCroft Garden when I was pregnant with our son, and the herbs naturally wove themselves in to our lives together. Just after my daughter was born, I also completed a three-year herbal apprenticeship at RavenCroft. The herbs had become a passion for both of us, and we were amazed by how they nourished and healed our family on a daily basis. We wanted to share what we had learned with other families, so we founded LearningHerbs.com. Teaching people about herbs became the heart of our work in the world.

Sensuality and sexuality have also been sources of deep nourishment and vital life energy for me throughout my life. At the heart of my ministry, which I call Trail of Beauty, are ceremonies and practices that celebrate the sacredness of being fully embodied and connected to sensation and the natural world. I delight in helping people fully inhabit their bodies and experience sensation. As I have delved more and more deeply into my own experience of sensuality and exploration of healthy sexuality, it has been natural for me to turn to the plants as allies and to weave these two passions together.

In preparation for writing this book, I gathered a group of friends and we went on a year-long journey together, experimenting with the aphrodisiac qualities of 13 herbs. These were herbs I had become curious about as I had been doing herbal research on aphrodisiacs over the course of the year before the book-writing project began. We experimented with a different herb each month, noticing how it impacted our bodies and our lives. The participants in this Aphrodisiac Circle are characters in this book. (They each chose a pseudonym to protect their privacy.) We'll look in depth at each of the herbs we experimented with, and I will share our experiences with you in the hopes of enhancing and enlivening your own journey.

I chose to undertake this intimate, vulnerable exploration with a small group of friends who I know and trust. There were 14 of us in the group, ranging in age between 30 and 65. Three couples participated and 10 of us were in committed partnerships, some exploring open relationship as part of that commitment. Several participants identify as bisexual. Nine of us were parents and one became a parent in the midst of the project. Several were going through periods of expansion and exploration in the area of their sexuality, and one was just rekindling the possibility of romantic and sexual exploration after many years of celibacy following the death of her husband. Four were healing from past sexual trauma and abuse, and one was just reeling from the ending of a multi-year partnership. Three of the women were in the midst of their transition through menopause.

Each of us began in a unique place, and each of us made discoveries along the way. Our small circle in no way represents the full diversity of human experience (for more information about each participant, see Appendix A), but what I know is that sexuality is a fundamentally *human* experience, bringing each of us to a naked, vulnerable place, regardless of race, class, gender, or age. Also, the herbs are potent and effective healers that are accessible to us all, and the herbs that we engaged with hold potential benefits for every body.

Just as the Aphrodisiac Circle went on an exploratory journey together seeking herbal support for greater sexual fulfillment and vital living, I have organized this book as a journey of personal exploration for you. Rather than following the Aphrodisiac Circle journey or focusing on one herb per chapter, I was inspired to take you through a series of experiences. Within the chapters you will find recipes and opportunities for cultivating the flow of erotic energy in your life.

I suggest you find a way to express and reflect on your learnings as you go along. Perhaps you would like to pick out a beautiful journal. Or maybe you would like a pad of drawing paper and some art pens or pencils. You can write or draw about your experiences and add to it as more emerges for you over time. Or perhaps you would like to sculpt with clay or express yourself through body movement or dance, or through song. You could make voice recordings. The important thing is to find a means of expression that resonates for you so you can honor your own unique journey. I encourage you to take time and make space for this in your life.

My herbal teachings are spread throughout the book (sometimes in the form of recipes, sometimes set apart as dedicated sections, and sometimes woven in with the flow of text) so that your herbal knowledge can grow organically, right along with your experience of your sexuality. I spread the teachings out and continually invite you into experiences because that is how I know effective learning happens—*slowly, one experience at a time.*

Each chapter contains a monograph for the herb that we explored in the Aphrodisiac Circle that I feel most aligns with the energy of that chapter. These monographs contain detailed information about each of these 13 herbs. You will find yourself flipping forward and backward in the book to consult these monographs as you consider whether a recipe is right for you. Each experience preparing an herbal recipe and taking herbs into your body will help you gain herbal skills and confidence.

Let's take our first step working with herbs right now by repeating that opening exercise of running a finger over our lips and bringing the plants into it. Let's imagine doing the same thing with a rose petal instead of just your finger. Participants in the Aphrodisiac Circle found this to be an absolutely exquisite sensual experience. In fact, if you happen to be reading this book at a time when you can pick yourself a rose (chemical free), I recommend this as your first step onto the herbal path to sexual fulfillment and vital living.

Go and pick yourself a rose. Place it in a vase or jar in a special place just for you, dedicated to your journey of sensual, sexual exploration. Place your journal, drawing paper, or clay here in this special place too. Once your rose is in its place, enjoy its delicate beauty, the evocative scent of it. Feel the softness of its petals. Now, pick just one petal. Choose your favorite one. Lightly and slowly brush the petal across your lips. Close your eyes and allow yourself to feel the sensation as fully and deeply as possible.

If it is not the right time of year to pick yourself a fresh rose, I invite you to enjoy the anticipation. Anticipation is, after all, another one of the delights of erotic experience. Our minds are one of our main sexual organs, our imaginations one of our most lovely erotic tools.

Over the course of this journey together, I am going to highlight and gift you with many tools to help bring more erotic, vital energy to your life. The recipes for herbal preparations and activities will help you deepen into sensation and connection with your own body, with your lover(s), with the plants, and with the natural world. Just as we are all at different places in our sexual journeys, different activities will resonate more deeply for each of you, and your level of wanting to engage with the plants will also vary. Whether you want to dip your toe in lightly or dive in as deeply as possible, you are welcome on this path.

Stepping onto the herbal path can be as simple as picking that rose, placing it in a special place, and running a petal over your lips. In the pages that follow, I will suggest other simple steps you can take. In order to prepare the recipes, you will need to gather some herbs. Some you may buy from a local herb shop or an online source. Others may grow right around you, and you will have the opportunity to be in direct relationship with them as you harvest the flowers, leaves, roots, bark, or seeds. I highly recommend engaging with the plants in these ways if it is possible for you. These experiences harvesting and preparing herbal creations are sensual experiences in themselves and can be a powerful part of the healing and nourishment available on this herbal path.

Over the course of reading this book, you will have the opportunity to explore what herbs are right for you at each moment of your personal journey, whether you need to heal and nourish your body or you are seeking to enhance your experience. There is a science and an art to discovering your perfect herb and preparation. The process has many parts, and we will be exploring them organically together, getting to know the plants and learning through sensual exploration and play. We will ask ourselves questions and listen deeply for answers. Our bodies are a great source of information about what tools, preparations, and activities are just right for us right now, so we will continually come back to a place of embodied sensation.

Here is a meditation to help you come into embodied sensation. You can use it anytime you want to bring yourself fully present and sensually alive:

Close your eyes, and take a few deep breaths, fully filling your lungs with air and feeling the resulting expansion in your body. Exhale completely so that your belly button naturally pulls inward. Allow your breath to return to a normal rhythm and begin to notice your body sensations. Feel the air on your skin. Is it warm or cool, still or breezy? Feel the places where your clothes or your hair brush against your skin. Feel those places where one body part is resting on another. Tune in to your internal landscape. Are there places in your body that are tight or tender? Breathe some loving energy into those places. Are there areas that feel expansive or soft? Tune in to your genital area. Notice what sensations you feel there in those private, tender places. How is your belly feeling? Is it in knots today or at ease? Your heart? Head?

Notice any scents that are present in the air today. I'm writing outside by a beautiful river in Twisp, Washington. I smell an earthy forest smell. And in the background I hear the gentle flow of river water over rocks, a constant, soothing lullaby. What are the sounds you hear around you? Do these scents or sounds lead to body sensations for you? Bring your awareness to those sensations. Breathe into them. Give yourself space and time to feel them.

When you are ready, open your eyes. Look around you, and find something beautiful in your environment. Rest your eyes there. Sink into the colors and textures, the pleasing shapes and patterns. Curl the corners of your mouth up into a smile and breathe into your heart as you rest in the beauty.

From this place, I invite you to reflect for a moment on what led you to pick up this book. The answer to this question will be different for each of you, and what I want you to know is that your unique answer is the absolutely perfect answer for you right now. Wherever you are on your journey of sensual and sexual empowerment is the perfect place for us to begin. Maybe you are heartbroken, scared, or shut down in some way. Maybe you are turned off and your turn-on feels very far away. Or . . . maybe you are ecstatic most of the time and just curious if this book can expand your pleasure even further.

I know, for me, living through this global pandemic has changed my daily experience of sensuality with others. Many more of us are suffering some degree of touch deprivation as we stay socially distant to protect each other's health. I know the lack of friendly hugs is impacting my nervous system. Going through a challenging time without being able to physically hold each other is something I hope we need never face again. The initial draft of this book was written before COVID-19 became widespread. Revisions are happening within the first year of social dis-tancing, and I find myself wondering if this book will serve as a reminder of the pre-COVID-19 world and help us remember the importance of touch and find our way back to ease and comfort with one another.

Whatever your reason, thank you for picking up this book, for stepping onto this path with me, for daring to prioritize pleasure—sensual, sexual pleasure—as a source of energy and joy in your life. The further I go down this road of seeking healthy sexual experience, the more convinced I become that this is a bold act. Bold because it challenges what our culture teaches us about our bodies and our very lives. Bold because it takes us to a core place—a place of tenderness and vul-nerability. A place where we can no longer hide behind masks. This is the place where I want to meet you. In that tender, raw place where your heart is open. Where you can barely breathe because you are feeling *sooooooo much*!

The pages that follow are me opening my heart and extending my hand to you, inviting you to revel in sensation and expand your capacity to feel and dwell in pleasure, joy, and gratitude.

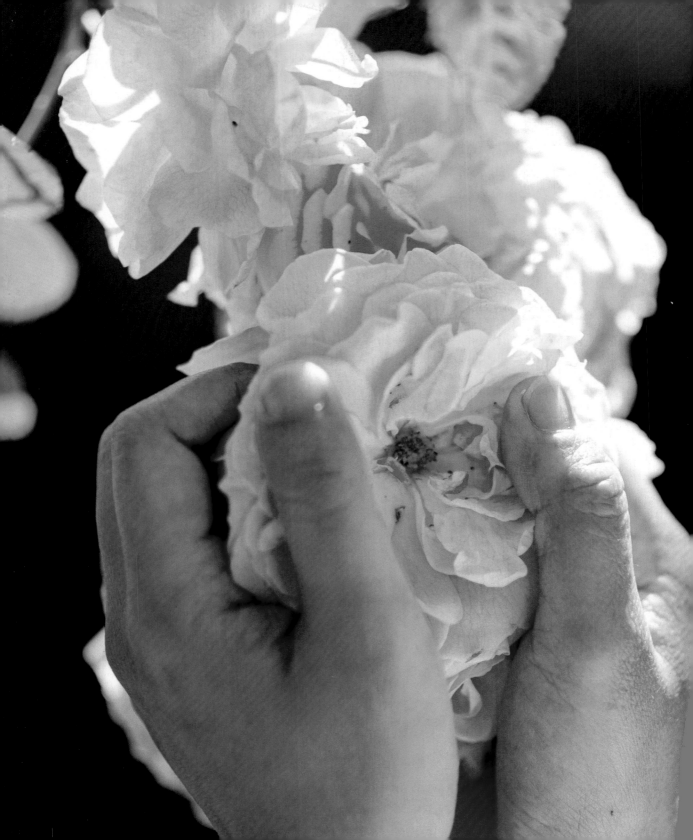

ONE

SLOWING DOWN

TO ENJOY

THE EROTIC

ENERGY

OF LIFE

Ah! That glorious, coveted feeling of falling in love! You know it, right? The boost of energy, the feeling that all is right with the world, the renewed confidence in ourselves. How about the nervous, excited anticipation about the next phone call? The tingling, electric energy that runs through our whole bodies at the slightest touch from our love.

What if we could consciously cultivate that feeling in our lives whether or not there is a person who is the object of our desire? I've been experimenting with that idea. I've been playing with ways to increase pleasure and sensual, erotic energy in my life. This energy is a precious resource. It is source energy that can be channeled not only into sexual expression but also into creative endeavors, like writing this book, dancing, or tending my garden. I've come to rely on having a healthy flow of erotic energy in my life.

Now, if you look up the word *erotic* in the dictionary, it will give you a definition like "arousing sexual desire." When I talk about this erotic flow, I am talking about something broader. It can, at times, feel sexual—when it centers in our pelvis—but it may also be more of a tingling sensation, a feeling of *aliveness* throughout our body. Cultivating this sensual aliveness is a key to finding sexual fulfillment and to overall vibrant living. When we have this flow of erotic energy in our lives, we feel more confident, more in our personal power, more able to face life challenges, and more able to bring our own unique gifts to the world.

So how do we cultivate it? That is the heart of what we will be exploring together in the pages that follow. I've collected many possibilities for you to explore and enjoy so that each of you can discover your own unique ways. One universal secret is to *slow down.* Slow down and consciously seek and create pleasurable experiences for yourself, and take the time to sink into sensation over and over again throughout each day.

You may feel like this is selfish or a frivolous use of time. On the contrary, I believe that people who are sexually fulfilled and sensually enlivened are peaceful, creative, and vital. Because of this, they naturally make important, positive contributions within their families and communities.

Intrigued? Then let's cultivate this flow of erotic energy together. Come, dare with my participants and me to act on the belief that sensuality and healthy sexuality are essential components of a life well lived. The first step is to set an intention for yourself, an intention that will encourage you to make space and time in your life to cultivate erotic energy. Taking time to set an intention is one way that we can slow down the relentless pace of modern life. Engaging in any exploration with intention will encourage us to be more fully present and tapped into the sensual, erotic energy of our experience.

Your intention will reflect where you are in your life right now. For example, Michelle, from the Aphrodisiac Circle, is menopausal and a survivor of childhood abuse. She is currently in a partnership that invites exploration of sensuality and sexuality. Her intention is to continue to open her heart and experience the strength and creativity she can gain through engaging vulnerably with a loving, strong, powerful male partner. Christina is a dancer who is enjoying her connection with the earth and is curious about herbs. She is also on a journey of healing from past sexual trauma. She is looking for ways to continue her healing and to make her life juicier. Joe feels like his connection with his wife, Cassie, is waning after 14 years of marriage. His intention is to "learn how and why I'm feeling less connected and find creative ways to hopefully rekindle our fire." Rachel has just ended an eight-year partnership and is looking to intentionally find pleasure again.

Whether you have a lover in your life or not, this book is about *you* and your journey of cultivating a healthy flow of erotic energy in *your* life for *yourself,* and your unique experience of what unfolds as a result. So take a moment right now and formulate an intention for yourself as you step onto this path.

Creating a Personal Intention

Rather than coming up with this intention from your mind, let's play with letting this intention arise from a sensually embodied place. Perhaps you will want to sit where you placed your rose or create a special place for yourself now.

1   Once you are settled, take some deep breaths, feeling the expansion and contraction in your body as you do so.

2   Let your breathing return to a natural rhythm and practice the meditation from the introduction, or run your finger over your lips to bring yourself to the present and into sensual awareness.

3   Ask out loud or in your mind, "What is my intention right now as I step onto this herbal path of sexual fulfillment and vital living? What am I cultivating in my life right now?"

4   Sit quietly and listen to what answers arise. I have found that my body is wise and allowing answers to rise up from this sensually embodied place is an insightful practice.

5   Write the intention(s) that arises and place it in the space you have made for yourself, a space dedicated to your own journey of sensual and sexual exploration and empowerment.

Let your intention be different from a goal. Be playful with it, holding it gently and without attachment, allowing it to take you on a journey. There is no pressure to make it happen. Just as the rose you pick(ed) will open, so much is about to open for you!

Aphrodi-Tea

INGREDIENTS

1 tablespoon dried tulsi leaf

2 tablespoons dried rose petals

Honey, to taste

HERBAL TIPS

✦ Teas are very basic herbal preparations. I loved the result of this recipe, and you can vary the taste and effects of herbal teas by varying the amounts of the herbs used and /or the steeping time. You may also get a different result using fresh herbs rather than dried. Experimenting and noticing subtle differences will help you grow your herbal knowledge and confidence.

✦ Generally, longer steeping times will increase the amount of herbal constituents being drawn into the water. This affects both the taste and effectiveness of the tea. Longer is not always better. Tulsi, for example, becomes bitter when steeped too long.

PREPARATION

1 Pour 1½ cups boiling water over the tulsi and rose petals (loose or using a mesh tea strainer).

2 Cover and steep 10 minutes.

3 Strain the herbs from the hot tea.

4 Add honey to taste.

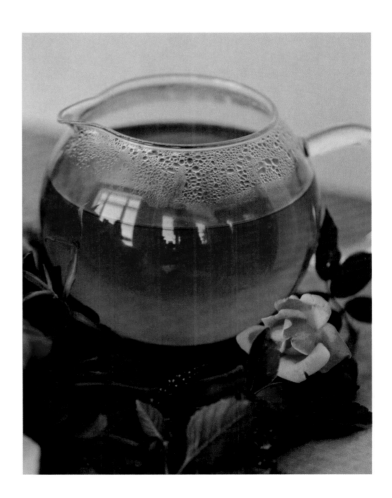

WHAT IS AN APHRODISIAC?

As I began to look at ways the herbs could support us in our quest for healthy sexual fulfillment, this question came to the forefront. When I thought about what I would like an aphrodisiac to be, I thought perhaps there were herbs that would somehow heighten my sensual experiences during sex, opening up doorways to more pleasure. In the course of my exploration, I also realized that some people are seeking exotic herbs or substances as aphrodisiacs to increase their own libido, or as love or sex potions to encourage less-interested partners to have sex with them or to help address their partner's "sexual issues."

Looking up the word *aphrodisiac* through Google gives us a definition like "foods, drinks, or drugs that stimulate sexual desire." Reading through the book *Herbal Aphrodisiacs from World Sources*, it seems that all sorts of things have been considered aphrodisiacs throughout time—from sweet potatoes to sunflowers to artichokes and apples. Why? What are these foods or herbs actually doing in our bodies to be considered aphrodisiacs?

Many herbal books will include *aphrodisiac* in their lists of herbal actions, but this does not tell us much about what the herb actually does in our bodies to stimulate sexual desire. It does not give us information about why we might choose this herb over another that is also listed as an aphrodisiac at this particular time in our lives. To gain more clarity about that, we can look more deeply into herbal actions and at the key constituents in the herbs. (An example of this is the phenylethylamine compound found in cacao. This is also a natural compound in the brain, which is released

when we are in love and during orgasm. So ingesting cacao can create similar feelings to those experiences.)

Let's take a deeper look at herbal actions that might stimulate sexual desire. Herbs that increase circulation or widen blood vessels can result in more blood being pumped to our pelvis, brain, and heart. Herbs can also be nourishing for our heart or our reproductive organs. They can be stimulating, restorative, or help to improve our mood. Perhaps the herb is demulcent and this slippery quality will help support our juiciness. Just the smells and textures of different herbs can help stimulate our senses.

It also may be that many herbs can support our quest for healthy sexual fulfillment without "stimulating sexual desire." Perhaps we just need an herb to help us relax after a busy, pressure-filled day. Or maybe we can call on an herb to help us heal so we are not distracted by pain or illness. There was one point during the study when perimenopause had me bleeding for weeks at a time. Taking vitex (a tincture of chasteberries) regulated my cycle, and that felt like an amazing aphrodisiac at that moment because it allowed me to come back to my sensual/sexual self.

Understanding just what you are hoping the herb will do for you is one key to choosing the right herb for your situation. Considering the actions of the herbs and looking at the constituents can provide valuable information. The experiences of others can help inform us as well. Ultimately, though, working with the herb yourself, making a preparation from a recipe and actually trying the herb in your own body, will give you the most information and help you develop your unique relationship with the plants. One thing that stood out for us in the Aphrodisiac Circle was that each of us had personal experiences with the herbs that varied significantly from those of other participants.

As you begin to work with the herbs, there are a few basic guidelines to keep in mind. An herb is a plant with edible or healing qualities, and they are powerful. It's important to treat them with respect.

✧ **Consider safety.**

The information in this book or any other book is no substitute for consulting with your health care provider if you are experiencing troublesome symptoms or have any special circumstances (like being pregnant, taking medication, or dealing with a chronic illness).

Always check dosage recommendations so you get a sense of how much of a particular herb to take to get the maximum benefit.

Read the plant monographs and especially the "Special Considerations" section to be sure the plant is safe for you at this time.

✧ **If you are picking herbs in the wild:**

Be 100 percent sure you have identified the plant correctly. This may mean using a field guide or online resource for plant identification and checking what you find with a knowledgeable herbalist.

Learn about sustainable harvesting techniques like taking only as much as you need and only the part of the plant you need and perhaps leaving the roots (or at least some of them) in the ground so the plant can continue to grow.

Make sure you are harvesting from a healthy area where pesticides are not sprayed.

✧ **If you are buying dried plant material from a retail source, be sure it was ethically wildcrafted or cultivated and has not been grown with the use of pesticides.**

There is lots of latitude for play and experimentation within these guidelines, and in my experience, interacting with the plants is easier than a lot of people think.

Cardamom Chocolate Mousse Torte _Rosalee de la Forêt_

INGREDIENTS

8 ounces bittersweet chocolate

½ cup coconut oil

½ cup honey

½ cup cocoa powder

1 (13.5-ounce) can coconut milk

2 eggs

1 tablespoon cardamom powder

2 tablespoons vanilla extract

sliced almonds and cocoa powder for the topping

PREPARATION

_1_ Preheat the oven to 350 degrees F.

_2_ Melt the chocolate and coconut oil in the top of a double boiler.

_3_ Remove from the heat. Add the honey and cocoa powder. Mix well.

_4_ Add the coconut milk and mix well.

_5_ Whisk the eggs in a small bowl.

_6_ Add the whisked eggs, cardamom, and vanilla extract to the chocolate mixture. Mix well.

_7_ Pour the mixture into a slightly oiled 9-inch pie pan.

_8_ Bake for 30 minutes.

_9_ When the torte is done, the top should be cracked but the middle should still be soft and wiggly.

_10_ Cool overnight in the refrigerator to allow it to set.

_11_ Sprinkle with slivered almonds and cocoa powder before serving.

HERBAL TIPS

✦ We may not really think of mixing up a dessert as making an herbal preparation, but herbalism can actually be that simple. Our food can be some of the best medicine if we consciously choose our ingredients and which foods we ingest.

✦ You might read through the cacao monograph in Chapter 12 to learn a little more about how cacao affects our bodies. Making it is also an opportunity to learn about cardamom and vanilla as herbs and why they may or may not be good allies for you.

✦ After eating it, take time to notice how you feel in your body. What experiences does it lead to? This is how you build your herbal knowledge—one experience at a time.

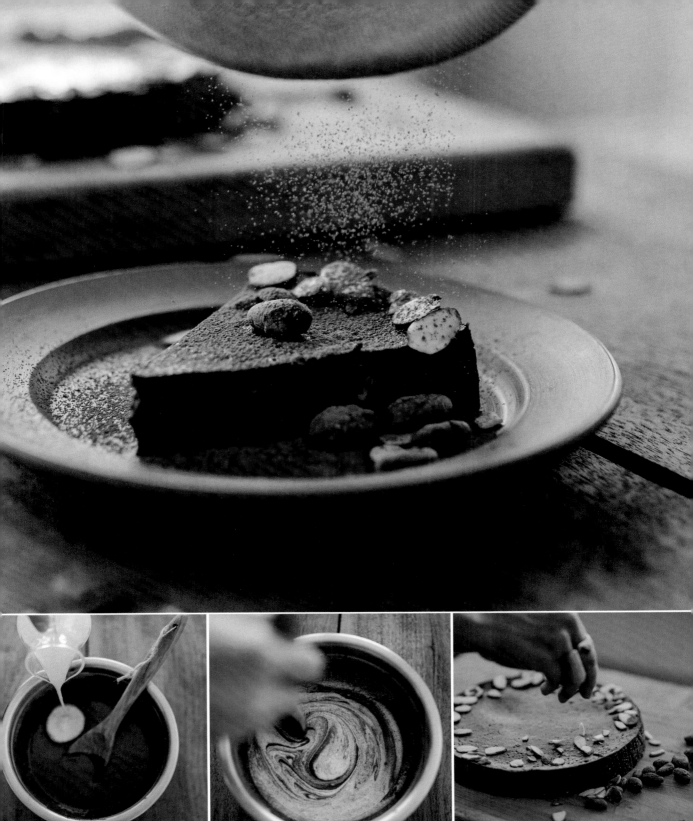

THE POWER OF INTENTION AND ATTENTION

Both setting intentions and bringing our full attention to an experience are key aspects of slowing down and enjoying the presence of erotic energy. Let's explore this idea as we engage in our first herbal preparation, the making of a cardamom chocolate mousse torte. The torte itself is delicious, and creating it can also be what I've come to talk about as an aphrodisiac experience. Let me explain.

Say you are making this torte for you and your lover to enjoy after a candlelit dinner together. Well, what if, instead of squeezing in making the torte between finishing up work, running errands, and perhaps talking on the phone with your mom while you do it, you actually set aside time for the torte creation process? Make an afternoon of it. Gather your ingredients together and set an intention for your time enjoying the torte with your beloved. Perhaps you would like it to be a sensual prelude to an evening of lovemaking, or perhaps you are making this torte just for you and want it to be a symbol of allowing yourself to really indulge in pleasurable experiences. Hold that intention as you create the torte. Make the intention an ingredient in your recipe. As you mix the ingredients, let yourself anticipate the fulfillment of your intention. The anticipation can be as delicious as the torte.

Bring yourself fully present and into your senses. Give the making of the torte your full attention. Smell the chocolate and the coconut oil as you melt them together. Enjoy the smooth richness of the combination. Taste a little bit of the honey before you add it to the mixture. Feel it on your finger; fully enjoy the sweetness on your tongue. Smell and taste the coconut milk. Enjoy the colors mixing together (I find the mixing of this torte to be beautiful). Smell the cardamom and the vanilla extract before you mix them with the eggs. Allow your senses to be fully stimulated by the torte ingredients. Again, enjoy the beauty as you mix the eggs with the chocolate mixture. While the torte bakes, put on some of your favorite sensual music and sit quietly and listen, or move your body to the music. Allow yourself to revel in your heightened sensations.

This torte needs to cool overnight to fully set. Lots of time to let the anticipation build. Let your sensual excitement smolder or grow. Perhaps

> *Imagine the rich, smooth taste on your tongue, in your mouth, sliding down your throat.*

call your lover and let them in on your secret; bring them into the experience of anticipation. Share your intention for the evening to come. Or write or find a poem or song to share with them or to read yourself as you enjoy the torte. Imagine the rich, smooth taste on your tongue, in your mouth, sliding down your throat.

Before serving the torte, bring yourself back into delicious sensation by enjoying the taste and feel of the slivered almonds and cocoa powder as you add this final touch to your masterpiece. Remind yourself of your intention. And take your time serving it. Build up to eating it. Enjoying its beauty. Taking in its scent. Taking that first bite, slowly, sensually onto your tongue. Feel it melt and fill your mouth with flavor.

Now you understand the power of bringing yourself fully present, tuning in to and heightening your senses, setting intention, and building anticipation. The experience of creating and enjoying this torte, as I have described it, is what I mean by an aphrodisiac experience. I invite you to slow down and bring yourself into these kinds of experiences throughout your reading of this book, and into as many areas of your life as possible. They are a primary secret for fully reveling in the presence of sensual, erotic energy and living a vital life.

Tasting dark chocolate
a ripe apricot
A luscious elixir—
Savor the expanding joy in your body.
Nature is offering herself to you.
How astonishing
To realize this world can taste so good.

When sipping some ambrosia,
Raise your glass,
Close your eyes,
Toast the universe.
The Sun and Moon and Earth
Danced together
To bring you this delight.
Receive the nectar on your tongue
As a kiss of the divine

— from *The Radiance Sutras* by Lorin Roche

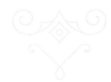

WEAVING PLEASURE
INTO DAILY LIFE

Bringing heightened sensual experiences into our daily life helps increase vital energy by cultivating a flow of erotic energy. One of my favorite ways to weave in pleasure is through simple rituals. Simple rituals are created through intention and attention. There is a quality of reverence and honoring to them, and yet they are simple in that they do not take a lot of time and energy for preparation. Michelle and Robert, a retired couple in a passionate love affair, created a simple ritual during our month when we focused on tulsi. Each morning Robert brought a cup of tulsi rose tea (Aphrodi-Tea, page 21) to Michelle's bedside. Taking the cup from him, she would feel the warmth on her hands and breathe in the luscious fragrance of the herbs, bathing herself in the calm support she felt them offering to her. Michelle and Robert consciously set aside time in their day for this ritual with the intention of creating a nourishing, sensual experience and connecting with the herbs. Michelle brought her full attention to her enjoyment of being gifted and enjoyment of the tea itself, reveling in each sensation.

Gabrielle created a simple ritual for herself during her exploration of cacao. Gabrielle's husband died in an accident when her two girls were still very young. The relationship had been a difficult one for her, and when he was gone, she chose to put her energy fully into her mothering, setting aside eroticism. Her girls are now grown women, and she came to the Aphrodisiac Circle as a way of reengaging with the sensual, sexual aspects of herself. She bought herself a big bar of 100 percent cacao chocolate and set aside time to savor a piece of it every day in February. She

describes taking time to play with it in her mouth, letting it become warm and thick and smooth, slowly releasing itself on her tongue. She said, "It felt private and special and fun to come to know this dark beauty. It woke me up. I felt more in touch with my body than I have in some time. I started an exercise program with a weekly walk in the mountains and paying closer attention to the other things I put into my body. The cacao was the bar of wholeness and intentionality."

Artemis wove cacao in to her life by creating a simple trail mix blend of cacao nibs with dried goji berry and almonds. Artemis is a single mom parenting three boys and is also diving deep into an exploration of sacred sexuality. This was a treat she could share with her boys, which also reminded her each time she ate it of her intention to live a sensual, vibrant life.

Simple pleasure rituals can look all sorts of ways, involving the herbs or not. I swim in the cold Pacific Northwest ocean three mornings a week. For me, this is an absolute sensual delight. I love feeling the sand under my feet, the breathtaking cold of the water on my skin, and then the warmth of the sun or my towel when I emerge. Engaging in ecstatic dance is a regular simple pleasure ritual for me as well. I love the feeling of simply allowing the music to move my body.

Even ordinary daily activities like doing the dishes can be places of heightened sensation and pleasure. Try it. Focus on the feel of the warm water and soap against your skin as you wash and rinse. Put on your favorite music and move your body while washing. Oh, and if the rose bush outside the window is blooming or the clouds are turning pink or the moon is up, then your sense of sight can be delighted as well.

Interacting with the plants can be another way of weaving pleasure in to daily life. Let's talk for a minute about the roses blooming outside the window while you were doing the dishes. Rose month was one of our favorite months. It was especially wonderful because wild roses are abundant where we live in the northwest. Everyone in the Aphrodisiac Circle agreed that being able to interact with the living, growing plants really increased our sensual connection with the herbs and helped them to feel like friends and allies.

Cassie found herself burying her nose in rose blossoms, harvesting petals to carry the scent home, and breathing in the aroma of rose tea. She loved how the scent helped awaken her senses and her feeling of play and joy in life. For Angela, the month was filled with stress, but she found delight in the blooming of the various rose bushes in her yard. She used cardamom rose oil on her skin every day and enjoyed the delicious taste of rose-infused honey (page 14) on a daily basis.

There are so many ways to add a little extra sensual delight to anything you do. The keys are slowing down, intention, and attention.

OPPORTUNITY FOR CULTIVATING EROTIC ENERGY FLOW

Daily Pleasure

Take a moment to consider how you might weave pleasure in to your own life.

1 Settle in and take a few deep breaths, feeling the expansion and contraction in your body as you do so.

2 Let your breathing return to a natural rhythm and practice the meditation from the introduction, or run your finger over your lips to bring yourself present and into sensual awareness.

3 From this place of embodied sensation, ask yourself if there is a simple ritual you would like to engage in regularly or if there is a daily activity that you can do while focusing on pleasurable physical sensation. Consider the answers that arise and choose one. Write it down if you like.

4 Choose a time to follow through with this idea, gather any materials you need, and do it daily for a week or more.

5 Reflect on the experience and express your insights so you integrate them. (Use the journal or drawing paper or clay you have set aside in your special place with your rose.)

Rose Honey

INGREDIENTS

Enough fresh rose petals to loosely fill an 8-ounce jar

8 ounces honey

PREPARATION

1. Chop fresh rose petals into small pieces.

2 Fill an 8-ounce jar (loosely packed) with fresh rose petal pieces.

3 Pour enough honey over the petals to fill the jar.

4 Stir to release any air bubbles (I like to use a wooden chopstick to stir).

5 Add more honey if needed to fill the jar. Cap with a lid.

6 Let sit on your kitchen counter for 2 weeks, stirring once or twice a day at least for the first week.

7 Enjoy as you would plain honey (the rose petals are edible, so no need to strain them out).

HERBAL TIPS

✦ You can use this same method to infuse honey with any number of edible flowers, including hawthorn, lilac, monarda, or lavender (you may only want to fill your jar ½ full with lavender flowers as they can be quite strong tasting). The honey draws constituents from the herbs while also taking on their aroma and taste, so you get herbal goodness in several ways while enjoying this treat.

✦ Honeys work well with aromatic and fruity herbs as the honey really takes on the smell and taste of the plants. Other herbs featured in this book that make delicious infused honeys include rose hips (remove seeds and fuzz from inside hips before infusing), hawthorn berries (strain the berries out before enjoying the honey; they have a large seed inside that is not edible), schisandra berries, and ginger root (grated). I recommend only filling the jar ½ full with each of these herbs.

✦ This is definitely one of my favorite herbal treats, and honeys are a beautiful way to infuse sensual herbal experience into your daily life. You can infuse the honeys and then just have them ready to add to your tea, spread on crackers or toast, or just eat by the fingerful any time you desire a sensual treat. You can have fun with licking it from your finger as well.

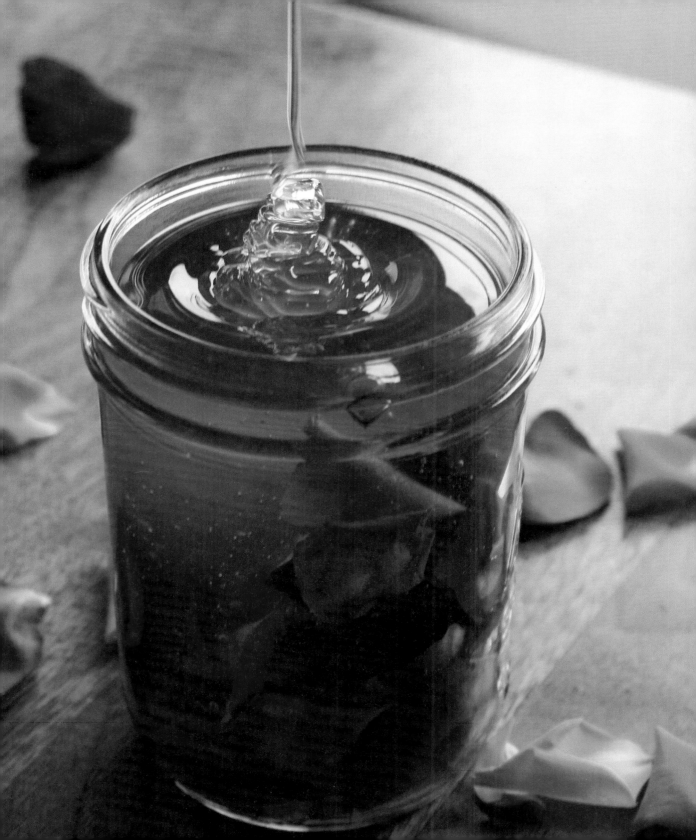

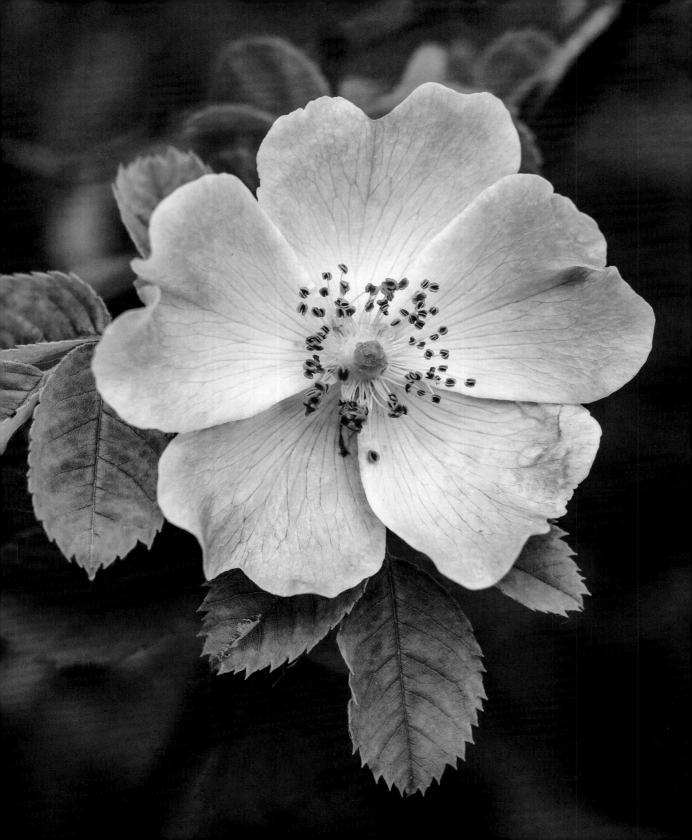

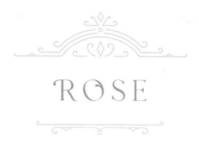

ROSE

Rosa spp., R. canina, R. rugosa, R. multiflora, R. nutkana

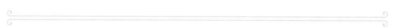

I love roses. Their intoxicating scent is one of my absolute favorite things about life on earth. I love their delicate beauty and the softness of their petals.

Roses have been seducing humans for thousands of years, stimulating our senses in powerful ways. We cultivate them for their beauty and gift them to one another to express our love and affection.

In her book *The Sexual Herbal*, Brigitte Mars calls roses the "supreme heart opener" and shares that "the open rose is a symbol for the opening heart and vulva."

How Do Roses Act as an Aphrodisiac in Our Bodies?

Roses calm our nerves and uplift our spirits. The aromatic quality of roses has the power to relax and restore us, easing anxiety and depression. In addition rose works as a neuro-protective, helping to protect our nerve cells from damage.[1] Two of the main constituents found in rose oil, citronellol and geraniol, interact with the AMPA receptors in our brain to help calm and protect the central nervous system.[2] The flavonoids found in roses interact with the GABA receptors in our brain to help relieve anxiety.[3]

A rose petal or rose hip infusion can help tone and regulate both the feminine and masculine reproductive systems. For women in particular, it can help strengthen our uteruses, regulate our menstrual cycles, and help relieve cramps.[4] Infusions also may help regulate hormones during menopause.[5]

Rose hips are a heart and circulatory system tonic, with powerful, risk-reducing antioxidant and anti-inflammatory effects.[6] Rose hips are also nourishing, with high vitamin and mineral content. They are especially high in vitamin C. Fresh rose hips contain about eight times more vitamin C than oranges (per 100 grams), and rose hips made into syrup or jam are equivalent to oranges in vitamin C content.[7]

Roses are also nourishing, soothing, and healing for our skin, both taken internally and applied externally.[8] Rosebuds, blossoms, and hips are moisturizing for irritated, sun-damaged, or aging skin, and rose water is an astringent skin toner with a beautiful scent and a wonderful addition to lotions, creams, and body oils.[9] Rose oils are nourishing for breast tissue and can help minimize stretch marks and wrinkles. Rose petal vinegar can be used as a douche, an after-bath splash, or a facial rinse. A rose petal facial or genital steam is both softening and moisturizing.

Herbal Shorthand

APHRODISIAC ACTIONS: *aromatic, emotionally uplifting, nervine, neuroprotective, nutritive, reproductive system tonic, restorative, soothing and healing for skin*

HIPS: *heart and circulatory system tonic, hormone regulator, nutritive*

OTHER ACTIONS: *analgesic, anti-inflammatory, antioxidant, astringent*

ENERGETICS: *cooling, drying*   TASTES: *sweet, sour*

NOTABLE APHRODISIAC CONSTITUENTS: *volatile oils, flavonoids, citronellol and geraniol / hips: vitamin C*

DOSAGE SUGGESTIONS: *Rose is a nourishing herb; both petals and hips are safe to consume as you would any other healthy food.*

SPECIAL CONSIDERATIONS: *Avoid using roses that have been sprayed with pesticides, including those from florist shops.*

Cheap rose essential oils are likely diluted or adulterated. It takes a huge quantity of roses to make a single ounce of essential oil, and it can cost hundreds of dollars an ounce. Rose Otto, which is rose essential oil diluted in good quality jojoba oil, can be a reasonably priced, high quality alternative.

A Bit about Rose Plants

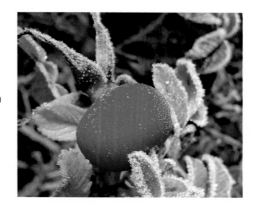

There are over 150 species of roses around the world. When searching for roses to use in your recipes, be sure the ones you choose are fragrant. That makes all the difference! Rugosa rose is a beautiful wild rose with a glorious scent. This species, native to east Asia, has made its way around the world, so you may well be able to find some not far from your own doorstep.

As with all roses, be mindful of the thorns when you go to harvest the petals. Thorns are how rose bushes wisely protect their precious bee-attracting flowers, just as our clear boundaries help us protect our own precious bodies.

Leave some flowers for the bees and when you come back to harvest in the fall or winter you will find the rose bush full with luscious rose hips, the fruit of the rose plant.

How to Use Rose

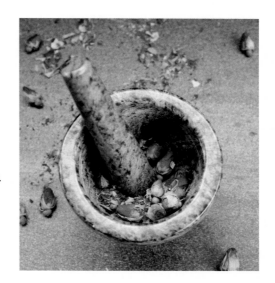

PARTS USED: *Petals, Fruits (hips)*

MAKE ROSE DRINKS: *Rose petal tea or infusion, fermented rose petal soda, rose juleps (rose petals steeped in cold water with lemon and honey), rose–petal infused tequila. Food-quality rose water can be added to smoothies or hot chocolate.*

Use rose water to enhance lotions and creams.

Use candied rose petals to decorate cakes.

Infuse rose petals in honey or vinegar.

Make a rose petal tincture.

Make a rose petal facial or genital steam.

Make a rose syrup.

Add dried rose petals to a potpourri mix.

Sprinkle rose petals on the bed or in the bedroom to create a beautiful, sacred, romantic space.

Participant Experiences

This month experimenting with roses was one of our most potent months. Most all of us got out and harvested rose petals, and several of us tended rose bushes in our yards. Being able to see and touch the growing plant and then make aphrodisiac preparations from the petals we harvested had us really falling in love with roses. Joe and Cassie played with rose drinks, infusing petals into tequila, brandy, and rum. Sarah and Artemis drank rose petal tea daily.

Sarah used rose petal powder in her body-care blends, enjoying a rose and oat powder body rub and rose honey skin masks. Lisa, Rachel, and Gabrielle all really enjoyed rose petal massage oil, and Christina noticed that rose petals in her bath made her feel "really special, like a goddess or queen."

Roses filled up our senses, bringing softness, gentleness, and ease and also igniting a sense of joy and play. The roses brought us into openhearted, loving connection with others. A rose oil massage offered loving comfort for Rachel even through the pain and grief she was feeling around ending her multiyear partnership. For Christina, roses brought unresolved grief to the surface for healing, allowing her to be more available for connection.

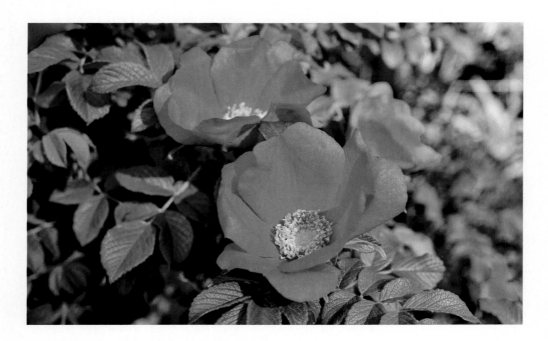

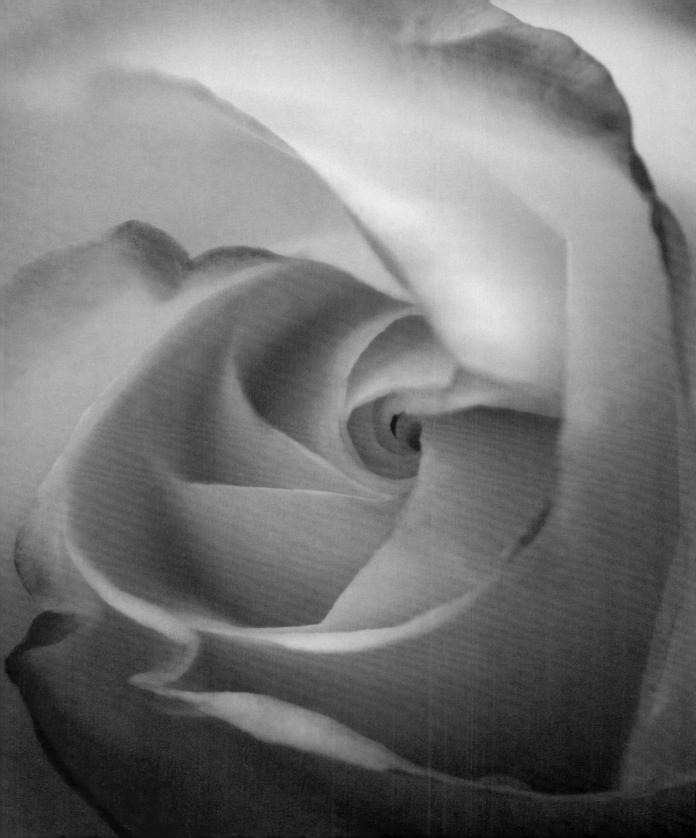

READING A MONOGRAPH

I have included plant monographs for 13 herbs in this book (one in each chapter). Monographs are commonly used by herbalists to convey detailed information about a plant in a way that is easy to access. As you learn to read a monograph, they become a valuable source of information when considering which herbs are right for you. Let's look at some of the key pieces of information they provide.

First, they include both the common and scientific name of the plant. Common names will vary from area to area, so identifying a plant by its scientific name is a way to be sure we are talking about the same plant. Looking up the plant in a field guide by the scientific name will give you the identifying characteristics of the plant and information about where you can find it growing.

Monographs will also tell you about the actions associated with the plant and about the plant constituents. Both of these pieces of information will help you understand how the herbs are likely to affect your body. In each of my monographs, I have highlighted the actions that seem to me to indicate how this herb can support healthy sexuality. I have taken a rather broad view, including actions like adaptogen (works in a general way to help normalize our metabolic processes, which increases our resilience in stressful times), nervine (calming for our nerves), and restorative. I have chosen actions that support our overall health and vitality, those that help to relax or enliven us, and those that specifically support our reproductive systems, heart, and circulatory systems.

Each herb has a number of active constituents that contribute to the effects it has on our bodies. In my monographs, I have highlighted a few constituents in each plant that contribute to healthy sexuality in some way. This book is in no way a comprehensive study of herbal constituents, but rather provides examples of how growing our understanding of plant constituents can provide a window into a plant's effectiveness. It is important to remember that when we are working with a whole plant, we are working with a combination of constituents, so any study of a single constituent provides only a partial understanding of the plant's effectiveness. Constituents may also have different effects in combinations than they have on their own. One beautiful thing about life on this planet is that life supports other life. Plants in their whole form often provide combinations of constituents for nourishing and healing other beings and in a form that our bodies can easily assimilate.

Monographs also provide an overview of how an herb is generally used. I researched my monographs by looking at herbal information from herbalists I trust like Rosemary Gladstar, K. P. Khalsa, Rosalee de la Forêt, and jim mcdonald. I also hired researchers who are more familiar with the realm of scientific studies to find scientific backing for the information I had compiled. I have summarized this information for you. I also included a section about how participants in my Aphrodisiac Circle experienced these herbs. Reading about others' discoveries and experiences can give you a sense of what you might experience yourself.

Considering your own constitution in relation to an herb's energetics is another good way to help narrow down which herbs might be perfect for you. For example, if you are someone who runs hot and dry, you will likely want to work with herbs that are cooling and moistening. You might also consider the nature of the situation you are working with in relation to the herb's energetics. If you are feeling cold and sluggish and are wanting more energy and vitality, look to herbs that are warming. If your sexual juices aren't flowing, moistening herbs may be particularly helpful.

Monographs also give information about why an herb may not be right for you. In my monographs you will find some of that information in the "Special Considerations" section. Some herbs are not appropriate to take during pregnancy or if you have a certain illness or are currently taking other medications. The energetics of an herb can also be an indicator that this herb is not a good choice for you. For example, if you are someone who runs hot, you may not want to add an herb like ginger to your diet on a regular basis as it could raise your body heat to uncomfortable levels. Herbal actions can also be a good source of information about why you might not want to choose a particular herb. For example, an herb like oatstraw can be blissfully relaxing, but it is also a diuretic, so drinking a quart of infusion just before sex may not be your best choice since you will likely have to get up to pee more than once during your sexual experience.

As you are making your choices, please also consider issues of sustainability. An herb like maca may be supportive for you, and you may choose to call on it for a period of time, but if you don't live high in the mountains of Peru, it is likely not the most sustainable choice. Is there an herb that grows right outside your door that can support you in similar ways? That one will be a better choice for long-term support. Monographs often provide information about where an herb grows so you can take elements like this into consideration.

Dosage and preparation suggestions are also included in monographs, giving you a sense of how to integrate this herb into your life. As you begin to do that, the real learning begins. There is no better source of information than your own personal experience with an herb. As you decide on a dose and preparation and take the herb into your body, take time to notice the effects you feel. Participants in the Aphrodisiac Circle were delighted by how empowering it felt to gain this body knowledge and develop a personal relationship with the various herbs.

BEING EMBODIED
AND INCREASING
OUR CAPACITY
FOR SENSATION

As you begin to slow down and notice sensual experiences throughout your day, you may find the focus on your body to be uncomfortable at first. Many of us spend the majority of our time in our heads and disconnected from our body sensations. We may find that we have been ignoring our physical sensations so we don't have to listen to what they have been trying to tell us. For instance, we may feel compelled to stay up in our heads so that we can continue to work in an unsustainable way, not allowing our bodies the rest they need. Give yourself time to integrate this new way of being. Start with one conscious experience and gradually increase the time you spend in sensation from there.

That simple sensory meditation from the introduction is a good beginning. Let's come back to a version of it now. It is a practice to return to time and time again. Sit quietly with your eyes closed and notice the places where your body is touching your chair or the floor. Notice any places where your body is touching something else. Notice the places where one body part is resting on another body part. Notice the feel of your clothes and hair against your skin. Is there a breeze? Is it hot or cold? Are there any smells in the air? Take a moment to sniff and notice what arises in you as you smell the air. Can you hear any sounds? What are they? How do they make you feel? Notice places in your body that are tight or stiff. Bring some breath or gentle movement to those areas. Stillness, deep breathing, and allowing are perfect tools to use any time uncom-

fortable feelings or sensations arise for you. Simply giving space for them to exist can allow these feelings to pass or can allow you to get in touch with what actions you can choose to take to alleviate them.

Practicing a meditation like this will help you tune in more and more to the subtle sensations in your body. Our bodies are an invaluable source of information and wisdom for us. We all know the feeling of nervous knots in our stomach. As we begin to tune in to the subtle sensations of our bodies, we can gain more insights into what our bodies are telling us about what we do and don't want to do, what makes us feel happy or nervous. I recommend beginning to listen to this wisdom. Just listen, at first. Notice what your body is telling you. Over time, you may find yourself making different choices, allowing yourself more rest and pleasure.

The herbs can also help us become more embodied and increase our capacity for sensation. Sarah found this in her use of kava tincture. During our year together, Sarah was in a time of expanding and deepening her relationship with her own sensuality and sexuality, exploring her own arousal and personal pleasure. She found kava to be an ally for this opening. Kava brought her into a slower pace of life and helped create ease and flow, as well as giving her a tingly feeling, a softness in her breasts, and an aliveness in her yoni. (*Yoni* is a Sanskrit word referring to the female genitalia.)

Lisa really noticed how participating in cacao ceremonies that included music and vocalizing helped her feel embodied and increased her capacity for feeling sensation. The ceremonies were held with intention and time and space to really sink into the effects of the cacao drink. The cacao plant and the hands that grew it were honored,

Ceremonial Cacao

Prepare this cacao drink for use with intention in a ceremony or ritual.

INGREDIENTS

3½ tablespoons ceremonial-grade cacao

Honey, cinnamon, and cayenne, to taste (optional)

PREPARATION

1 Shave the cacao into small pieces with a knife or blender.

2 Bring 1 cup of water to near boiling (do not overheat because it will cause the oils in the cacao to separate).

3 Put the cacao in a blender and pour hot water over the cacao. Blend until fully melted and integrated.

4 Add honey, cinnamon, and/or cayenne to taste.

5 Pour it into your favorite mug and drink slowly, savoring each mouthful.

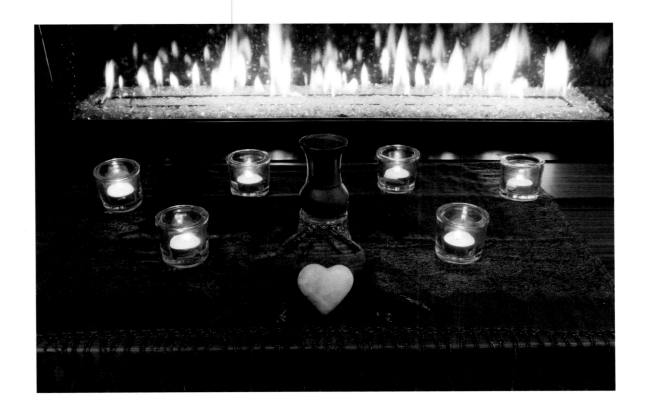

and the cacao was sipped slowly, savoring each mouthful. Lisa said the experiences led to "a beautiful opening in my heart and mind. During one, I was overcome with love for my grown son and reveled in the memories of so many shared moments of deep connection with him over the years. In each ceremony, I felt deeply connected to my loved ones and open to fresh perspectives and insights. At the same time, I felt deeply connected to my body and to sensation." Following the ceremony, her mind continued to feel relaxed and both movement and touch felt exquisite for hours on end.

OUR GENITALS: What's in a Name?

Choosing the words we use to refer to our genitals is both empowering and important. The words we learned growing up may very well reflect the culture of sexual repression and shame our parents and their parents grew up within. Consider for a moment the words that you have heard to refer to the male and female genitals. Make a list of all of them. What words did you grow up using? What words do you use now? Do you use different words with your lover than you do with your doctor?

Let's do a little exercise:

1 Using the sensory meditation or another technique, bring yourself into a sensual, embodied state.

2 Pick one of the words from your list. Say it out loud.

3 Notice any sensations that arise in your body. Notice any emotions that arise as well. Are these the sensations and emotions you would like to feel in relation to your genitals?

4 Explore other words on your list in the same way. Notice if there are some that you would like to use more than others. Some you would like to use in certain circumstances. One that feels most right for how you want to think about your own genitals.

For the past 20 years, I have been primarily using the word *yoni* to reference my genitals. I am a lover of words, and I have loved this word since the first time I heard it. I love the way it feels in my mouth and how it resonates in my mind. My limited understanding of the word is that it is a Sanskrit word with a sacred element to it that refers to the vagina and vulva together. I have loved those feelings of wholeness and sacredness. As I have used the word *yoni*, those have become the main elements I feel in relation to my genitals. This word has grounded me in a reverent way of connecting with my body and my sexuality.

The word *yoni* came to the West with the early translations of the Kama Sutra into English. It is one of the words I have chosen to use for the female genitalia in my text because of these feelings of wholeness and sacredness. I do want to acknowledge that there is more to this word than I know, since it comes from sacred cultural traditions in India. I am using it here only in the limited way it is used in the West.

I also use the words *pussy*, *vulva*, and *vagina* in my text. Regena Thomashauer's book *Pussy: A Reclamation* reclaims the use of the word *pussy* as a positive and powerful word for female genitalia. *Vulva* and *vagina* are the commonly accepted Western scientific words for the genitalia, so I've included those too.

For men, the Sanskrit word *lingam* is the companion to *yoni* to refer to the male genitalia, with *penis* being the Western, more scientific option. *Cock* is another commonly used term for this feature of the male anatomy. I use both *penis* and *cock* in my text but have chosen not to use *lingam* since it is so much less common in Western literature at this time.

I encourage you to choose words to reference your genitals that encompass the way you most want to feel about your body and your sexuality. For me, I like the feelings of reverence and wholeness I associate with the words *yoni* and *lingam*. I like the playfulness and adventurousness I associate with the words *cock* and *pussy*, and I like the ease of the commonly accepted terms *vagina*, *vulva*, and *penis*. The important thing, I think, is to become comfortable using words to refer to our genitals so we can talk with ease and share and learn about our sexuality.

NATURE CONNECTION

As you slow down and sink more into sensation, it is likely you will also be increasingly drawn to the natural beauty that surrounds you. You may find yourself pausing to really take in the stunning colors of a sunset or the delightful fragrance of a wild rose. Your connection to the plants and the natural world will begin to deepen, and you may find yourself slowing down even more and your senses becoming increasingly heightened. This is a beautiful feedback loop that I have noticed in my own life.

Joe's experiences with roses provide a wonderful example of this. He and Cassie visited me during that month, and we went out and harvested rose petals together. We spent a good hour out with the rose bushes, gathering and talking, listening to the birds, taking in the beauty around us. Back at home we made necklaces from rose buds, and Joe remarked on how relaxing and nourishing it was to spend that time creating beauty. Over the course of the month, he felt a sense of ease in his life, a coming into a gentler part of himself. He enjoyed opening to the complexity of roses in all the varieties around him. He found roses to be a great excuse for getting out and feeling sensual.

Christina and Gabrielle were also drawn outside by the roses. Christina was drawn to start taking care of a rose bush, really cultivating a relationship with this plant and rose energy. She loved that roses were so abundant and freely available. Gabrielle didn't think she liked roses much, but it turned out that, like cacao, roses offered her another portal into reconnecting with

her sensuality. After her month of connecting with the bush in her yard, she wrote:

I know my rose bush now and her blooms are the color of coral, reddish, orangish, salmon, and terra-cotta. A vibrant color of ocean life, sun, and autumn. She brought me unmistaken expressions of love, admiration, purity, mysticism, longing, regret, devotion, whimsy, hope, focus, and fun. I look forward to playing with her again when her hips are set and when she blooms again next year.

Whether you're currently with a partner or not, a sensual connection to the natural world can be a beautiful aspect of a vibrant life. One man I spoke with described a practice he calls "earthing," which involves simply lying naked on the earth. This gives him a feeling of being grounded and anchored

> *As you love and accept your natural sensual and sexual nature, truly healthy sexual expression will begin to unfold.*

and helps him tap into a resonance with the earth. "We are nature," he said, "and our inherent natural essence is to be sensual/sexual beings." Perhaps it will be the roses that draw you outside, or your tulsi or lavender plants. Perhaps just the softness of the fresh, green grass at the end of a stressful day. Pleasurable sensation can draw you out, and from there your connection to nature and acceptance of your natural self will begin to grow. As you love and accept your natural sensual and sexual nature, truly healthy sexual expression will begin to unfold.

List of Sensual Delights

Let's wrap up this chapter by making a list of things you *love*, things that bring you immediately back into pleasurable sensation and gratitude for being alive in a human body.

1   Take out your journal or a beautiful piece of paper, and find your favorite pen.

2   Settle in and take a few deep breaths, feeling the expansion and contraction in your body as you do so.

3   Let your breathing return to a natural rhythm and practice the meditation from the introduction, or run your finger over your lips to bring yourself present and into sensual awareness.

4   Ask yourself, "What sensory experiences (sights, sounds, smells, tastes, etc.) absolutely delight me?"

5   As the answers arise, write them down.

Post your list somewhere you will see it every day. Even if you don't directly experience something from the list, the act of reading it over can help reconnect you with your intention to live a more pleasure-filled, vibrant life!

This is my list: the smell of roses, ocean waves / smell of salt in the air, warm sand, feeling of sun on my body, tree leaves against blue sky, flowers, warm chai, soft blankets, taste of halibut, sensual touch, sunsets, being naked outside, knitting with beautiful yarn, gardening, rocking chairs, porch swings, window seats, and good stories.

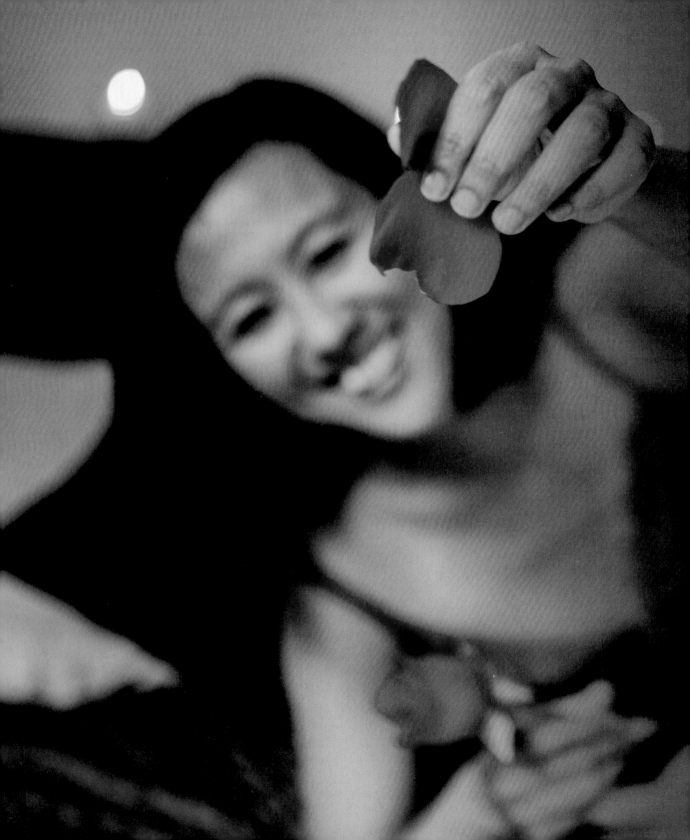

TWO

CREATING
ENVIRONMENTS
WHERE
LOVE AND EROS
FLOURISH

The word *aphrodisiac* is derived from the name Aphrodite, the Greek goddess of love. She is known for creating environments where love and eros can flourish. I *love* that. Finding ways to make my home a place of beauty and sensual delight is a continual source of joy for me. I have cultivated lush gardens where flowers are blooming around me throughout much of the year, creating beauty for both my eyes and my nose. Herbs like mint and oregano are plentiful and within easy reach of my doors so that I can also delight my mouth all summer long. Right now, I am sitting in my lounge chair outside, writing to the soothing sound of birdsong and feeling the warmth of the sun on my arms and legs.

Inside, I have chosen paint colors and inspiring art to cover my walls in beauty. I love the well-made wooden Amish furniture we chose for our living and dining rooms. There are many cozy sitting areas in my home that are dressed up with colorful quilts, soft pillows, and blankets. And my husband gave me a large lambskin that I lay out in front of our woodstove hearth in the winter. The smells of fresh, home-cooked meals and herbal teas fill the air, while my favorite music or the sound of my children's voices and laughter delights my ears.

Some things that help to create this kind of environment change with the seasons. I create mini altars in my house, bringing out objects of beauty that correlate with the seasons as they change. In the spring and summer, I bring in fresh flower bouquets. In the fall, gourds and winter squash become beautiful decorations. In summertime, my windows are flung wide to let in the fresh air. In winter, the fire in the wood stove creates warmth and beauty. Each season has its special, sensual magic.

This home I live in now, at 52, is the result of me having cultivated this practice of creating an environment where love and eros flourish over the course of many years. It reflects my particular tastes and the things that bring me joy. I have lived in much smaller places and with many fewer resources. For a while my outside space was limited to a container garden on the tiny patio deck of my apartment. When I was pregnant with my son, we lived in a friend's RV in their yard. We loved that place because cleaning involved wiping down the small kitchen and vacuuming the aisle between the kitchen and dining table. We spent most of our time outside in those days, enjoying the beauty of the natural world. Wherever you are and however much you have, you can make choices to bring more sensual delight into your everyday living space. I encourage you to act from inspiration. Bring in a bouquet of wildflowers, light a candle on your bedside table, or make yourself a soft place with blankets and pillows that is dedicated to pleasurable sensation. Do one small thing at a time, taking delight in each transformation, no matter how large or small.

EMOTIONAL ENVIRONMENTS WHERE LOVE AND EROS FLOURISH

The emotional environment in our homes is perhaps even more important than the physical environment. When I think of an emotional environment where love and eros can flourish, I imagine a space where people feel accepted, loved, and cherished just as they are and where people are open and honest with each other without being judgmental. I imagine being wrapped in a warm hug.

Setting an intention for that kind of environment in your home can be a powerful first step to creating it. For a while I had a simple ritual of lighting a tea candle on my hearth (stove) and setting out a card stating my intention of my home being a "safe, welcoming, and nourishing place for family and friends." I would do this each month on the day of the new moon. Often, I would add a beautiful flower or two to my mini altar. Intentions can also be written in beautiful script and hung for all to see. Having them out and visible definitely helps make them more effective.

Beyond setting the intention, it is also important to learn and cultivate skills that help us relate with others in healthy ways. My favorite tool for this is the work of Marshall Rosenberg on Nonviolent Communication. His book and educational materials give lots of practical ideas for listening to one another, expressing empathy, and making clear requests. Just learning to listen to one another and validate each other's experiences before responding can be life changing. After some work with Imago Dialogue, my husband and I have come to love the phrase "You make sense to me." It is a way we can validate each other's thoughts and experiences, even if we have a different opinion. We also have learned to repeat back what the other is saying and ask, "Am I getting you?" and "Is there more you would like me to understand?" As we listen to each other in these ways, we find we feel heard, validated, and emotionally safe.

There is also tremendous, groundbreaking work being done right now in the area of consent culture. The heart of this is that each person's body is their own and sacred. The work here is about learning to make clear requests of others, to respond to requests with a true yes or no, and to be conscious of respecting each other's physical and emotional boundaries. This creates a foundation of clarity and respect that goes a long way toward creating a loving, trusting environment.

We can call on the herbs for support as we endeavor to create this respectful, loving atmosphere. Relaxing nervines like milky oats, kava, or tulsi can be taken in tincture form to help keep our nerves steady as we navigate relationships with those closest to us. Hawthorn can be another ally, helping to protect and open our hearts. My friend and herbalist Lauren Morgan said, "I like

to think that the thorns on hawthorn help to cut through to the truth of the matter, invoking the truth of heart, and slicing away all else. Hawthorn helps us to be in an openhearted, expansive state while also keeping us in our boundaries with a proper amount of protection and discernment. An ally of safe love!"

Another aspect of the emotional environment that Aphrodisiac Circle participants identified was playfulness. This element can often get lost as we are learning and practicing new relating skills, but if cultivated can be incredibly helpful in creating the ease necessary for learning and integration. Frequent expressions of gratitude and appreciation for each other's efforts and qualities can be a helpful underpinning for playfulness to flourish. Smiling and being willing to laugh at yourself and appreciate your "failures" as steps toward growth are also wonderful ways of cultivating a playful environment.

PERSONAL CARE AND PREPARATION

Within an emotionally healthy environment, we can also nourish and care for our physical bodies so our bodies themselves become environments where love and eros flourish. This flourishing happens when we are happy and our bodies are healthy. Bringing ourselves to this state and continually cultivating it is foundational for vital living, so this is a theme that will be built upon through the entire book.

This kind of care has multiple physical, mental, emotional, social, and spiritual components. For example, on the physical level, we want to be sure we are eating well and getting plenty of sleep

Expressions of Gratitude and Appreciation

Taking the time to appreciate your partner, your children, your housemates, or yourself is an important part of creating a loving environment in your home. You can do this activity when you are filled with love and joy or when you are upset and wanting to shift the energy in a positive way.

1 Using breath, sensory meditation, or other tools, bring yourself to a place of embodied sensation.

2 With your eyes closed, picture the person you want to appreciate. Ask yourself, "What has this person done lately that has made my life more wonderful? What qualities does this person embody that I appreciate?" and/or "What do I love about this person?"

3 Listen for the answers that naturally arise and find a way to express them. You can write them in a beautiful card and leave it for this person to find, send them in an e-mail, or tell them in person. I find this last option to be the most moving. Take a moment with this person, look them in the eyes, and gift them with your gratitude.

4 Notice and reflect on the positive energy that is generated for both people in this exchange.

5 Make this a habit, offering appreciation multiple times in a day or week!

and exercise. For mental health, we can seek ways to engage our mental capacity and creativity so we are always learning and growing through our daily experiences. Emotionally and socially, we can cultivate joy and a feeling of having adequate support by investing in family ties, friendships, intimate relationships, and professional help from a therapist or coach. A spiritual practice like meditation or prayer can also be an invaluable part of our personal care. Overall, we want to live lives that include plenty of rest and play, as well as meaningful work. Each of these components is worthy of in-depth exploration (whole books have been written about each one) and will look differently for each of us as we find our own way with them.

For now, let's begin to explore some ways that the herbs can support us in tending our bodies as environments where love and eros naturally flourish. Like exercise routines or meditation practices, herbs can help support our health and happiness when used regularly as nourishment or tonics over time.

One of my favorite ways of doing this is with daily herbal infusions. There are many herbs that are packed with vitamins and minerals and that work on a nourishing level. Some of my favorite herbs in this category are oatstraw, nettle, red raspberry, kelp, and red clover. These herbs are staples in my diet. I create a nourishing herbal infusion with a mix of them every day for each member of my family, and we think of them as our multivitamin, since vitamins and minerals are easily assimilated into our bodies when taken in the form of tea.

My absolute favorite nourishing and also aphrodisiac herbal infusion is a Golden Oat Infusion made with oatstraw and oat tops. This infusion calms my nerves, nourishes my body with vitamins and minerals (especially calcium), and is particularly nourishing for my reproductive system, heart, and blood vessels.[1] For men, oats also liberate testosterone and improve sperm motility.[2] There are definite physical reasons that we have a saying about "sowing our wild oats."

Cassie and Joe found the routine of drinking Golden Oat Infusions daily to be transformational for their sex life. Cassie had been struggling for years with vaginal dryness, but with the oatstraw, she noticed lots of natural vaginal fluid that really enhanced her pleasure during their lovemaking. She noticed that it heightened all the sensations around her vulva, clitoris, and G-spot, and that she was able to stay wet throughout the course of their lovemaking. Joe had been struggling with painful ejaculations. With the oatstraw he found the consistency of his semen was less viscous and felt his reproductive system was lined with more fluids. These factors led to smoother flow of ejaculate, less anxiety around ejaculation, and incredibly pleasurable orgasm. He said, "I would have never guessed how much one little herb would have made such a huge difference in our love life. It's fair to say that oatstraw helped me become a better lover because I am now able to stay present when we are intimate. It's hard to describe how transformational this herb has been for me. Instead of being fearful of whether I'd experience sharp pain, I can relax into the moment, and now, every time I come feels like juicy, flowing pleasure. Wow! What a difference!"

Integrating a nourishing herb like oatstraw into your diet is very safe, and like Cassie and Joe, you may experience profound effects, or the effects may be more subtle, a sense of ease or relief from anxiety. If you are experiencing any ongoing symptoms like painful ejaculations, it is always a good idea to check with a qualified health care practitioner to get the care you need. More ideas about steps to take to find the right course of action for your particular case are covered in Chapter 11.

Another herb I would like to highlight here is hawthorn. Hawthorn is a heart tonic that works on many levels. Not only is it nourishing for our physical hearts, it provides care on emotional and spiritual levels as well. During the month before our experimentation with hawthorn, my husband and I had been experiencing some relationship challenges. Taking a spoonful of Autumn Blush Cordial (page 39) nightly for a month felt soothing and comforting for my tender heart

Golden Oat Infusion

INGREDIENTS

1 ounce oatstraw (or a combination of oatstraw and oat tops)

HERBAL TIPS

✦ Nourishing herbal infusions (strong herbal teas) are made by combining one ounce of herbs with one quart of boiling water and letting it steep for at least four hours.

✦ These kinds of infusions for daily nourishment should only be made with nourishing herbs like those mentioned earlier. It may make sense to prepare tonic herbs (like hawthorn) in this way for a specific period of time. Many herbs have medicinal qualities that are too strong to be infused or at least are not meant for daily consumption.

✦ A nice rhythm to establish is making your herbal infusions before you go to bed, letting them steep overnight, and drinking them throughout the following day. Or making them at breakfast time and drinking them at dinner.

PREPARATION

1 Put the oatstraw (and tops) into a quart jar.

2 Boil 1 quart of water, and pour it over the oats to fill the jar and cap with a lid.

3 Let steep for at least 4 hours and not more than 12 hours.

4 Strain, reserving the liquid and composting the oats.

5 Drink iced, warmed, or at room temperature, depending on your preference (I like mine iced!).

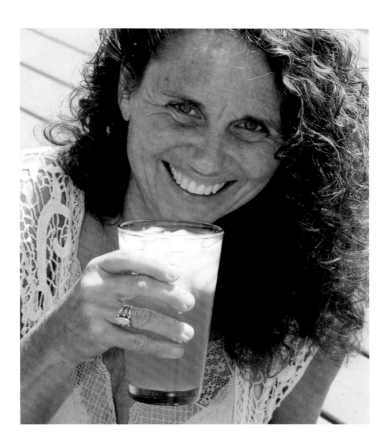

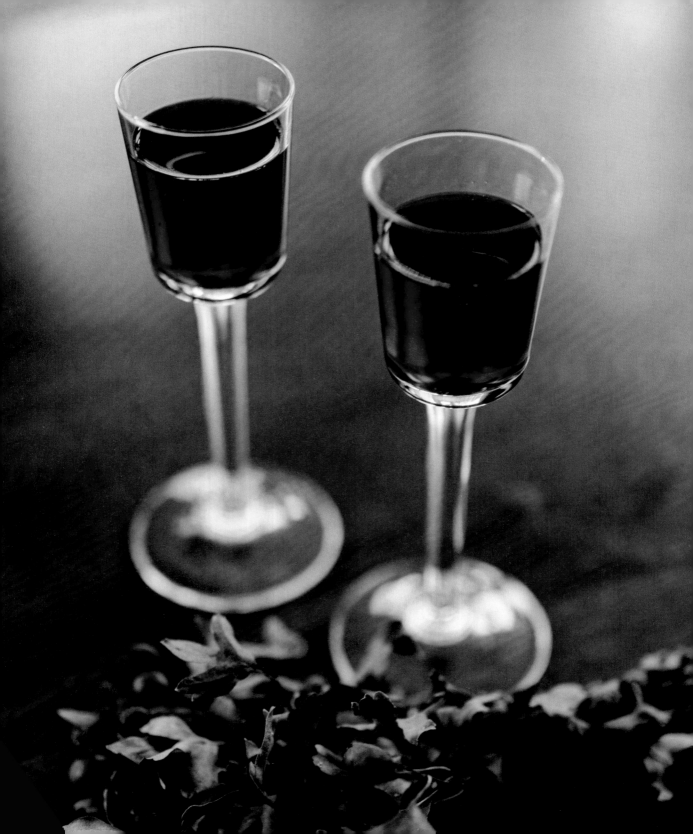

Autumn Blush Cordial

INGREDIENTS

1 teaspoon minced fresh ginger

3 crushed cardamom pods

5 cherries (can be fresh or frozen, sweet or tart)

2 teaspoons cacao nibs

2 tablespoons dried rose petals

1 vanilla bean, cut in half lengthwise

1 cinnamon stick

Zest from one lemon

1 sweet apple, coarsely chopped

⅓ cup pomegranate seeds (optional)

½ cup hawthorn berries (fresh or dried)

2 tablespoons dried hibiscus petals

½ cup honey (or to taste)

Approximately 4 cups brandy

PREPARATION

1 Place all the spices and fruit in a quart-sized jar. This cordial is very amenable to substitutions, so enjoy experimenting.

2 Add the honey and then fill the jar with brandy.

3 Stir and be sure all the ingredients are completely covered with liquid.

4 Infuse this for 4 weeks on your kitchen counter, stirring or shaking daily for at least the first week.

5 Strain and enjoy in small, regular quantities (a nightly ounce for a month is nice).

HERBAL TIPS

✦ Cordials are sweetened alcohol extracts often made with brandy, but other base alcohols can be used instead to balance flavors. Cordials are generally made from fresh ingredients, while elixirs are made from dried, but the line between the two has become blurred over time.

✦ Both the honey and alcohol are extracting constituents from the herbs and other ingredients through the process of infusing this cordial. You get the benefits of these constituents when you drink the cordial. Plus, it tastes divine.

and helped ease the tensions that had developed between us. Christina had been struggling with lingering hurt from past heartbreaks. She felt her daily use of hawthorn tincture slowly but surely wash away this pain, leaving her open to the possibility of a new romance. Having a healthy and open heart is definitely a key to preparing our bodies for flourishing love and eros.

Herbs like oatstraw and hawthorn work to nourish us slowly over time to help cultivate the conditions within our bodies for love and eros to flourish. Other herbs, like cacao or kava (or a combination of the two) can be used just before engaging in intimate experiences to create sensually arousing effects. Christina noticed tingling in her lips and genitals during and after a kava/cacao ceremony, and I found this combination helpful for preparing my vagina for more internal sensation during penetration. After the month of exploration with cacao, James noted that he wanted to be more conscious in his use of this herb, realizing that just by eating it, he was choosing to engage with erotic energy.

STRENGTHS AND DOSAGES

Nourishing Herbs: *This class of herbs can be consumed in high quantities. We call on them primarily for their vitamin and mineral content to bring nourishment to our bodies. (oats, rose)*

Tonic Herbs: *Tonic herbs are generally taken in specific dosages, in a regular rhythm for a specified length of time. They will likely have slow acting effects that increase and settle in over the period of time they are taken. Some tonic herbs can be taken regularly for months or years. Others may be more effective when taken regularly for a while and then stopped altogether or just given a rest for a period of time. (eleuthero, fenugreek, schisandra, hawthorn, ashwagandha, maca, tulsi, cacao, ginger)*

Medicinal Herbs: *These are herbs that are taken more like medicine. They likely contain some powerful constituents and may have distinct, immediate (or relatively quick) effects, and it is important to pay careful attention to the recommended dosage as they may be harmful if taken incorrectly. (damiana, kava)*

I offer these categories as a general way to think about the strength of different herbs and to make decisions about dosages, but it is important to note that there are no hard and fast rules here. For example, tonic and nourishing herbs can be used medicinally if they are taken in higher doses. Also, different herbalists might choose to categorize the herbs differently, putting ginger under medicinal herbs, for example. Your own experience of the herb in your body will be your best source of information about strength and dosage that is right for you.

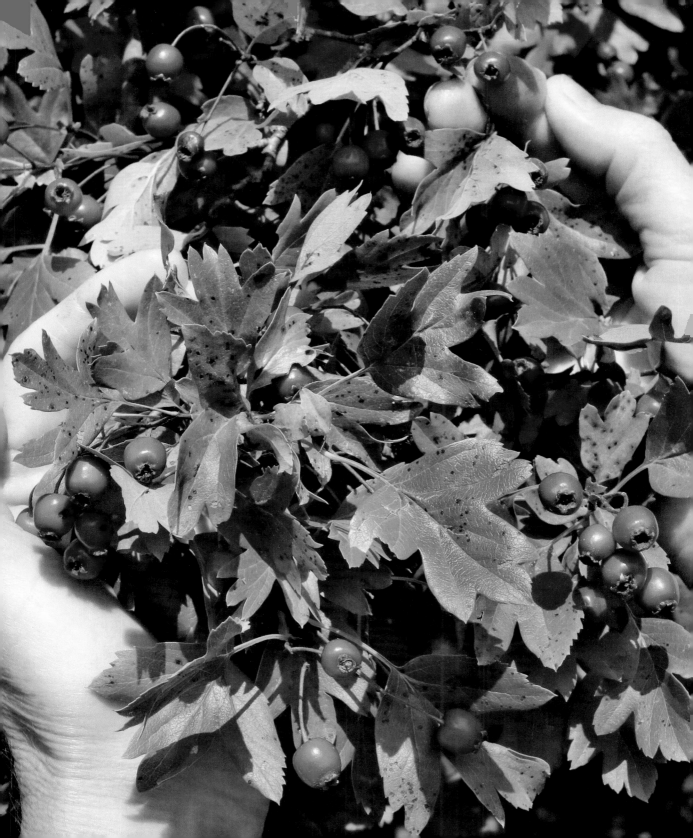

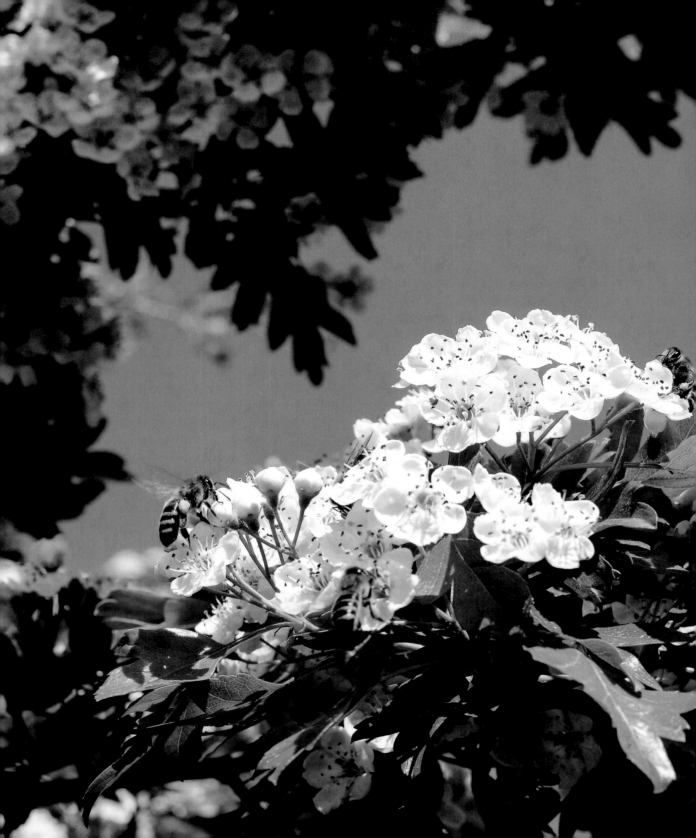

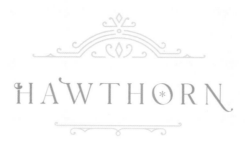

HAWTHORN

Crataegus monogyna, C. laevigata, Crataegus spp.

Hawthorn, with its tiny, abundant white flowers and deep red berries, is a tree that is dear to my heart. Hawthorn flowers have a sort of musky smell that reminds me of sex, and to me, they feel both soothing and playful. The berries are a source of deep nourishment, especially for our hearts. When walking among hawthorn trees, I feel playful love, care, and protection.

Back where I used to live in Carnation, Washington, I would harvest hawthorn flowers and berries in a wetland area. There was a beautiful grandmother tree there, and in the early summer I loved to slip into the cool hiding place beneath her branches and listen to the hum of bees collecting pollen from all those beautiful, tiny, white flowers. I would return in the late summer to gather berries from the same location.

How Does Hawthorn Work in Our Bodies?

Hawthorn is all about heart health. Rosemary Gladstar calls it the supreme cardiovascular tonic.[3] When used consistently over time, hawthorn berries (and particularly the flavonoids within them) nourish, strengthen, and tone the heart muscle and its blood vessels.[4] Quercetin, one of hawthorn's main flavonoids, has been shown to suppress abnormal heart rhythms.[5] When used as a tonic, hawthorn also improves our circulation by dilating our arteries and veins and clearing blockages so our blood flows more freely.[6]

When you go to pick the hawthorn flowers and berries, you will notice that this plant offers an incredible abundance of both, but that it also has some serious thorns protecting them. Just as these thorns protect its flowers and berries, hawthorn has a way of helping us on an emotional level, protecting our heart while helping it to open so we can feel safe entering into relationships.[7]

This heart protection also happens on a physical level. Luteolin, a flavonoid abundant in hawthorn, has been shown to be a smooth muscle relaxant and entire scientific papers have been written about its heart-protective properties.[8] Hawthorn contains another powerful flavonoid, vitexin, which also has been shown to protect the heart.[9]

I also find hawthorn to be soothing for my nervous system and emotionally uplifting. Brigitte Mars, in her book *The Sexual Herbal*, calls hawthorn a relaxing nervine that can help relieve depression, anxiety, and insomnia, helping us to reestablish serenity.[10]

A Bit about Hawthorn Plants

Hawthorn is a tree in the rose family that is native to the temperate regions of the Northern Hemisphere in Europe, Asia, and North America.

There are over 280 species of hawthorn, which can all be used similarly.

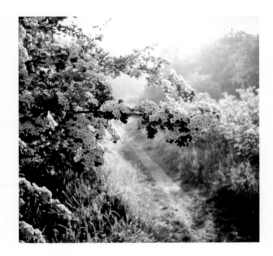

Herbal Shorthand

APHRODISIAC ACTIONS: *cardiotonic, cardioprotective, emotionally uplifting, nervine, vasodilator*

OTHER ACTIONS: *antioxidant, astringent, digestant, diuretic*

BERRIES: *antioxidant, anti-inflammatory*

ENERGETICS: *slightly cooling, neutral*

TASTES: *sour*

NOTABLE APHRODISIAC CONSTITUENTS: *flavonoids including quercetin, luteolin, vitexin*

DOSAGE SUGGESTIONS: *Hawthorn is a tonic herb and should be used in medium doses over a specific period of time. (A medium dose could look like a dropperful of tincture or a cup of tea several times a day or a nightly ounce of hawthorn cordial.)*

SPECIAL CONSIDERATIONS: *If taking heart medication, consult with a doctor, and do not use if you have diastolic congestive heart failure.*

Large doses of hawthorn leaf and flower can cause stomach upset.

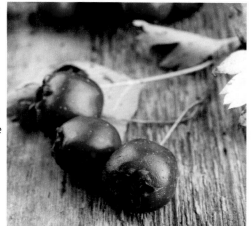

How to Use Hawthorn

PARTS USED: *leaves, flowers, and berries*

To get the tonic effects of hawthorn, you will want ways to make it part of your daily diet for a specific period of time. Some delicious ways to do so:

Make a berry honey to spread on your morning toast. **(recipe on page 14)**

Add a handful of dried hawthorn berries when you make soup stock.

Make a lovely iced tea from a nourishing infusion with hawthorn flowers and/or berries to drink on a hot day. **(follow general infusion instructions on page 37)**

Make a flower- or berry-fermented soda, which is equally delightful. **(recipe on page 292)**

Make a berry cordial—one of my personal favorites! **(recipe on page 39)**

Participant Experiences

We found hawthorn to be a delicious, gentle tonic that is deeply grounding and healing. Whether drinking hawthorn infusions, taking dropperfuls of tincture, or sipping Autumn Blush Cordial, we noticed this herb helping to wash away past hurts and heartaches and helping us build emotional resilience. Participants used words like steady heart presence, self-compassion, forgiveness, soothing, softening rough edges, centering, heartwarming, libido charging, passionate, openhearted, courageous, empathic, and playful. Artemis said, "Hawthorn is a warm hug."

SETTING UP A SPACE FOR INTIMACY

Imagine your lover leading you into a room lit by the soft light of a dozen candles. The sultry voice of Paula Cole singing "Feelin' Love" delights your ears. There is a gentle scent of roses in the air, and pink and red petals are spread across the white comforter on the bed. A bouquet of peonies rests on the headboard. On the bedside table you glimpse warmed massage oil, a bowl of homemade chocolates, an assortment of feathers, and a fur massage mitt. Your lover has taken time with their appearance, dressing sexy just for you. Their hair is shining, their skin glistening, and their eyes are dancing with delight as they turn and smile at you . . .

Taking time to set up a space in preparation for intimacy is an act of love. It can be part of your foreplay, helping to build the anticipation of what is to come, just like when making the Cardamom Chocolate Mousse Torte in Chapter 1. As you begin to set the stage, imagine your time with your lover. Think of them and all their favorite things. Look for ways to delight each and every sense. Perhaps you begin the evening with a beautiful meal including sensual foods—figs, sauces that can be slowly drizzled, and a salad or dessert decorated with edible flowers like calendula, rose, or hawthorn. This can also be a time to pull out one of those herbal honeys (maybe a hawthorn one) to tend and open your hearts. Play your favorite sensual music. Sound permeates our bodies and can relax, arouse, and open us in magical ways.

Scent can do that as well. Do you have a favorite perfume for your own or your lover's body or do you prefer their natural, human scent? Both can be exceptionally erotic. Herbal perfume making is a true art unto itself. I am including a simple spray variety here for you to play with. You can also scent the air of your love nest with incense or by using a hydrosol mist.

Knowing about what increases or decreases your arousal and what elements you enjoy in an intimate environment is important whether you are currently exploring sexually with another or not. If you are currently single, you can set up a beautiful space dedicated to your own sensual or sexual self-pleasuring. This space can be a source point for increasing the erotic flow of energy that leads to both confidence and creativity.

Creating a space for intimacy can also be a step toward manifesting a lover if you would like to attract someone into your life. You are literally creating a space that you can welcome someone into. The source energy you generate from sensual pleasure in that space will lead to you moving in the world with the confidence and ease that will attract others. And being clear about what enhances your own arousal and being willing to communicate about it will help you get your sexual needs met as you enter into new relationships.

> *Taking time to set up a space in preparation for intimacy is an act of love.*

Identifying Elements of Arousal

1   Using breath, sensory meditation, or other tools, bring yourself into a place of embodied sensation.

2   Allow your mind to drift to a memory of a time when you were highly aroused. What elements were in place that led to that arousal?

3   Does another memory come to the surface? Do you notice any similarities or differences in the elements that were present?

4   Whether you have memories of times of high arousal or not, you can also bring your awareness to each of your senses individually. Are there particular sights, smells, sounds, tastes, or feelings that increase or decrease your arousal?

5   Ask yourself some questions. Do you need the house to be free of other people or is a private room with a locked door enough for you to be able to relax into arousal? Does it help to have things neat and tidy? Is it important for you to have completed your work for the day? Do you like it if both you and your partner have just showered, or do you love the smell and feel of a sweaty body just after a workout? Is there anything else you can identify that affects your level of arousal? Perhaps you love roses and candlelight. Perhaps you really don't.

6   Write these elements down in two lists: those things that increase your arousal and those things that decrease it.

7   Use these lists to help set yourself up for erotic encounters. Manage the things that you have control over and consider sharing these lists with your partner and asking them to share theirs with you. Gifting each other with this information can help you become more effective at creating environments for one another that help lead to sexual fulfillment.

8   As you continue through this book and your life, you will learn about more things that excite you or turn you off. Keep adding to your lists, and keep sharing them!

note: *Hold these lists loosely. Not all of the things on your list need to be managed every time you want to make love. Sometimes spontaneity is more important for a hot sexual encounter. Perhaps the laundry is still on the floor, but your partner is dressed sexy and stretched out on the bed waiting for you. Let the laundry wait and focus on your sexy partner!*

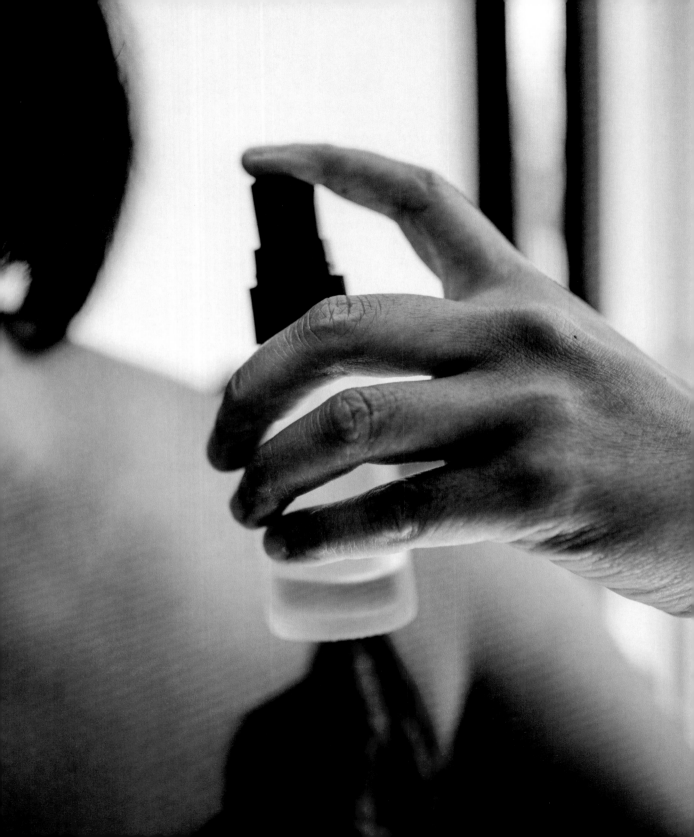

Evoke Perfume

Karin Rose

INGREDIENTS

¼ teaspoon vanilla-infused vodka or vanilla extract

2 drops vetiver (*Vetiveria zizanioides*) essential oil

1 drop ylang-ylang complete (*Cananga odorata*) essential oil

1 drop bergamot (*Citrus bergamia*) FCF essential oil

1 teaspoon Everclear (at least 95% alcohol—this is needed for ylang-ylang proper dilution of 0.8%)

SUPPLIES

10-milliliter glass spray bottle

Tiny funnel

PREPARATION

1 Measure each ingredient into a tiny glass or ceramic bowl.

2 Use the funnel to pour your blend into your 10-milliliter glass spray bottle.

3 Gently roll the bottle between your palms while setting an intention.

4 Let it sit (upright) for a week to harmonize.

5 Shake the bottle gently before use.

6 Spritz the mixture on your hair and body, as desired.

HERBAL TIPS

✦ Herbal perfume making and aromatherapy requires some learning and skill. Essential oils are wonderful for scent but are made from huge quantities of plant material. It is important to explore safety precautions for using essential oils in proper dilution to be used on your skin. This recipe has been carefully formulated with safety in mind.

✦ If you want to play with formulating your own perfumes, there are some online resources at Mountain Rose Herbs and Aromatics International. A great source for safety considerations is Robert Tisserand and Rodney Young's book *Essential Oil Safety* second edition (this is a better and more in-depth version).

Herbal Incense

INGREDIENTS

Damiana Mana Incense

1 tablespoon damiana leaf powder

1 tablespoon schisandra berry powder

1 teaspoon marshmallow root powder

Tulsi Rose Incense

1 tablespoon rose petal powder

1 tablespoon tulsi leaf powder

1 teaspoon marshmallow root powder

Kava Santo Incense

1 tablespoon kava root powder

1 tablespoon palo santo powder

1 teaspoon marshmallow root powder

PREPARATION

1 Stir the powders together until they are completely combined.

2 Slowly add approximately 1 tablespoon of water to the mix, 5 to 10 drops at a time.

3 After each addition of water, use the back of a spoon to mash the powder and water together. At first the mixture will look crumbly, and eventually those crumbles will begin to form a dough. You're looking for a fairly dry dough, just wet enough that it holds together without crumbling apart but definitely not runny.

4 Once the mixture can hold together, pinch off a small piece and form it into a cone. I've found that taller, skinnier cones burn best.

5 Set the cones on a flat surface and allow them to dry for about 5 to 7 days. If your cones are not burning well, give them a few more days to dry. You can also dry your cones in a dehydrator or on low heat in an oven.

6 To burn a cone, first place it on a fire-safe surface. Light the tip and allow it to burn slightly until the tip burns red and it is smoking freely.

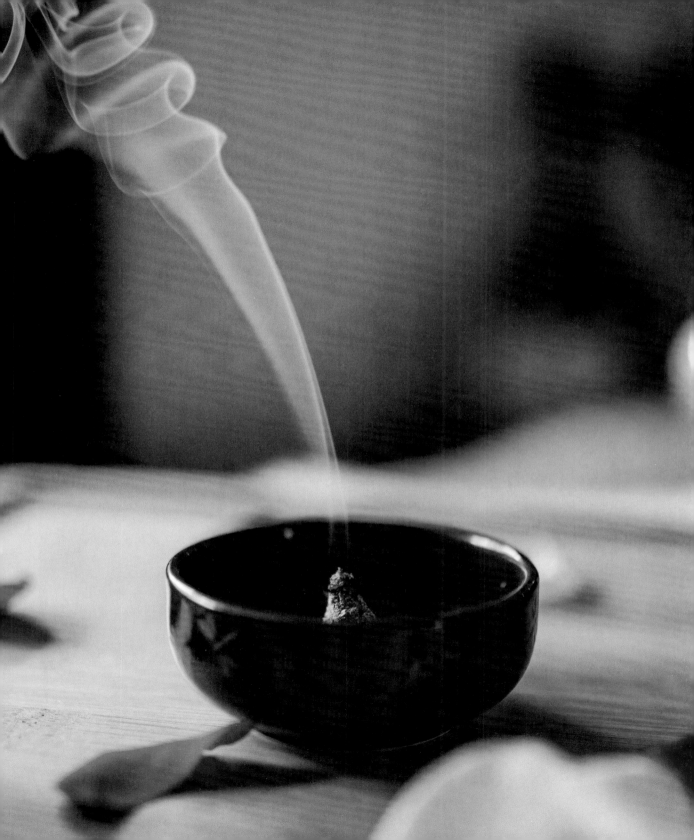

Hydrosol Mist
Air Fresheners

INGREDIENTS

Heart's Breath

Rose hydrosol and hawthorn flower hydrosol (equal parts of both)

Surrender

Tulsi hydrosol and lavender hydrosol (equal parts of both)

HERBAL TIPS

✦ For directions on making your own hydrosols, see the recipe for Sweet Spot Facial and Yoni Mist on page 99. Purchased hydrosols are often more fragrant than those made at home and are probably preferable as air fresheners.

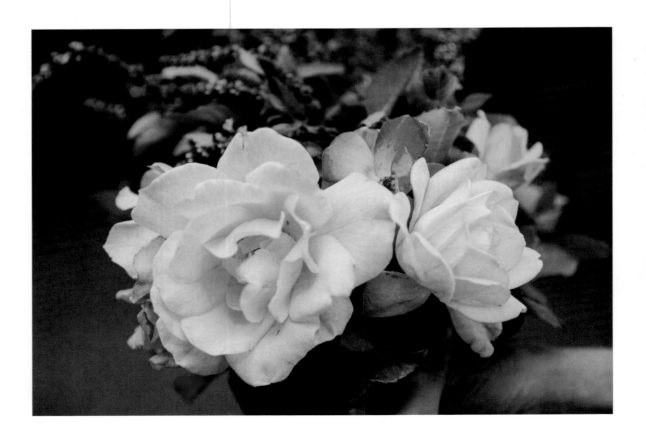

ENTERING INTIMATE SPACE WITH CONSCIOUS INTENTION

Any time we enter intimate space with ourselves or with another, we are entering into vulnerable, tender territory. In doing so, we open ourselves up to one another. We risk being seen naked, and when fully aroused, out of control. Our body's capacity to give and receive pleasure is an exquisite and precious gift, and sharing our bodies with one another is a profoundly loving and generous act. Entering intimate space with conscious intention is a way of honoring these truths.

Please take a moment to let the words from the last paragraph sink in. Let them settle not just in your mind, but deeply into your body. Let your breath carry them down into your lungs and heart. Down into your belly, your core. Down further into your pelvis, your genitals. How does your body feel with these ideas resonating inside of it? Take a few deep breaths here and imagine entering intimate space with this understanding. Imagine your lover shares this understanding. Does anything change for you about how it feels to enter intimate space?

For me, when I get present to the vulnerability and the profound gift of giving and receiving pleasure, I am moved to approach intimate space with awe and reverence, and with the intention of nourishing and honoring both myself and my lover. Entering intimate space consciously and with intention is a key to creating fulfilling and beautiful intimate experiences.

Part of this consciousness includes laying some groundwork before choosing to be sexually intimate. Be sure you are on the same page about birth control. What protection will you be using to support your readiness to bring a child into the world? Also, in order to both nourish and honor your partners, please be completely honest about any STIs you are carrying and take necessary precautions not to pass them on. Creating intimate space where we are free from worry is essential to creating an environment where love and eros flourish.

If you are entering intimate space with a new lover, I encourage you to take it slow and together consider a number of questions before engaging sexually:

✦ **What will it mean to you if we have sex?**

✦ **What expectations will you have of me after?**

✦ **Do you have other partners or lovers who will be impacted by our choice to enter into a sexual exploration together?**

✦ **What are your agreements with them?**

After exchanging answers to these questions, I encourage you to ask yourself, "Are my heart, head, and body all in alignment about this choice?" If all are a full "Yes!", then that is when to consider entering into sexual exploration together.

As you do so, you may want to create an even more specific intention for the moment you are coming together with another. Perhaps you are feeling depleted and want your time together to be nourishing. Perhaps you want to explore a particular aspect of your sexuality like G-spot stimulation or separating orgasm from ejaculation. Being honest with ourselves and sharing our wishes with our lover can help us co-create an intention for our time together and set the stage for a beautiful unfolding of intimate connection and experience.

LIFESTYLE

Of course, in order for any of the ideas put forward in this chapter to come to fruition, you need both time and space to follow through with them. Love and eros need time and space to flourish, and both of these often feel in short supply in our modern lifestyles. Luckily eros is also fed by obstacles. The fact that you picked up this book and have read this far indicates that you are prioritizing the flourishing of love and eros in your life. As you continue to do so, you will begin to grapple with and overcome whatever obstacles are standing in your way, and the rewards will be all that much sweeter for having done so.

Simon and Rebecca noticed over the course of our year-long exploration how the lifestyle they had created for themselves did not leave much time and space for intimacy. Managing their home farm and running their business required long days and was continually stressful. They were hosting business guests in their home much of the time, and their young daughter was on a schedule where she was staying up even later than them. Their participation in the Aphrodisiac Circle led to conversations about their longing for more time for intimate connection and exploration. They loved their work, and yet they ended up making the challenging decision to downsize their business and re-create their lifestyle to allow more time and space for intimacy, play, and joy.

Similarly, Angela had a surprisingly stressful year. She faced many health challenges, an unexpected need to move from her home, and ultimately to change her job as well. She found that the stress decreased her ability to relate in a physically sensual way and strained her relationship with her husband. The herbs and our exploration supported her through these challenges, helping her stay in her body and encouraging her to prioritize sensuality and sexuality. She credits the herbs with helping her see the beauty through the chaos and love herself despite feeling so much self-doubt. By the end of the project, she felt that the breakthroughs she had experienced and her shift to a more fulfilling livelihood would ultimately lead to a life with more space and health to cultivate sensuality and eroticism.

It makes my heart happy to report these stories. I love it when people find their way to happier, more vibrant lives. One of the things I love most about my own life is that I have a lot of flexibility in my schedule. Since my husband and I co-own our business, we are responsible for directing our own time. For many years now, I have scheduled in time for the things that help me thrive—things like sleep, exercise, eating well, dancing, and yes, sex. My husband and I set aside multiple times in our busy weeks for intimate connection with each other. We hold that time sacred, and arrange our schedules around it. My husband is a night person, I am a morning person. We find we connect best in the late morning / early afternoon. This is also a time when our daughter is out of the house at school, so we can fully sink into our experience with each other, without interruption.

I encourage you to think about your own life and how you can set yourself up to have the kinds of experiences you want. Can you set up your bedroom in a way that invites and inspires intimate connection? Are there other spaces in your home or yard that can serve as cozy love nests? If you have a partner, can you schedule some time to meet up for intimate connection? Maybe a long lunch hour? Or perhaps you are both night owls and can connect before falling asleep, or take

OPPORTUNITY FOR CULTIVATING EROTIC ENERGY FLOW

Envisioning Your Space Where Love and Eros Flourish

1   Using breath, sensory meditation, or other tools, bring yourself into a place of embodied sensation.

2   Imagine yourself in a place where love and eros are flourishing for you. What do you see in the space? What do you smell, hear, and taste? Is anyone here with you? What sensations do you feel in your body? How do you feel emotionally? Is the space large and open or small and womblike? Is it inside or outside? What else do you notice about this space?

3   Write about or draw the space you envisioned.

4   Using breath, sensory meditation, or other tools, bring yourself back into a place of embodied sensation.

5   Ask, "What is one element of the space I envisioned that I can bring into my everyday life right now? Is there some lifestyle shift I can make that will give me more ease of access to that kind of space? Am I willing and ready to make that shift, or is there something I need to do first?"

6   Take an action, no matter how small, to begin creating the time and space in your life that you desire.

7   Celebrate and enjoy the fruits of that action.

8   Repeat steps 4 through 7 over and over again, slowly over time, and enjoy the slow, steady transformation that results.

some long, leisurely mornings in bed. Two hours or more will give a feeling of relaxation and ease so you can really sink into sensation and connection. This may seem like an impossible amount of time to devote, but we have noticed that time spent in this way creates more ease, efficiency, and creativity throughout the rest of our lives.

If you do not currently have a lover in your life, set yourself up for self-pleasuring time or time to be alive in your senses. Creating a lifestyle that invites more pleasure can be the beginning of surprising, positive changes throughout your whole life.

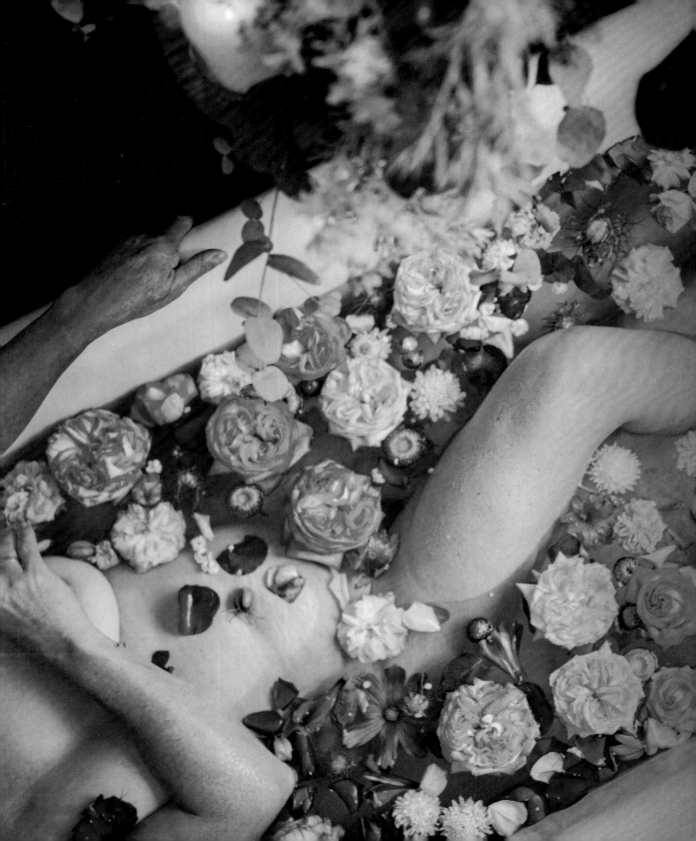

THREE

FALLING IN LOVE WITH YOUR BODY

tep with me now into the beautiful, sensual space you've begun creating for yourself. Step in and slow down. Give yourself time and permission to fall in love with your body. This body, your own wonderful body, has carried you here through uncountable moments of sensual experience. The feeling of smooth silk or soft cotton against your skin, the taste of that cardamom chocolate mousse torte, the aroma of rose petals, the sight of green tree leaves against a pure blue sky, the sound of birdsong. Each delicious, pleasurable sensation is a gift of being alive in your very own human body.

Take a moment to fully appreciate the miracle of your body. Your legs and feet for carrying you from experience to experience. Your bones, muscles, ligaments, tendons, and the way they fit together to allow for movement. Your heart pumping blood through your circulatory system, a network of veins branching through every part of your body.

Your lungs taking in oxygen, and your respiratory system distributing it. Your mouth, belly, intestines—your miraculous digestive system—that allow you to experience the delight of all different sorts of foods, and turn them into nutrients that provide you with the energy you need to move through your life.

And I haven't even yet mentioned the body systems associated with sexual pleasure and reproduction. Our bodies are built for pleasurable sexual sensation and also to facilitate the miracle of growing new life and giving birth. Healthy sexuality is your birthright, one of the greatest gifts of being alive in a human body. Appreciate your unique genitalia—penises and vaginas, and all the nerve endings and wiring that lead to pleasurable sensation in these organs and throughout your whole body. Appreciate scrotums and ovaries and the sperm and eggs within them. Whether they currently hold the capacity to create new life or not, appreciate the miracle of this co-creative potential. Appreciate the womb and its soft, beautiful, nourishing, and nurturing qualities.

HONORING YOUR RELATIONSHIP WITH YOUR BODY

Each of our magnificent bodies developed within a soft, nourishing womb space, and each (whether we feel it or not) is worthy of honoring. I hope that reading through those body appreciations led each of you to some feelings of joy and gratitude, and I am imagining that for some of you it brought up feelings like sadness, shame, or anger as well. Many of us have grown up in a culture

that taught us to relate to our bodies as shameful, ugly, or unlovable. Please take a deep breath right now and acknowledge whatever feelings surfaced. Perhaps you can even give yourself permission to express them in some way. Let some tears flow, let your body shake, punch a pillow, or wrap yourself in a soft blanket. Giving these feelings space to exist and be expressed is both vulnerable and deeply honoring, and though you may not feel it yet, it is a step toward a healthy relationship with your body and toward vibrant living.

Many of us in the United States are dissociated from our bodies, living mostly in our heads. This can happen for a wide variety of reasons. Perhaps you are in school or have chosen a career that has you working at a computer most of the day, and you just don't have much time for movement or connection with your body. Chronic pain can also lead to dissociation as can suffering sexual trauma or other physical abuse. More and more of the women I talk with report having been sexually abused at one point in their lives, and the Me Too movement has brought to light just how prevalent such abuse is in our culture. Many men, too, have experienced sexual trauma and abuse in their lives. Michelle, Christina, Angela, and Joe from the Aphrodisiac Circle are all survivors of childhood sexual abuse. Even if you have not experienced abuse, you have likely been exposed to damaging messages through mass media or may have experienced body shaming from peers or adults in your life. Most people I've met are somewhat dissociated or are dissatisfied with their body in some way.

Because of this, the process of beginning to honor and love your body is likely a tender one that will call for care and compassion. It may challenge you to question some beliefs that you didn't even know you were carrying. The herbs are here to nourish and support you through it. Several Aphrodisiac Circle participants found maca to be a powerfully grounding and supportive herb. Joe described it as helping him feel more centered and whole, more in touch with the truth of who he is. Cassie and Joe found that maca combines well with cacao. It is a tonic herb that works best when taken regularly over time, so perhaps you can integrate this maca/cacao drink into your daily routine for a while as you uncover and honor your journey.

Another herb that can support people through emotional healing is eleuthero. Christina found that this herb effectively supported her trauma healing process. It helped her feel grounded and move past chronic pain so she could come home to being in her body. She took a capsule dose of eleuthero daily during the month we were experimenting with it. This is a simple way to integrate this tonic herb into your life. You will find other eleuthero recipes like Date Treats (page 236) and Dream Cream smoothies (page 234) later in the book.

Christina and Joe found drinking a daily Golden Oat Infusion (page 37)to be helpful in this way as well. Christina writes that "recovery from childhood sexual trauma and abusive adult relationships is a primary focus of my current journey with sensuality. Oatstraw helped me feel a greater sense of calm and deep resilience for handling stress. I felt more relaxed and drawn to prioritize self-care for stress relief more often." Joe found oatstraw to have a subtle soothing effect on his anxiety related to intimacy and his body image, which he came to understand over the course of the year is associated with his childhood sexual trauma. He said, "For years I've had anxiety about being nude in front of my partner for fear of being shamed because my body doesn't look like those buff guys in the magazines. Oatstraw softened the edginess of my anxiety and helped me open and acknowledge that I was experiencing this fear. It helped me come to a place of feeling more at ease, open and accepting of my body exactly how it is. Of course, it's not a magic pill—it also requires a willingness to go into the sensations to better understand them—but oatstraw was definitely a helpful aid in my healing process."

Each of us has had a unique journey to get to exactly where we are in our relationship with our body and our personal exploration of our sexuality. Finding a way to physically honor your own process, past and present, can be very grounding. You can use your journal, drawing paper, clay, a voice recording, or dance, whatever means of expression resonates for you to honor your own unique journey.

Acknowledging your current relationship with your body and what led you to this place is the first step toward falling in love with your own unique and precious body. You may want to return to this exercise again and again over the next few weeks, adding more pivotal experiences that come to the surface for you. This will help fill out your personal story of your relationship with yourself as a sensual and sexual being.

Remembering pivotal moments related to your sexuality can make you feel quite vulnerable. So let me invite you into a nourishing moment, turning once more to the herbs. Let's step into a soothing bath.

Seda Blanca Bath

INGREDIENTS

1 cup rolled oats

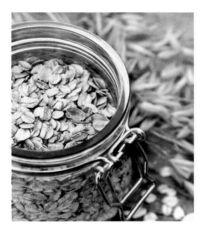

PREPARATION

1 Fill a muslin bag with the oats.

2 Draw a bath (or step into a shower), taking the bag of oats into the water with you.

3 As you soak, squeeze the bag and enjoy the silky smooth, milky texture that the oats add to the water. You can also rub the bag along your skin to feel this silkiness even more directly.

BATH NOTES

✦ Breathe deeply, enjoying the softness of this bathing experience. The silkiness of the oats on your skin can be a way to revel in the pleasurable memories, and sinking into the hot milky water can help soothe places where you are feeling tenderness or pain and bring you into places in your body where you have been shut down. Close your eyes and relax, allowing the oats to work their magic, calming and nourishing you and your body. Allow yourself to feel whatever emotions are emerging.

✦ Learning to hold myself while fully feeling my emotions has been one of the most empowering skills I have learned. We tend to think that if we let ourselves feel our sadness or fear, our anger or hopelessness, that we will never find our way back to joy, happiness, hope, and faith. In reality, when fully honored and felt, intense emotions often pass fairly quickly, and as we move through them, we find a new sense of freedom and ease and heightened feelings of hope and joy. A soothing Seda Blanca Bath can help with this holding, feeling, and moving through emotions. As we do so, our lives may begin to shift in substantial and often unexpected ways.

✦ Perhaps you already have ways of nourishing yourself when you need to move through difficult things or revel in pleasurable feelings. Whatever your methods are, I encourage you to practice them regularly in the days and months to come as you continue on your journey of embodiment and sexual empowerment.

Honoring Your Unique Relationship with Your Body

1   Settle in and take a few deep breaths, feeling the expansion and contraction in your body as you do so.

2   Let your breathing return to a natural rhythm, and practice the meditation from the introduction, or run your finger over your lips to bring yourself present and into sensual awareness.

3   Allow experiences from your past to arise that feel like they were pivotal moments for you in your connection to yourself as a sensual/sexual being. There is no need to remember all the pivotal moments, just be with the ones that are arising easily today.

4   Take time to physically honor these experiences in a way that feels good to you. (You might use your journal, drawing paper, or clay.)

Joe from the Aphrodisiac Circle shared this poem, Presence, that arose for him out of this exercise.

Be a man! Do it right! Make her come!
Deep down the voice inside churns
Like a meat grinder, leaving me mashed
Confused, unable to discern who I am
If I listen to its never-ending cry I will miss
Soft tenderness
Subtle shiver
Quiet yearning
Ecstasy
The yearning to be free!
But the voice is strong
Years of conditioning and servitude
Do not break easily
I breathe
And try again . . .

5 Settle back into embodied sensual awareness using breath and meditation or a method that works for you.

6 Ask yourself, "What has come of these experiences? How would you describe your relationship with your body right now?"

7 Take a few deep breaths as you acknowledge your personal truth.

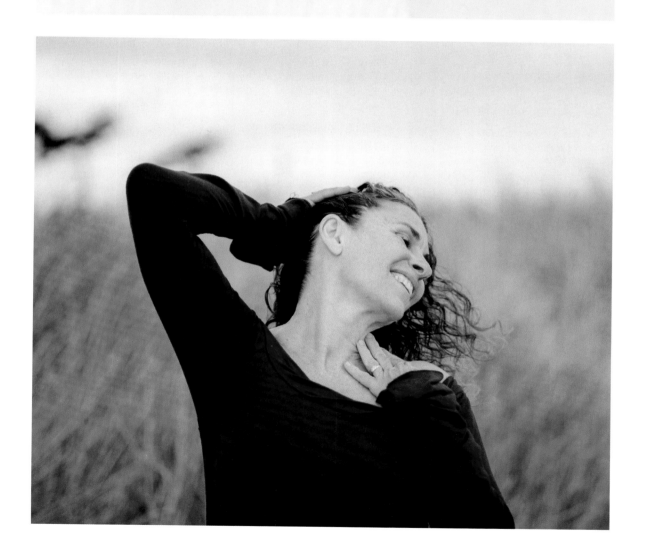

AshwaMacaMocha Shake

John Gallagher

INGREDIENTS

Root Blend

Yield: Enough powder
for 7 shakes

¾ ounce ashwagandha root
powder (approximately 4
tablespoons)

¾ ounce roasted dandelion
root powder (or Dandy Blend)
(approximately 3 tablespoons
plus 1 teaspoon)

¾ ounce beetroot powder
(approximately
3 tablespoons)

1 ounce maca root powder
(approximately 4 tablespoons
plus 1 teaspoon)

1 ounce cacao powder
(approximately
9 tablespoons)

Shake

8 ounces crushed ice

4 ounces of your favorite
creamy beverage (milk,
coconut milk, etc.)

1 banana

3 tablespoons (or one 3-ounce
scoop) Root Blend

PREPARATION

Root Blend

1 Put the powdered
ingredients in a mason
jar with a lid and shake it
really well. This is your
mix for the week.

Shake

1 Blend shake ingredients
with 8 ounces of water in
a blender or in a mason jar
with a hand blender.

2 Pour the shake into your
favorite glass, and enjoy!

HERBAL TIPS

✦ The "mocha" in this recipe
is created by adding cacao
powder with roasted
dandelion root.

✦ Roasted dandelion root
is available through
Mountain Rose Herbs. You
can also use Dandy Blend,
which is a caffeine-free
herbal coffee substitute
that is widely available.

✦ Beetroot powder has a
myriad of health benefits
and colors the shake a
velvety red. For a zero-
sugar option, Mercola
makes fermented beetroot
powder.

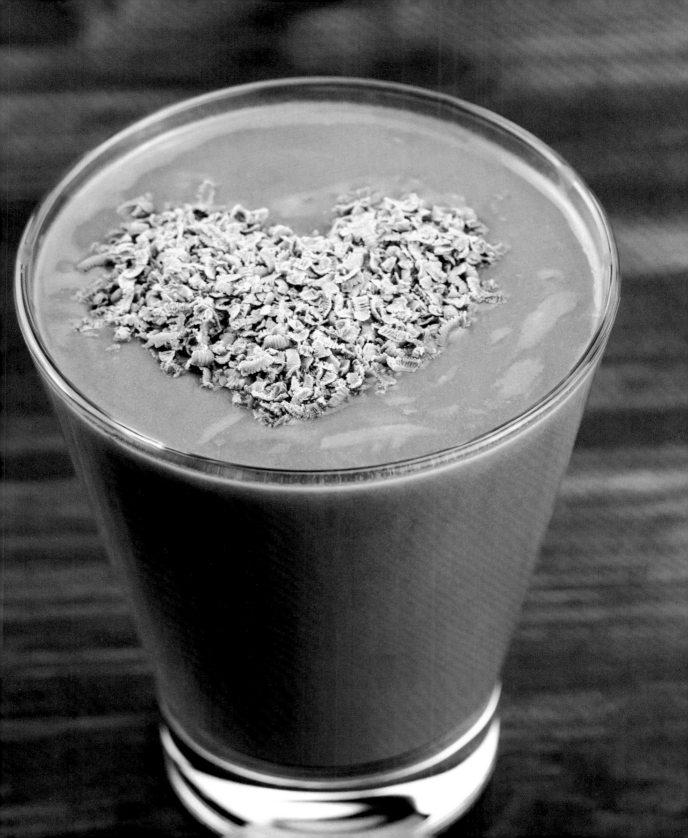

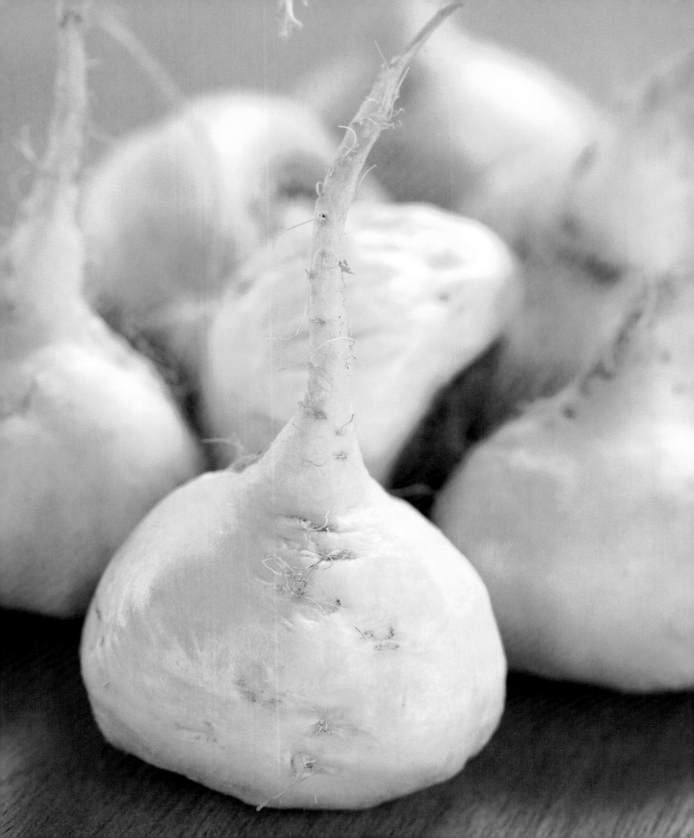

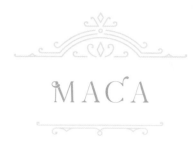

MACA

Lepidium meyenii, syn. L. peruvianum

If you are lucky enough to get it fresh, maca can be eaten much like sweet potatoes. It has a butterscotch flavor. Maca root is more available to most of us dried and powdered. This powder makes a delightful addition to smoothies and herbal treats like Maca Butter Barz (page 304).

How Does Maca Work in Our Bodies?

Maca has been called a superfood. It is packed with beneficial nutrients, including essential fatty acids (omega-3 and omega-5), vitamins B1, B2, B12, C, and E, calcium, iodine, and iron. So it is a wonderful nourisher for our bodies, helping to increase strength and stamina.

Because of its nutrient profile, maca has a wide range of positive effects on sexual function, sperm production, female reproductive function, memory, depression and anxiety, and energy, as well as reducing benign prostate enlargement, osteoporosis, aging, and metabolic syndrome.[1] Maca acts as a hormone balancer and adaptogen, which means it can help our bodies adapt to stress, helping to normalize our bodies' endocrine and metabolic processes via positive effects on our hypothalamic-pituitary axis, which leads to positive effects on our adrenals, thyroid, and pancreas.[2]

Sexually speaking, maca may increase our bodies' production of estrogen, testosterone, and progesterone, thus enhancing reproductive health.[3] It can help support women's bodies during menopause, addressing symptoms like hot flashes, night sweats, mood swings, and vaginal dryness.[4]

Maca also enhances libido and improves fertility in both sexes.[5] A combination of maca with Chinese chive seed provides positive effects on male sexual function.[6] It also increases the quality and motility of sperm.[7] Maca has a significant effect on performance and perception of general and sexual well-being in adult males with erectile dysfunction.[8]

In the grand time scale of herbal usage, maca has only recently found its way to the "modern world" and thus is just beginning to have molecular research to support all the experiential claims of this powerful plant. The current research has discovered a group of bioactive compounds found only within maca, called macamides.[9] Studies show that macamides have neuroprotective effects and cannabimimetic actions, meaning they act similarly to *Cannabis* in the body.[10] One of maca's most notable impacts on our biochemistry is its ability to break down and thus release anandamide in the body. Anandamide (also known as "the bliss molecule") is an endocannabinoid made in the body.[11] The breakdown of anandamide has been shown to boost mood and decrease fear, releasing feel-good qualities into the body. Macamides may also act on the central nervous system by regulating the release of other neurotransmitters.[12]

Herbal Shorthand

APHRODISIAC ACTIONS: *adaptogen, emotionally uplifting, hormone balancing, improves fertility, nutritive, restorative*

ENERGETICS: *warming, moistening*   TASTES: *sweet*

NOTABLE APHRODISIAC CONSTITUENTS: *essential fatty acids (omega-3 and omega-5), vitamins B1, B2, B12, C, and E, calcium, iodine, iron, macamides[13]*

DOSAGE SUGGESTIONS: *Maca is a tonic herb and should be taken in medium doses on a regular basis for a specific period of time. (A medium dose could look like 5–20 grams dried root daily or a dropperful of tincture 3 times daily.)*

SPECIAL CONSIDERATIONS: *High doses may cause insomnia.*

Also, use this herb with a high level of conscious choice. It has been used traditionally among the Andean people for over 1,000 years, but there have not been enough clinical trials to scientifically support all the health claims currently attributed to it. There is a possibility that the health benefits of maca have been exaggerated to increase sales.

Another issue to be aware of is that Peruvians are struggling to meet the global demand, and maca being cultivated in other areas for mass production may include the use of fertilizers and pesticides, which may affect the phytochemistry and composition of the plant. So please be especially careful in checking your sources if you choose to experiment with maca. Make sure it is not being grown with fertilizers and pesticides and that it is being grown in a sustainable way.

As you feel into the benefits of adding this herb into your diet, consider carefully if it is one you want to include on an ongoing basis. For sustainability reasons, it is always preferable to call upon a dooryard herb, one that grows in your own bioregion, for ongoing use. However, you may choose to call on an exotic herb for a time if the health benefits are significant. I would like to encourage you to do your research and make an informed choice.

A Bit about Maca

Maca is a turniplike plant that grows at high altitudes (12,500–14,400 feet). It is grown in the Andes Mountains in Peru and Bolivia and also in Brazil. Different varieties have roots of various sizes, shapes, colors, and sweetness.

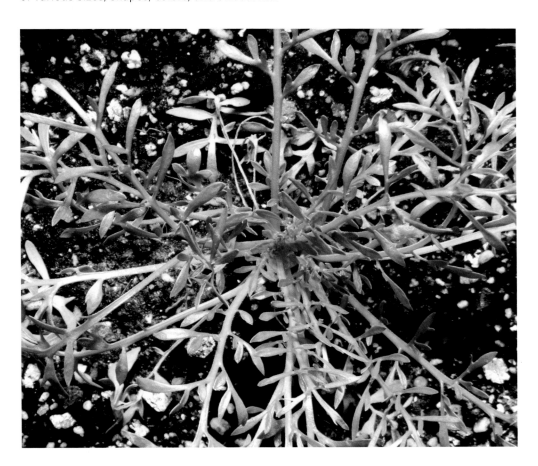

How to Use Maca

PARTS USED: *roots*

To get the tonic effects of maca, you will want to take it regularly for an extended period of time. You can take it in capsule or tincture form or add the root powder to smoothies or other foods.

Maca root is cooked, baked, fermented as a drink, and made into porridge.

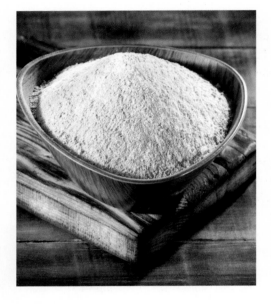

Participant Experiences

Those of us who experimented with maca found it to be grounding while also giving a steady energy boost. Rebecca was hoping maca would help with her menopausal symptoms but did not find the hormonal changes to be positive. The smell made her queasy, and maca threw off her digestion. Other friends have reported quite the opposite, swearing by maca to balance hormones and help with hot flashes and night sweats. I am currently taking a daily dose of maca and am enjoying its grounding effect. I find my hot flashes are fairly mild.

Robert remembered taking it in capsule form during a period of time when he was training hard for rowing. He found that it "raised his base energy so he didn't crash so much after hard work." Similarly, Cassie found that maca was very supportive for her through a stressful period at work. It gave her an energy boost and also heightened her libido.

Both Joe and Sarah noted that maca helped them to feel more centered and promoted a stronger sense of self. Joe said he felt "rooted and empowered" and "enjoyed a sense of grounded depth in [his] sexuality."

LEARNING TO LISTEN TO YOUR BODY

Another step you can take on this tender journey of falling in love with your body is to learn to listen to your body's wisdom. We have already started to practice this by coming into a sensually alive, embodied place at the beginning of each of the exercises in the book so far. Now, I'm going to offer you a way to take this a step further.

Find a comfortable place where you can be quietly alone for a few minutes. Sit or lie comfortably, close your eyes, and take some deep breaths, breaths that fill your belly first, then slowly progress upward into your chest. Feel your belly and then your chest expand on your inhale and contract as you exhale, your belly button moving away from and then toward your spine. Do this 10 times and then relax into a normal breathing pattern.

Now imagine a time when someone you love greeted you warmly with a hug. Notice the sensations in your body as you re-experience that memory. Bring words to what you feel. A relaxation of your muscles? Maybe a smile comes to your lips. Maybe there is a tingling feeling in your arms or belly. There is no right answer. Just notice and bring words to your own experience. This is how you feel when your body wants something—when you are feeling a yes to what is happening or being offered to you.

Now take five more of those deep breaths. Then imagine you are walking down the street and you cross paths with someone you are angry with or scared of. Someone who has done you wrong or hurt someone you love. Again, notice the sensations in your body, and bring words to them. Maybe there is a tightening of your mus-

cles, a gritting of your teeth, a churning in your stomach. Remember there is no right answer. This is about learning how to read your own body's cues about what it likes and doesn't like. This is how you feel when your body does not want something—when you are feeling a no to what is happening or being offered to you.

This information from your body can be vital as you navigate life. So often, we make decisions from information in our heads alone, while valuable cues from our body go unrecognized or ignored. Relying on reason alone, we may find ourselves agreeing to things we don't actually want or are not good for us. As we get clear about when we are feeling a yes or a no in our bodies, we begin to claim our personal sovereignty.

A next step on this journey is to learn to speak and receive a no. How often do you say yes when you want to say no? How gracefully can you receive a no from someone else without taking it personally? Let's practice with a friend. Have them make requests of you that you will say no to. (Both of you knowing that you will be saying no helps relieve some of the sting that can happen with a genuine no.) When you say no, have them respond with "Thank you" or "Thank you for taking care of yourself." Do this over and over so you get used to what it feels like to say no to someone and having your no honored and respected. Now, ask your friend to say no to you as you make requests, and thank them in return. Feel what it is like to have someone say no to you and to be grateful to them for it.

Take these practices into your life. When someone asks something of you, take a moment to breathe and feel the cues from your body. Take a risk to honor what you are feeling and respond with an authentic yes or no. Notice how people respond. How often are your yes's and no's honored? How do you respond in each case? Now, when you make a request of someone, begin checking with them. Let them know you want their authentic yes or no. Really honor their no when they give it to you. See how your relationships begin to change. Sharing and respecting our authentic yes's and no's is key to honoring and respecting ourselves and each other.

Is any of this easy? Will you learn it and get good at it overnight? No. It is vulnerable to interact in this way. It takes practice and it takes courage, so let me introduce you to another herb, one that some of us in the Aphrodisiac Circle dubbed the "courage berry." This is the schisandra berry. It is quite extraordinary, really. I've only tasted them dried, and it is like nothing I've ever tasted before. All five tastes are contained in one of these berries: sour, sweet, pungent, salty, and bitter. You can eat them fresh or dried for an energy boost, and as we found, a boost in courage. I had fun sharing them with each member of my family and watching their reactions as they experienced all five tastes at once. My favorite way to enjoy them is as an iced tea (Five Springs Tea). It's a much milder taste experience and still has profound effects.

It is vulnerable to interact in this way. It takes practice and it takes courage.

GETTING TO KNOW YOUR BODY

With schisandra as an ally for courage and those visceral experiences of what a yes and a no feels like in our bodies, let's step into a process for getting to know our own bodies better. Imagine how empowering it would feel to have a pleasure map for your and your partner's body. By listening to your body's yes's and no's as you experience touch, you can discover just how you like to be touched where and when and for what purpose (to heighten pleasure or calm yourself, or . . .). There are so many different touch sensations possible, from hugs to gentle stroking, massaging, patting, tickling, slapping, or pinching—the list goes on and on. Each sensation can be pleasurable, annoying, or unbearable at different times and for different reasons.

Creating a pleasure map involves exploring different kinds of touch on different areas of your body, noticing your body responses, and bringing words to what you discover. While we can and do learn from the pleasure of lovemaking, setting aside time for pleasure mapping outside of lovemaking can be very helpful since you can focus more fully on your own body and what you are learning.

A simple herbal massage oil can help facilitate this exploration. Almond oil infused with rose (page 74) is my current favorite for erotic massage. I love the delicate scent and the way the almond oil moisturizes my skin while creating just the right glide for massage strokes.

Five Springs Tea

INGREDIENTS

1 ounce schisandra berries

HERBAL TIPS

✦ In general, when you want to extract constituents from harder plant material like dried berries, roots, or seeds, I would recommend making a decoction (simmering the plant material in boiling water for at least 20 minutes), but I find these schisandra berries infuse the water quite well without boiling. You can use the same measurements and make a decoction for a stronger tea.

PREPARATION

1 Put the berries in a quart jar.

2 Fill the jar with 1 quart of cool water.

3 Infuse in the refrigerator for at least 2 hours (more time gives a stronger flavor).

4 Strain and enjoy!

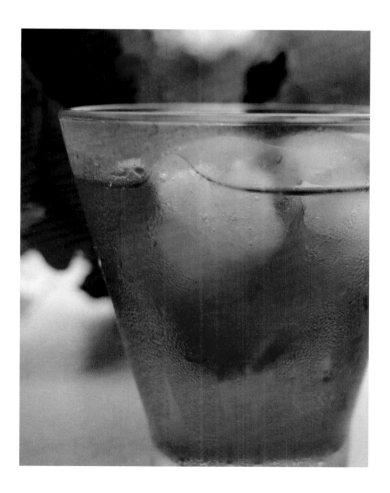

Love's Touch Massage Oil

INGREDIENTS

1 cup finely chopped fresh (or ½ cup dried) rose petals

1 cup almond oil

5 to 10 drops of Rose Otto (optional, for added scent)

PREPARATION

We will be making this oil in a slow cooker. You will need a pot or jar that will fit inside the slow cooker without touching the sides. I like to make mine using the top of my double boiler. It fits perfectly into my slow cooker without touching the sides or bottom.

1 Put the rose petals and oil in the top of a double boiler or in a jar. If using dried roses, cover with a lid. If using fresh rose petals, leave uncovered or cover with cheesecloth secured with a rubber band.

2 Place a small folded cloth or towel on the bottom of your slow cooker.

3 Place the pot or jar with the oil on top of the towel.

4 Put enough water in the slow cooker to reach ¼ way up the side of the pot or jar.

5 Set the slow cooker to warm and leave the slow cooker lid off.

6 Allow the oil to infuse on warm for 48 hours, refilling water as needed. (Be sure to fill water up before going to bed and then first thing in the morning.)

7 Using a fine mesh strainer, strain the petals from the oil, reserving the oil and composting the petals.

8 Store the oil in an easy-pour jar, and use the oil within 3 months.

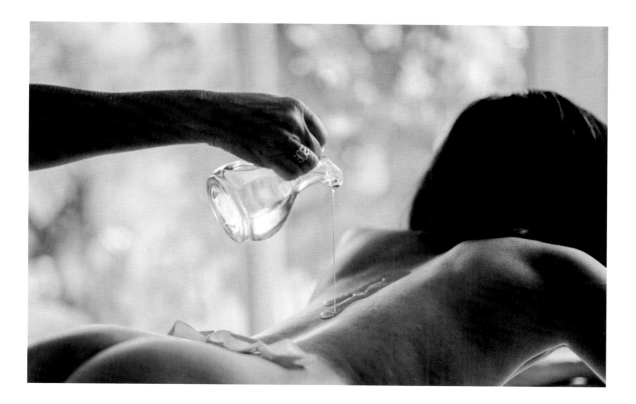

HERBAL TIPS

✦ Herbal oils are tricky to make because they can easily become rancid if too much water gets into the oil or if it gets too hot. To prevent your oil from becoming rancid, do the following:

Make sure your hands and all your implements are perfectly dry. (Water can cause rancidity.)

Infuse oils for only a few hours or days.

During and after infusing, cover your oil with cheesecloth or paper towel instead of a tight lid to allow excess water to evaporate.

Use slow, gentle heat. Heat helps to extract plant constituents into the oil, but high heat will cause your oil to go rancid.

✦ Finely chopping your plant material will increase the surface area and help create a stronger infusion.

✦ When making any kind of infusion (water, oil, vinegar, alcohol, etc.), it is important to keep all of the plant material completely covered with liquid to prevent mold.

✦ Without the Rose Otto, this makes a delicately scented oil. The amount of scent will depend on the fragrance of your rose petals. Good quality rose essential oil (that has not been adulterated) can cost hundreds of dollars per ounce. I suggest using Rose Otto as an alternative. It is good quality rose essential oil diluted in jojoba. Please feel free to do your research and choose your own way of adding scent to this oil.

You can engage in a pleasure mapping activity on your own or with a partner. One thing I've learned for myself is that the deepest levels of pleasure arise when I am feeling safe and relaxed. I begin to feel this way when my partner is present with me and gifts me with slow, firm touch on my arms, back, belly, and legs. Hair stroking also feels deeply relaxing for me. What kinds of touch help you feel safe and relaxed? Begin your pleasure mapping here. Using the oil, explore some different strokes. Perhaps circular strokes on your belly or a soothing back rub. What pressure feels nice? Soft, gentle strokes or something more firm? Give yourself permission to experiment, and remember to listen to your body's cues about its yes's and no's. This touch is just for *you*, for your own process of discovery.

Take time to record your results in your journal, or draw, speak, or dance them. Bringing words to your experiences is powerful because it allows you to ask for what you want and need.

As you sink into the feeling of safety, you can move into exploring touch that initiates and then gradually heightens your level of arousal. There are whole books and courses on this topic, and your pleasure map will grow as you continue to learn. One of my favorite books is Sheri Winston's *Women's Anatomy of Arousal*. In it she explores pleasurable touch in depth, giving lots of ideas for how to build arousal for maximum pleasure. *Taoist Secrets of Love: Cultivating Male Sexual Energy* by Mantak Chia and Michael Winn is a similarly wonderful book focused on the male anatomy.

Our whole bodies are wired for pleasure. As you explore touch, gently coaxing your body into arousal, stay tuned in to your body, listening for yes's and no's. A gentle slap here and there might bring a surge of excitement. Gentle patting can help bring energy to any area of the body. Gentle squeezing and releasing of leg and arm muscles can feel pleasurable, as can soft blowing of air or gentle kissing in sensitive places like ears, bellies, and inner thighs. Perhaps you need a firm touch at first and enjoy a gentler touch later on or vice versa.

Does the type of touch you enjoy change as your arousal increases?

As you move into exploring genital touch, you may want to try one of these herbal lubes (pages 77 and 78). There are many areas of our genitals that enjoy sensual stimulation. For women, the clitoris, including its whole shaft, head, and legs, is one such area. There are sponges that swell as the yoni is pleasured—the vestibular bulbs, the perineal sponge, and the urethral sponge. The urethral sponge swells as the G-spot (the rough, ribbed area along the upper wall of the vagina) is stroked. The cervix is another spot that can be gently stimulated for pleasure. Giving energy and attention to these deeper vaginal areas can also stir emotional energy that has been stored in your body. As the energy is stirred up, you may need to release it through tears or movement or sounding. These can be deeply healing experiences. Inner vaginal stimulation can also bring orgasm, and stimulation of the G-spot may lead to female ejaculation.

For men, the area on the front of the cock very near the tip can be particularly sensitive. Gently rubbing this area with the thumbs or fingers can feel glorious. Gently holding or lightly tickling the scrotum can bring pleasure as can massaging the area between the scrotum and the anus. The entire shaft of the cock delights in being stroked as well. Men have another pleasure spot within their anus that corresponds to the location of

Slippery When Wet

This slippery herbal lube is great for genital massage.

INGREDIENTS

½ cup aloe vera gel

2 teaspoons dried fenugreek seeds

2 teaspoons dried, cut, and sifted marshmallow root

2 teaspoons dried, cut, and sifted kava root (optional)

HERBAL TIPS

✦ In this recipe you are infusing the demulcent and other herbal qualities into the aloe gel by allowing the plants to rest in the aloe overnight.

✦ Please use high quality, pure aloe gel. Some varieties of aloe prove too sticky for lube.

PREPARATION

1 Put the aloe gel into an 8-ounce mason jar.

2 Stir in fenugreek, marshmallow, and kava.

3 Cover and allow to sit overnight.

4 Strain and enjoy!

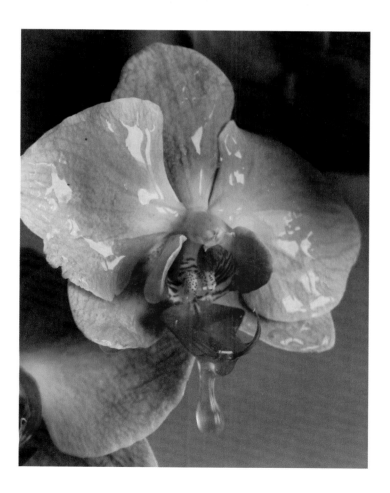

Aphrodite's Kiss

Rosemary Gladstar

This luscious herbal lube can also be used as a nourishing body oil.

INGREDIENTS

½ cup cocoa butter

½ cup coconut oil

1 cup almond oil

¼ ounce dried rose petals (⅔ cup)

¼ ounce dried hawthorn flowers and leaves (½ cup)

10 cardamom pods

Vitamin E oil (about 25 drops)

HERBAL TIPS

+ Herbal oils work well as a base for many body-care products like lotions and body butters. In this recipe the oil is heated and only infused for one hour. If you want to pull more constituents from the plants into the oil, you can increase the infusion time.

+ While petroleum-based oils are not recommended for genital use, these natural oils can work well for many bodies.

PREPARATION

1 Warm the oils in the top of a double boiler until they are thoroughly melted.

2 Add the herbs to the melted oil mixture. Let them macerate in the oil over very low heat for about one hour.

3 Strain the oil while it is still warm.

4 Stir in the vitamin E oil.

5 Pour into a small jar, and refrigerate until solid.

6 Remove the jar from the refrigerator, and store at room temperature for later use.

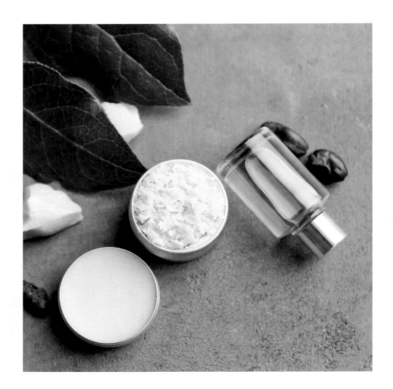

their prostate gland. With adequate lubrication, anal penetration and internal massage with a finger or toy can feel amazing for a person of any gender.

I encourage you to look at books and other resources that can give you even more ideas for different ways to touch and be touched. I have found the diagrams in *Women's Anatomy of Arousal* and *Taoist Secrets of Love* to be particularly helpful for getting a good sense of genital areas to stimulate. As we explore, our bodies become wonderlands of pleasure and delight. While there are similarities about what stimulates erotic pleasure, each of our bodies is wired slightly differently, and we can crave different kinds of stimulation at different times. There is no one right pleasure map and no one-touch formula that will bring maximum pleasure to yourself or your partner every time. Increasing your knowledge and expanding your touch vocabulary allow for more means of expressing your love and joy for yourself or another. Enjoy the exploration!

HONORING YOURSELF AND YOUR UNIQUE DESIRES

Learning about your body and exploring what kinds of touch you like is one aspect of fully honoring and respecting yourself and your body. It is part of allowing yourself to want what you want, your own unique desires. There is definitely power in allowing and naming the truth of who we know ourselves to be with all of our desires. At the same time, especially when it comes to our sexuality, it is important not to box ourselves in through labels. Our understanding of ourselves and our desires is always evolving and changing for all kinds of reasons. When it comes to claiming our identity as sexual beings, we may consider aspects of ourselves like our gender, our sexual orientation, and our sexual desires. Recognizing that our truth in any of these areas can change over the course of our lives can bring ease to our exploration.

Let's consider gender. We are each born with male or female genitalia or some combination of both, but the presence of a penis or vagina is in no way the end of the story for gender identification. You may feel comfortable and at peace with the gender identity that matches your genitals, or you may want or feel compelled to explore the gender spectrum to find an identity that more closely matches your experience of yourself. Allowing yourself to explore and find your own truth is an honoring and empowering gift you can give yourself.

Regardless of what gender identity resonates for you and regardless of your genitalia, you may at different times feel more masculine or more feminine. I like to think of masculinity and femininity as two types of energy. Masculine energy is more dominant, penetrating, and focused on doing. Feminine energy is more submissive, receptive, and focused on being. Both are equally powerful and important, and regardless of our gender, we have access to both types of energy. We can and do call on aspects of these energies at different times for different reasons. We can identify as female but find ourselves calling on our masculine energy more often than our feminine energy or vice versa. This can change over the course of our lives without meaning anything about our core gender identity. Practicing love and acceptance of ourselves and others as we explore masculine and feminine energies and varying gender identities brings peace and allows us to settle into ourselves just as we are.

Another aspect of ourselves as sexual beings that deserves exploration and honoring is our sexual orientation. This is an exploration of who we feel sexually attracted to, and the relationship style that resonates most deeply for us. Again, I'd like to bring ease to this topic by allowing ourselves to wonder and explore and to know we can change our minds. We often think of sexual orientation as fixed. People are heterosexual or homosexual, polyamorous or monogamous, bisexual, or even pansexual. We think we have to choose, and we may even have beliefs about one orientation or another being right and others being wrong. I find a lot more ease in thinking of these orientations as continuums upon which we can locate ourselves at different times in our lives.

Participants in the Aphrodisiac Circle identified with a variety of orientations and were exploring different relationship styles. Some were heterosexual and monogamous. Others bisexual. Several were exploring polyamory. Our group was a safe place to openly express our current truths in these areas.

Honoring our sexual and relationship style preferences is one aspect of honoring our sexual desires. Another aspect is learning the types of touch we enjoy and communicating about this with our sexual partner(s). There are all sorts of other sexual preferences and desires we can explore and communicate about as well. You may want to have a glass of Five Springs Tea (page 73) on hand for courage as we delve into this topic. Sometimes our sexual preferences or desires can feel embarrassing or wrong. For many people, even admitting that they have sensual and sexual desires feels uncomfortable. We live in cultures of sexual repression and unhealthy sexual expression.

So, let's bring some ease to this topic. Let's bring ease by allowing ourselves to wonder and explore, to fantasize and know we need never act on our fantasies, and most importantly, by knowing that our preferences and desires can and likely will change over time. Is there something you think you would like to explore but haven't been willing to voice to your partner? Maybe you want to sink into a Seda Blanca Bath (page 61) and allow yourself to be comforted and soothed as you let your mind open and wander. Would you like to have your skin tickled with a feather? Would you like to try dressing up in some new and sexy way? Maybe you've been wondering how anal stimulation would feel. Or maybe you have always kept the lights off during sex and want to try turning them on so you can see your partner's body or allow them to see yours. All kinds of things can be erotic and intriguing to us, and as long as we explore them in mutually consensual ways—

HETEROSEXUAL ⟷ BISEXUAL OR PANSEXUAL ⟷ HOMOSEXUAL

MONOGAMOUS ⟷ OPEN RELATIONSHIP STYLES ⟷ POLYAMOROUS

Challenges with Mutual Consent

Exploring our desires in mutually consensual ways can be trickier than it sounds for all kinds of reasons. I'd like to highlight a couple of those reasons here. First, if there is a power differential between the people involved, the person in a less powerful position may say yes when they mean no because of fear of what might happen if they refuse. This kind of power differential is present if people are in roles like boss/employee or teacher/student. A healthy sexual experience is very unlikely in these kinds of situations. Another kind of power differential can involve physical strength. If you know you are in a position where you have power over another person, you will want to put extra effort into establishing full consent so that you are truly exploring together. As I have begun to delve into social justice issues, I realize there is also a power differential involved when white people are engaging with people of color. Acknowledging and navigating these complexities is an important part of full consent and taking good care of one another.

Something else to know is that when our bodies are aroused and we are feeling filled with desire, it can be especially hard to hear a no from our partner. We may try to coerce them into a yes or we may fail to hear their hesitation and jump at their tentative yes's instead of checking in and giving the time necessary for a full yes or no to emerge. The more excited you are, the more tempting it may be to override your partner's no. Even if they said yes initially and change their minds in the midst of an exciting exploration, it is critical to honor their no.

Maybe you are super excited to try out your new fantasy of tickling your partner's skin with a feather, but as you begin to do so, they feel their body tense up and ask you to stop. The more excited you are, the more it may be tempting to override your partner's no, to remind them that they said yes initially, and try to coerce them into letting you continue with your agenda. Fully honoring and respecting ourselves and each other requires that we give ourselves and each other full permission to change our minds at any moment—no matter how excited we are. We might really need a Seda Blanca Bath or a cold shower to take care of ourselves in our disappointment after such an experience, and yet we will give thanks next time we engage with our partner and feel the relaxation in their body because they have new and deeper trust in the fact that their boundaries will be honored, and maybe they will even ask you to get out that feather and try again.

Honoring Women's Hormonal Cycles

As a female, my connection to my beauty, my sensuality, and my sexuality naturally changes over the course of the month, depending on where I am in my menstrual cycle. Honoring these changes throughout the month has proved a powerful practice in honoring and loving myself. For me, the days leading up to my period are often times of intense emotional swings. The first two days of my bleeding cycle are days when my energy is very low. In contrast, the week after my bleeding stops is often when I feel the most energetic and optimistic. Ovulation is a time of high sexual charge.

If you are a menstruating woman, can you track patterns like these as you move through your monthly hormonal cycle? I would like to encourage you to find ways to honor these different times of the month, and especially your period or moon time. Consider taking a day or a morning off and allowing yourself to stop and go inward while your blood is flowing. This idea was revolutionary for me and many women that I know. For many years, I was part of a moon lodge community. The lodge was a place we could go to rest or be creative during that time of month. We had a gift basket there and would leave each other nurturing presents. Often, when women allow themselves to stop in this way, they discover that keeping up with their normal routines, performing, or trying to be sexy is just exhausting during this time of the month. Many women in our lodge community found that taking time off to honor the truth of how they were feeling led to a decrease in cramping and mood swings associated with their periods.

Finding ways to honor your natural cycles is a beautiful way to expand your capacity to listen and respond to messages from your body, and doing so can lead to profound, positive changes throughout your experience of your life.

Pssst—Special note to men:

Supporting the menstruating women in your life so they can take time to honor their moon time is a sweet gift you can offer to them. You may want to ask them questions to learn more about what their monthly cycle is like for them. Ask them if they have cramping associated with their moon time and ask them to rate their pain on a scale of 1 to 10 so you can understand the intensity. Ask them what other patterns they notice as their hormones shift throughout the month. And the most honoring questions you can ask may be "What can I do to support you during the challenging times? What do you most want or need from me?" This kind of curiosity may at first feel strange to women, but if you are confident and earnest in your desire to support them, it will likely be met with wonder and gratitude.

honoring our own and each other's yes's and no's—they can lead to healthy sexual experiences.

Admitting your desires to yourself is a beautiful gift. You can allow yourself to enjoy your desires through fantasy, even if you never move beyond that, and you may decide that some of your desires are better left as fantasy. Choosing to explore your desires in the physical realm may require courageous communication and negotiations. (We'll explore this through a partner exercise in Chapter 6.) For your desires to lead to healthy sexual experiences, it really is essential that you explore them in mutually consensual ways. This means that both you and your partner(s) are engaging willingly and without coercion.

Whether fantasizing or exploring in the physical realm, honoring your sexual desires is part of falling in love with your body. We have taken some huge steps in this chapter. Steps toward claiming and owning our sexual desires, our sexual orientation, and our gender identification; learning about our bodies and what kinds of touch we enjoy; identifying pivotal moments in our development as sensual and sexual beings and honoring our unique history. Before we move on, let's take a couple of deep breaths together and sink into the possibility of simply allowing ourselves to love what we love and want what we want.

CLAIMING YOUR PLEASURE AS PERSONAL SOURCE ENERGY

When we do this, allow ourselves to want what we want and take *mutually consensual* steps to fulfill our desires, lots of positive energy is generated.

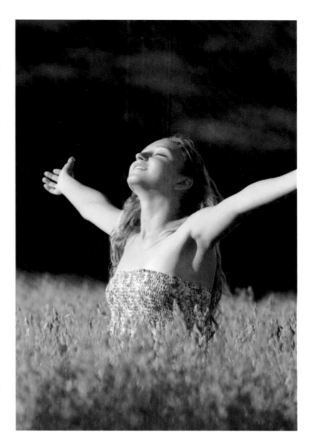

This energy feeds our confidence and creativity. What I've found is that my pleasure is a renewable energy source that powers my work in the world. In our culture, people deny their pleasure for all kinds of reasons, from time pressure from work or child raising, to religious beliefs, to beliefs that sex is primarily an obligation to fulfill the needs of their spouse. The list goes on, and the result is the same: we cut ourselves off from this natural source of energy.

So I would like to invite you to engage in a simple ritual for yourself, a ritual to honor your body and claim your pleasure as personal source energy.

Ritual to Claim Your Pleasure as Source Energy

1   Prepare a sugar scrub and get your favorite body lotion. (See recipes at the end of this chapter.)

2   Settle in and practice a sensory meditation to bring yourself present and into your body.

3   State your intention aloud: "With this ritual I am honoring my body and claiming my pleasure as personal source energy."

4   Sink into a bath or revel in the delight of a shower. In your bath or shower, honor and nourish your body by gently massaging the sugar mix into your skin using your hand or a shower mitt. Take your time, noticing areas of particular sensitivity, and fully enjoying moments of pleasure. When you rinse, allow the water to wash away any negative feelings you have about your body along with the herbal mixture.

5   After you step out of the bath, dry yourself with a soft towel and appreciate your clean, beautiful body. Feel the new smoothness of your skin.

6   If you have one, step in front of a full-length mirror and allow yourself to gaze at your own wondrous body. Speak aloud some words of appreciation and affirmation about what you see. We are so patterned to look in the mirror and notice the things we don't like, the things we would like to change about how we look or feel. This practice is about breaking that habit and honoring your body instead.

7   Rub body lotion into your skin, moistening and nourishing it. Allow yourself to feel the pleasure of taking care of yourself in this way.

8   Now lie down and let that pleasure energy course through your body. Feel it in your feet, up your legs, in your genitals and whole pelvic bowl, in your belly, chest, arms, hands, shoulders, neck, and up into your head. Recognize this pleasure energy as source energy. Claim it for yourself—to fuel your creative work in the world or simply as a source energy for vital living.

9   Finish your ritual with a poem, perhaps the one shown here. It's one of my favorites! (You will have to modify it a bit if you are male.)

Total Permission to Say Yes to Life
I give myself TOTAL PERMISSION TO FOLLOW MY HEART –
to listen to my desires,
to love myself completely,
to make myself happy and joyful,
to be deeply fulfilled,
and live in purposeful ecstasy.
My body is an Open and Receptive temple for Divinity, Joy, Bliss,
Fulfillment and Soulful Purpose to embody within.
I give myself COMPLETE PERMISSION to turn myself on,
to bathe in love,
and to embody the grace and wisdom of feminine divinity.
I am an Activated Goddess –
Overflowing with an abundance of Love, Joy, Bliss, Self-Love, Wis-
dom, Life Force Energy and Soulful Healing Creativity.
I say YES.
I say YES to Fulfillment.
I say YES to Heart Wisdom.
I say YES to Authentic Desire.
I say YES to Joy.
I say YES to Creativity.
I say YES to Sensuality.
I say YES to My Soul's Purpose.
I say YES to Sexuality.
I say YES to Abundance.
I say YES to Freedom & Liberation.
I say YES to LIFE.

— Wahkeena Sitka
(http://wahkeenasitka.com)

Simple Sugar Scrub

INGREDIENTS

½ cup rose-infused almond oil
(or plain almond oil if you don't
have any infused with roses)

¼ cup sesame oil for skincare
(not culinary type)

1½ cups granulated sugar

PREPARATION

1 Combine ingredients by stirring them together.

2 Store in a wide-mouth jar.

3 To use, simply use your hands or a washcloth to rub the scrub onto your skin. Rinse with warm water.

Kimberly's Love Your Body Lotion

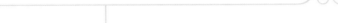

INGREDIENTS

¾ ounce beeswax

⅓ cup coconut oil

¼ cup Balm of Gilead almond oil
(cottonwood bud–infused oil)

¼ cup rose-infused almond oil

¼ cup calendula-infused
grapeseed oil

⅓ cup chamomile hydrosol

⅓ cup rose hydrosol

⅓ cup aloe gel

1 Melt the beeswax in the top of a double boiler. Add the coconut oil and stir until melted.

2 Add the infused oils and stir until everything is liquified. Remove from heat immediately.

3 Pour the mixture into a blender and allow it to cool while you combine the remaining ingredients in a measuring cup with a pour spout.

4 This is the tricky part of lotion making—combining the oil and water:

a. Allow the oils to cool to just a bit above room temperature.

b. Turn the blender on, and bring it up to high speed.

c. Pour in the liquids while the blender is spinning.

d. As soon as the blender "chokes," turn it off.

e. Use a spatula to gently stir any remaining water into the oils.

f. Blend again on low for about a minute to smooth out the mixture.

5 Pour the mixture into lotion-storage jars

HERBAL TIPS

✦ You can buy infused herbal oils for this recipe (Etsy can be a good source) or make them yourself. If you make them yourself, remember that it is important to follow the tips about preventing oils from going rancid in the Love's Touch Massage Oil recipe (page 74).

✦ For me, making this lotion is a year-long project that begins with harvesting the cottonwood buds in January or February. I fill a mason jar halfway with cottonwood buds, then pour oil over the buds to fill the jar. Then I stir and cover the jar with paper towel, using a rubber band to secure it (this allows any water to evaporate out). I stir daily for at least one week, and then allow the buds to stay in the oil until early December, when I make this lotion as a holiday present. Then, I strain out the buds, use the oil in my lotion recipe, and put the now resin-coated jars into the cabinet for next year's batch. (Cleaning them is almost impossible.) If you don't want to wait a whole year for your lotion, you can strain the oil after it sits at least six weeks or use one of the heated methods for quick results.

✦ Cottonwood oil is an exception to not letting oils infuse for a long period of time. Cottonwood is a natural preservative, and I have had success letting it infuse for months.

✦ I gather rose petals in the spring and calendula in the summer. I infuse these oils outside in the summer sun for three days or use the technique described in the Love's Touch Massage Oil recipe (page 74).

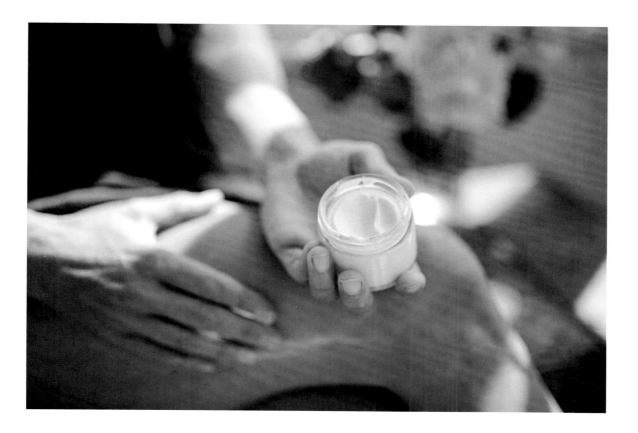

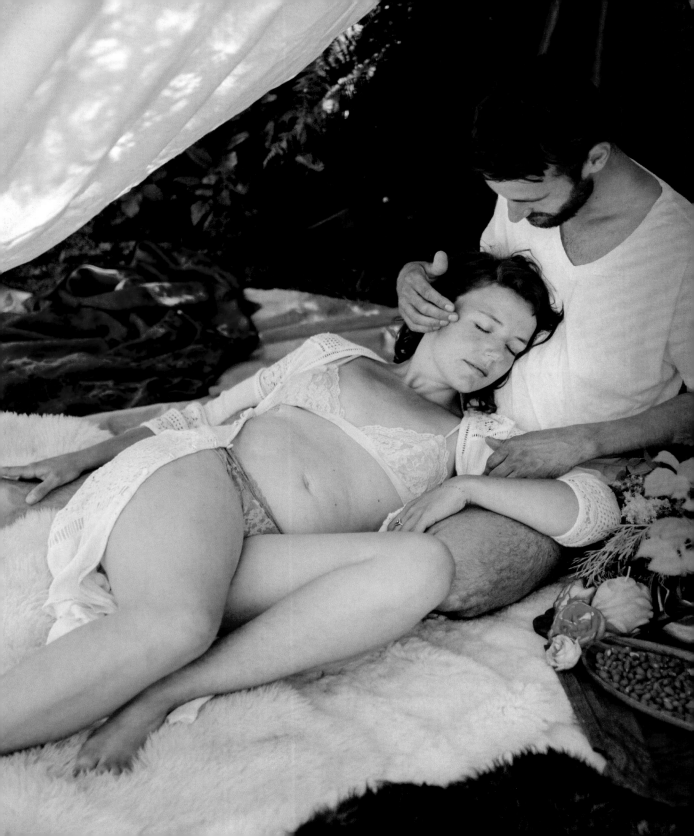

FOUR

THE

JOY

OF

PAMPERING

Imagine you and your partner coming home after a moonlit walk. Before opening the door, your partner pulls you into an embrace and whispers in your ear, "Tonight is just for you." When you walk through the door, you hear soft, sensual music playing and catch a hint of tulsi scent in the air. There is a trail of rose petals leading to the bathroom.

You've been working so hard the past few months, completing a major project with your co-workers. Your partner leads you into a candlelit bathroom and pours bubbles into the bath water. As you sink into the bath, tears begin to flow as you realize just how exhausted you are. Your partner begins to massage your sore neck and shoulders. You close your eyes and relax into the massage, letting their fingers work the tension from your muscles, gently stimulate your scalp, and run lovingly through your hair. "Just rest," your partner whispers. "I'm going to get the bedroom set up for the rest of your massage."

This is what pampering is all about. Treating ourselves and our partners extraordinarily well, adding that special touch, that bit of extra sweetness and care. It can be as delicious and energizing to give as it is to receive. Pampering is a way of cultivating pleasure and is a beautiful way to replenish or build our energy. There are so many ways to pamper ourselves or our loved ones. The key is to discover what nourishes and delights you and/or your partner and then give it with no strings attached.

Take a moment to really consider that idea of "no strings attached." Imagine that scene I just described with your partner expecting that you will engage in sex after the massage in order to fulfill her or his desires. How does that change the experience? If you're even wondering if that expectation exists, would you be able to fully relax? Or, what if you felt like because you were getting pampered, your partner would expect pampering in return? How would that change your experience? Did either of those thoughts occur to you as you read?

While it is fine to set up trades with your partner, there is a whole other level of relaxation and healing that can occur when the pampering is fully and completely a gift. Giving in this way is one of my core life practices and has led me to multiple rich learning opportunities. Each time I accomplish it successfully, I am struck by what a gift it is for me, this letting go of expectations of compensation or reward. There is so much pleasure for me in being generous and in making a positive difference in someone else's life! When you have given in this way, be sure to take a moment to really delight in that pleasure.

There are a few things I've noticed that make this kind of giving possible. One is to consciously ask myself before I give if I am expecting anything in return and then noticing if I do have expectations. In that moment, I can choose to either communicate the expectation or let it go. (Either choice is much cleaner for the relationship than giving with a silent expectation behind the gift. That choice makes it very unlikely that your expectation will be fulfilled and leaves the door open for disappointment and resentment.) Letting it go simply means consciously making the choice not to have that expectation, and then fully and completely dropping it from my mind.

Another key for me is believing in a much bigger level of reciprocity that is happening in the universe. I believe that I get back even more than I give, though it may not come in the form I imagine or expect. I have found this to be true in my life. So many people are so generous with me in so many ways! Noticing this helps me let go of specific expectations. I do not spend time tracking who owes me what according to what I have done for them. This opens up a tremendous amount of freedom and ease and leads to feelings of gratitude and abundance.

The last secret I will tell you about all of this is that I can give in this way because I practice what we started talking about in Chapter 2: I take exquisite care of myself. As I honor my physical, emotional, psychological, and spiritual needs in a myriad of ways in my daily life, I get filled up to overflowing with positive energy. When I live like this, I can give to others from the overflow and still be filled up myself. At the very least, I make sure I am sufficiently resourced so that I can fill myself back up after giving to others.

CREATING AN HERBAL PAMPERING SPA

One beautiful way of tending to your own needs and filling yourself up is by creating herbal spa time for yourself. Herbal spa time can be as simple as relaxing into a bath with aromatic, nourishing herbs or can look like spending a day tending your body with a variety of herbal preparations. It is a way of pampering yourself that allows you to tend to your physical body as well as your emotional and psychological well-being. It need not take a lot of time, space, or money, and is perhaps even more important when any of those things feel in short supply. Your spa time will allow you to rest and consider even more ways of nourishing yourself.

The first step will be to block out some time in your busy schedule. Set aside an afternoon or even a whole day if you can manage it. Even setting aside an hour for yourself will be nourishing if you are short on time. Planning ahead will help with this. I find that if I block out time in my calendar a few weeks or even a month in advance, I will likely be able to plan around it. You will need some time to gather ingredients and make your preparations anyway. Be sure to enroll other members of your household in your plans so you are sure to have a quiet, private space for your spa time.

The idea of preparing spa treatments for yourself may feel overwhelming. Breathe into that. Feel it. And then create a different possibility. This preparation time can actually be part of the nourishment. Perhaps choose just one or two recipes for your first spa. Choose recipes that are affordable for your budget, sound fun to try, and feel possible to you. Set an intention for your day and for the preparation time. Enjoy exploring the recipe possibilities as a way of building the anticipation. Gather or order ingredients and enjoy receiving them—little gifts that will contribute to your nourishment.

Pampering is a beautiful way to replenish or build our energy.

Bring your full attention to your preparations, engaging your senses as we did with that cardamom chocolate mousse torte. Each step of the process can be an aphrodisiac experience and part of your nourishing spa experience. If you like, you can supplement your spa preparations with premade products. There are lots of wonderful ones available, and you can engage your senses as you explore these products and enjoy gathering and receiving them.

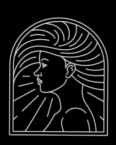

HERBAL SPA
PREPARATIONS

— ◇ ◇ ◇ —

Luscious Locks

INGREDIENTS

1 tablespoon coconut oil (melted)

1 tablespoon avocado

1 tablespoon honey

2 drops of your favorite essential oil (optional)

PREPARATION

1 Mix the ingredients together in a small bowl.

2 Work the mixture into your hair using your hands.

3 If your hair is long, put it up with a barrette to keep oil off your clothes.

4 Allow the mixture to remain in your hair for at least an hour.

5 Rinse your hair and let it dry.

Mineral Rinse

INGREDIENTS

½ cup rolled oats

PREPARATION

1 Put the oats in a mesh bag and submerge the bag in 4 cups of water.

2 Squeeze the bag with your hands to release the milky softness into the water.

3 Remove the bag and compost the oats. (Rinsing the bag immediately will make for easier clean up.)

4 Pour oat water into your already wet hair in the shower or over the sink, and work the liquid in with your hands.

5 Let the oat water rest in your hair for 5 minutes and then rinse it clean.

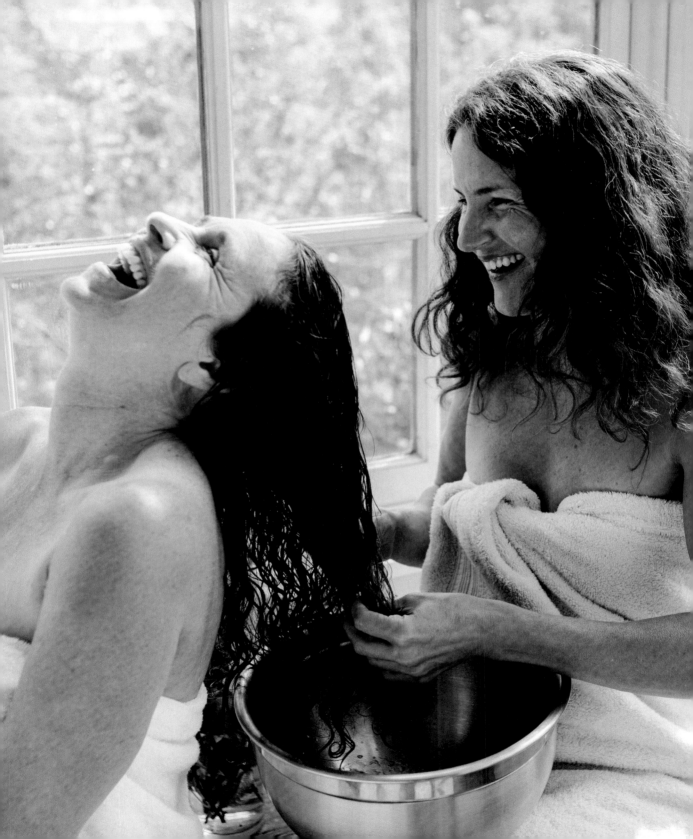

Miracle Grains *Rosemary Gladstar*

INGREDIENTS

2 cups white clay

1 cup finely ground oats

¼ cup finely ground almonds

⅛ cup finely ground dried
lavender flowers

⅛ cup dried poppy seeds

⅛ cup finely ground dried rose petals

PREPARATION

1 Combine all the ingredients. Store them in a closed-top container.

2 To use, mix 1 to 2 teaspoons of the cleansing grains with a small amount of water to make a paste.

3 Gently massage the paste onto your face, and rest with it on until the clay dries.

4 Rinse it off with warm water.

Rose Honey Mask

INGREDIENTS

¼ cup dried rose petals
(1 tablespoon rose petal powder)

2 tablespoons honey

PREPARATION

1 Use a coffee grinder to grind rose petals into a fine powder.

2 Add honey to a small pot and heat gently over low heat.

3 Add powdered rose to the warm honey and stir together.

4 Remove from heat and transfer the mixture to a small dish.

5 Use your fingers to apply the mixture to your face. Leave it on for 10-20 minutes.

6 To remove the mask, gently wipe your face with a warm washcloth or combine this treatment with the Facial de Fleur (on the next page) and steam the honey into your skin. Use a washcloth to remove any excess honey after the steam.

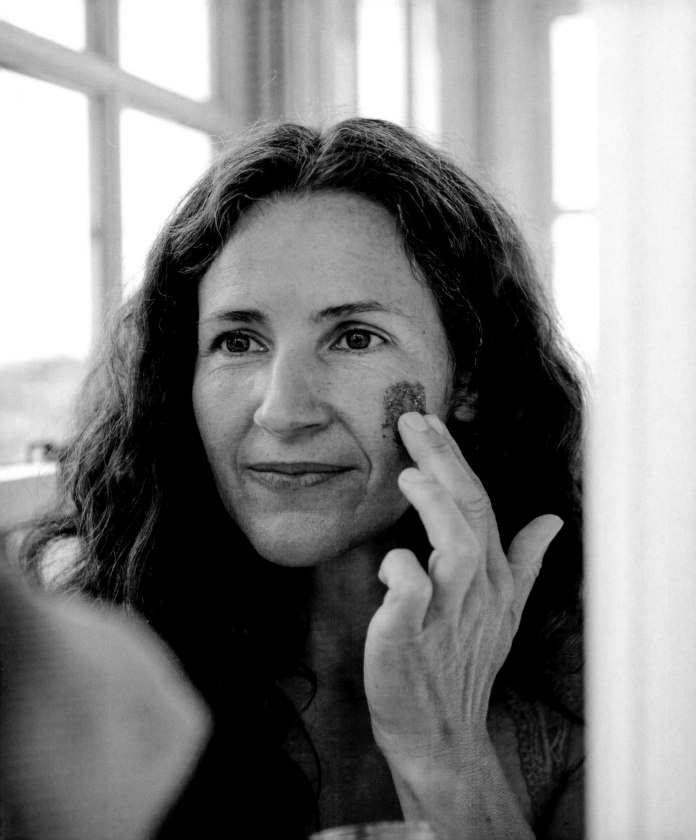

Facial de Fleur

INGREDIENTS

2 tablespoons dried
chamomile flowers

1 tablespoon dried lavender flowers

3 tablespoons dried rose petals

2 tablespoons dried fennel seeds

6 whole fresh or dried
calendula flowers

PREPARATION

1 Place herbs/flowers in a large bowl and pour 3 cups of boiling water over top.

2 When the steam is a comfortable temperature, place your face over the bowl and create a tent around your head and neck with a bath towel to keep the steam in. Stay under the towel for 3 to 15 minutes, depending on your comfort level.

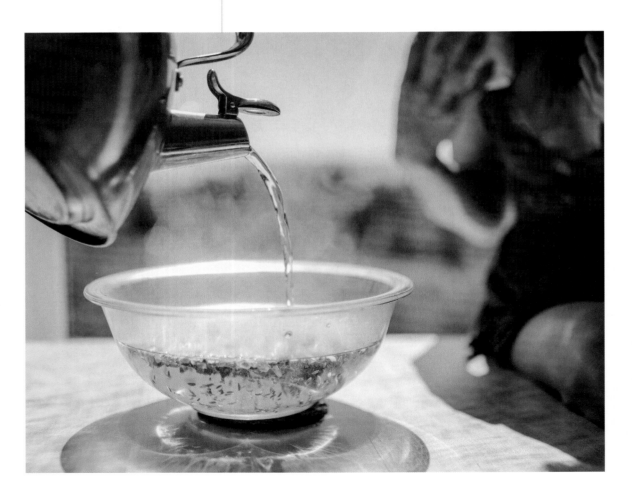

Sweet Spot Facial and Yoni Mist

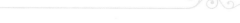

Rose, chamomile, or calendula hydrosols make a lovely, nourishing mist.

INGREDIENTS

1 cup of dried flowers or petals, or 2 cups fresh

PREPARATION

If creating your own hydrosol, do the following:

1 Place a shallow glass bowl upside down in the center of a large soup pot, and place another slightly deeper bowl on top, right-side up. (There should be enough room to place the soup pot lid upside down so the lid handle hangs in the center of the top bowl.)

2 Evenly distribute the fresh or dried herbs around the bowls stacked in the center of the pot. If any of the flowers fall into the top bowl, just pick them out and place them evenly around.

3 Pour 2 to 3 cups of water over the herbs, being careful not to get any water in the top bowl. The water should just cover the herbs.

4 Place your lid upside down over the pot so the lid handle is hanging down toward the center of the top bowl (ideally there is space between the lid handle and the basin of the top bowl). Bring your burner to medium-high heat, and turn down to low immediately when the water begins to simmer. Aim for a steady and very gentle simmer, just enough to get the water evaporating steadily toward the lid and dripping down into the bowl.

5 Just as the water begins to simmer, place enough ice cubes in the upside-down lid to almost cover the surface. This will help the steam condense and drop into your top bowl. As the ice cubes melt because of the heat, remove the water with a turkey baster or by carefully lifting the lid to the sink, dumping it out, and placing it back on the pot for the next load of ice cubes. Do this until the bowl is full and/or the water in the pot is almost gone.

6 Remove the top bowl from the pot when it is full or the water is almost completely evaporated from the bottom of the pot, and set it aside to cool.

7 Pour into a spray bottle for misting.

Love Your Body Lotion (page 86)

This makes a great face cream.

Basic Balm

INGREDIENTS

½ ounce beeswax

¼ cup jojoba oil

5 drops vitamin E oil

PREPARATION

1 Set out your lip balm tubes or jars, and remove lids.

2 Melt the beeswax in the top of a double boiler (and cacao butter for Chocolate Kiss, below).

3 Add oil(s) and stir until liquified.

4 Remove the mixture from the heat.

5 Stir in the vitamin E oil (and essential oil and cacao powder for Chocolate Kiss, below).

6 Pour the mixture into lip balm tubes or small jars and allow it to cool and harden.

7 Store the balm in a cool place to prevent melting.

Chocolate Kiss Lip Balm

INGREDIENTS

0.3 ounces beeswax

0.2 ounces cacao butter

¼ cup rose-infused sweet almond oil

1 teaspoon cacao powder

4 to 10 drops Rose Otto for scent (10% rose in jojoba oil)

10 drops vitamin E oil

PREPARATION

Step 1: *Making rose-infused almond oil:*

Use the recipe for Love's Touch Massage Oil (page 74) or:

1 Loosely fill a mason jar with fresh, finely chopped rose petals and cover them with enough almond oil to fill the jar. Stir, making sure the rose petals are completely covered with oil.

2 Place a paper towel over the top of the jar with a rubber band to secure it, and let it sit in the sun for 3 days. Bring it inside at night and stir daily.

3 Strain through a clean cheesecloth, reserving the oil and composting the petals.

Step 2: *Follow the preparation instructions for Basic Balm.*

Hot Lips Lip Balm

INGREDIENTS

¼ cup schisandra and ginger-infused jojoba oil

½ ounce beeswax

5 to 10 drops vitamin E oil

5 to 10 drops sweet orange (*Citrus sinensis*) essential oil

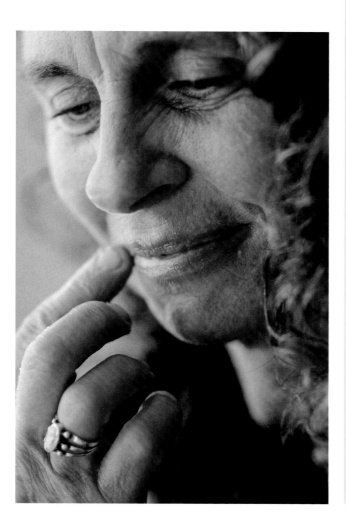

PREPARATION

Step 1: *Making the infused oil:*

You will make this oil in a slow cooker. You will need a pot or jar that will fit inside the slow cooker without touching the sides. I like to make mine using the top of my double boiler. It fits perfectly into my slow cooker without touching the sides or bottom.

1 Put ¼ cup dried schisandra berries and ¾ cup jojoba oil in the top of a double boiler. Cover with a lid.

2 Place a small folded cloth or towel on the bottom of your slow cooker.

3 Place the double-boiler pan with the oil on top of the towel so that it is not in contact with the bottom or sides of the slow cooker.

4 Put enough water in the slow cooker to reach ¼ way up the side of the pan.

5 Set the slow cooker to warm and leave the lid off.

6 Allow the oil to infuse on warm for 24 hours, refilling the slow cooker with water as needed. (Be sure to fill the water up before going to bed.)

7 Add ¼ cup freshly grated ginger to the oil, and allow to infuse for another 12 hours.

8 Strain the herbs from the oil, reserving the oil and composting the herbs.

Step 2: *Follow the preparation instructions for Basic Balm.*

Divinity Soak

INGREDIENTS

3 tablespoons cacao nibs

2 tablespoons dried tulsi leaves

10 cardamom pods, lightly crushed

1 tablespoon powdered ginger root

2 tablespoons rose buds or petals

2 tablespoons hawthorn flowers

1 cup Epsom salts

PREPARATION

1 Mix the ingredients together.

2 Put the mixture into a muslin bag and take it into the bath with you, letting the herbs infuse into the water through the bag. The bag is important because it prevents the cacao nibs from staining the bottom of your tub.

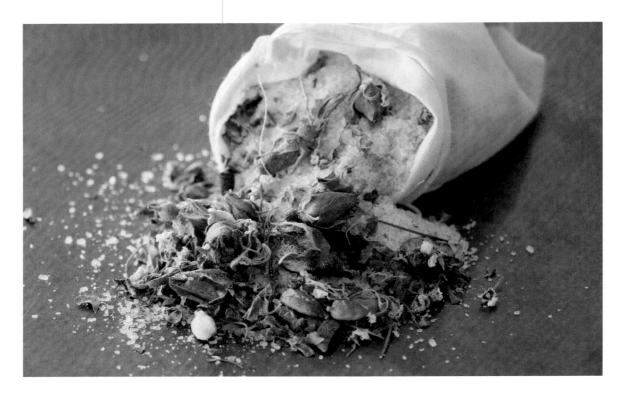

Rose Glow Body Scrub

INGREDIENTS

½ cup powdered oats

½ cup powdered rose petals

PREPARATION

1 Using a clean coffee grinder, mini blender, or a small food processor, coarsely grind/chop the oats and rose petals separately. (The roses will take fewer pulses before they are broken down.)

2 Grind the ingredients finer if you wish to use this mix for your face, or leave them a little coarser for a full-body scrub.

3 Mix the powders together.

4 Keep the powder mixture stored in an airtight container for easy sink or shower use.

5 To apply, get your body or face slightly moist, and sprinkle the scrub over your wet skin. Rub the scrub into your skin in circular motions or as preferred. Rinse off with warm water or a warm washcloth for a silky and glowing result.

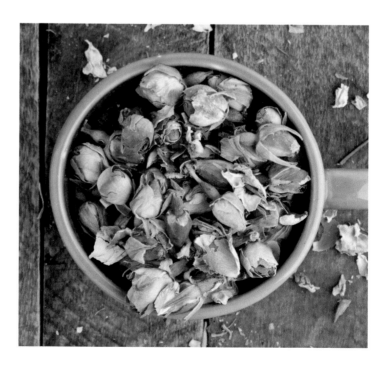

Tulsi Rose Body Butter

INGREDIENTS

¾ cup carrier oil (jojoba, almond, apricot kernel, etc.)

¼ cup fresh, chopped tulsi leaves (or ⅛ cup dried)

½ cup fresh, chopped rose petals (or ¼ cup dried)

100 grams shea butter

100 grams cacao butter

5 drops lavender essential oil (*Lavandula angustifolia*) or Rose Otto (optional, for added scent)

HERBAL TIPS

✦ Any of the methods described for making rose herbal oil infusions are effective for most any oils. Feel free to use the one you like best—slow cooker, double boiler, or a jar in the sun.

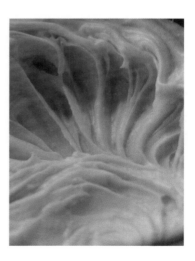

PREPARATION

To make the infused oil, you can use the slow cooker method described in the Love's Touch Massage Oil recipe (page 74) or use a double boiler on the stove. If using a double boiler, place the carrier oil and tulsi leaves in the top of a double boiler. Heat the ingredients until they are fairly warm to the touch. Turn off the heat and let it stand. Every couple of hours, reheat the oil and then let it stand. Continue this for 24 to 48 hours (heat it before you go to bed and then again first thing in the morning). Be sure to heat the oil slowly and avoid letting the temperature get overly hot.

1 Strain the rose petals and tulsi leaves from the warm oil using a fine mesh strainer or cheesecloth. Compost the plant material. You will need ½ cup of oil for this recipe. Extra oil can be used as a bath or body oil or saved for another recipe.

2 Place the shea and cacao butters in a double boiler, and heat until melted.

3 Remove it from the heat, and add ½ cup of the infused tulsi oil and lavender essential oil. Stir well.

4 Refrigerate until the mixture begins to harden and looks opaque.

5 Whip the mixture vigorously using a cake mixer or immersion wand. (You may have to let it warm a bit if it became too hard in the refrigerator.) It should be light and fluffy when done.

6 Transfer the mixture to jars. Store in a cool place (for up to one year). If it gets too warm, the mixture will decrease in volume but will still be fine to use.

7 Spread the body butter on warm skin, preferably just out of the shower or bath.

Pampered Petals
Yoni Steam

Yoni steams have a long history of use. They are nourishing for the exterior vulva lips that the steam can reach. Please be careful to let the steam cool enough so that you do not burn these sensitive tissues!

INGREDIENTS

Flowers can be fresh or dried.

½ cup chamomile flowers

½ cup rose petals

6 cups water

PREPARATION

1 Boil water, remove it from the heat, and pour it into a bowl.

2 Add chamomile flowers and rose petals.

3 Squat over the bowl to steam your yoni, or sit on a stool with a hole in it and a blanket covering your bottom half and the stool to keep the steam inside.

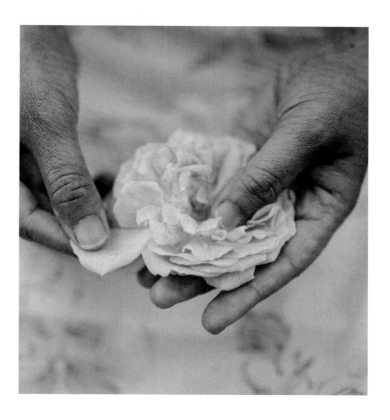

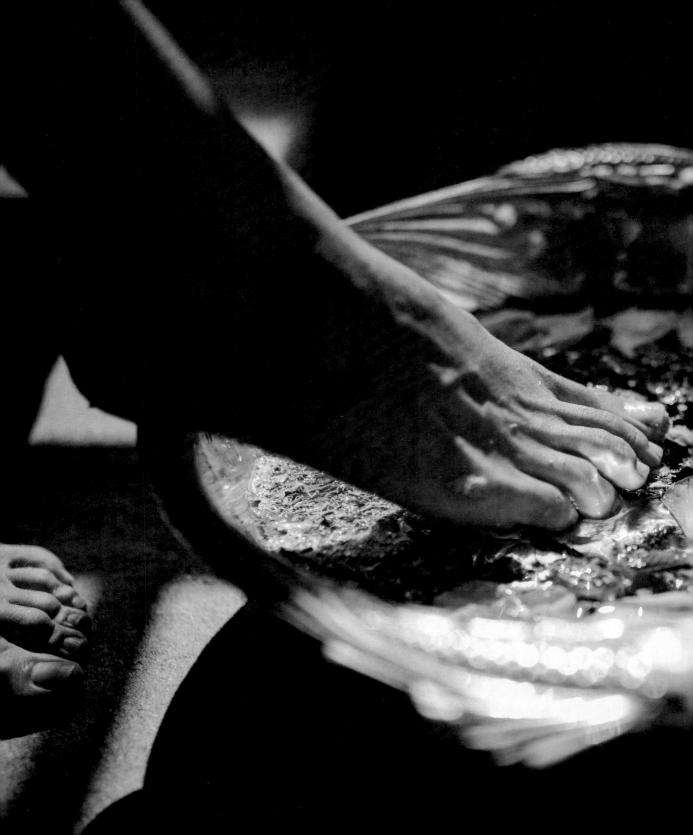

Pampered Sole

INGREDIENTS

All these herbs can be fresh or dried.

½ cup rose petals

½ cup lavender flowers

½ cup tulsi leaves

½ cup chamomile flowers

PREPARATION

1 Boil 8 to 12 cups of water.

2 Place the herbs into a foot tub, and pour boiling water over top.

3 Add cool water until it is just the right temperature for your feet, and enjoy soaking for as long as you like.

4 Follow the foot bath with a scrub with a pumice stone and then Love Your Body Lotion (page 86).

On the day of your spa, make sure to linger over each step you have prepared for yourself, enjoying the silky feel of the hair mask as you massage it into your hair, the smell and feel of each of the facial products. As you sink into your herbal bath, really enjoy the sensation of being submerged in the warm, scented water. Feel your tension melt away, and allow yourself to meditate on the self-care you need physically, emotionally, socially, and spiritually in order to be filled to overflowing with positive, turned-on energy. As you continue with your spa day, let ideas flow about how you can meet those needs even in the midst of your busy life.

These herbal pampering creations can be part of meeting those needs on a more regular basis. They do not need to be saved just for spa days.

Consider how you might integrate a few of your favorites into your regular routines. I do a hair mask once a week, a short facial treatment daily, and a foot bath whenever my feet call for one. Artemis found that the simple routine of spraying her body with rose hydrosol helped her connect to her beauty and sensuality. Sarah used her oat and rose body scrub regularly in her showers and so appreciated the smoothness and firmness of her skin. Another of her favorites was a rose water and oat mask on her face, which left her skin feeling delightfully smooth. These kinds of routines led to her feeling healthy and vibrant. Weaving ways of delighting and pampering yourself into your everyday life can help you feel more attractive and more vibrant as well.

SELF-PLEASURING— EXPANDING CAPACITY FOR PLEASURE

We can take our personal pampering and self-care into the realm of sexuality with self-pleasuring. This can be a wonderful way of finding out more about what your body likes and doesn't like. It can also be healing and empowering, providing you with sexual satisfaction when you are not with a partner. It is freeing to experiment and learn without worrying about a partner's reactions and astounding to find out how fully you can please yourself.

Let's pause here for a moment. I want to acknowledge two things. First, I realize that bringing pampering into the realm of sexuality through self-pleasuring may conflict with your religious or spiritual belief system. If that is the case for you, please give yourself permission to skip over this section. Second, though it may not conflict with your belief system, you may feel some level of shame or guilt around the idea of self-pleasuring. If that is the case, I encourage you to lie still and take some deep breaths, just letting the truth of that be present for you and being curious about the possibility of it transforming. Give yourself permission to go as slowly as you need to with these suggestions. Remember, this is about pleasure. When we stay with our truth and lean into pleasure, things have a way of shifting and changing in beautiful, unexpected ways.

Set aside time and space for your self-pleasuring, just as you did with the herbal spa or as you might if you were expecting a lover. Look back at Chapter 2 for ideas. Think about each of your senses and how you want to set up your space for your personal delight. Straighten up the room, putting a beautiful comforter on the bed and maybe even scattering some rose petals for yourself. Choose music you love. Scent the room with incense or your hydrosol mix. Bring in chocolates or strawberries or some other treat that feels decadent and delicious to you. Perhaps you want to take a few moments to drink an aphrodisiac tea. I'll give you the recipe for one of my favorites on page 110. Bring in silky or soft fabrics or brushes to run over your skin, and your favorite sex toys. Dress sexy. Have your rose massage oil and herbal lube next to the bed. Turn off your cell phone, dim the lights, and lock the door. This time is just for you.

From here, once you have set the perfect scene for yourself, your self-pleasuring session can unfold any number of ways. Follow your pleasure! Sometimes, I've set up a self-pleasuring session for myself, only to find that my body is calling for rest, and I spend the time sleeping. Other times, maybe there are tight places in my body or I am feeling tender and raw emotionally, and I just want to spend the time tending myself. There is no way to do this wrong. Bring your journal or art supplies so you can bring expression to your new learnings when you are finished.

Self-pleasure practices can be very genitally focused and goal oriented, a directed effort to release sexual tension in our bodies. This kind of release is extremely pleasurable, but notice also that it is a release of pleasurable sensation. Orgasm often ends our lovemaking or self-pleasuring. We each have a threshold of how much pleasure we can tolerate, and going over into orgasm can be a relief as the pleasure has built to the point we can tolerate. As we expand the possibilities of what self-pleasuring can look and feel like, we also have the opportunity to expand our capacity for pleasure so that we begin to feel more pleasure for longer periods of time. This idea of setting a space for yourself sets you up to expand the realm of what is possible. Let's continue to explore possibilities of how your session could unfold to increase your self-pleasuring vocabulary. The most important thing, though, is to follow your own intuition and your own body.

You might begin in a comfortable position with your eyes closed, doing some deep breathing all the way down into your belly, and even filling your pelvic bowl with your breath. Notice that with your eyes closed, you are aware of where your body is in space. This is another one of our senses beyond the five we generally think of—our sense of proprioception. Notice the places where your body is touching the bed or the floor, where one body part is resting against another. Breathe into any tender areas, soothing them with your breath. Is there any place where you are feeling a pleasurable sensation? Does the fabric of the comforter feel nice against your skin? Breathe into that sensation. Begin to move your body in ways that increase your pleasure. Movement is another one of our senses and can lead to exquisite pleasure. Perhaps the music you chose is encouraging you to move in a certain way. Allow your body to explore movement that feels good in this moment.

Begin to add touch. Remember the ways you identified that you like to be touched when you mapped your body for pleasure. Give yourself just the kinds of touch you love and need right now. Touch to calm yourself and relax, or touch to begin to build pleasure in your body. Run your hands or a soft piece of fabric over your legs and arms, your belly and chest, your face and ears,

your back and butt, and yes, your pussy or cock. Perhaps you want to add some massage oil as you run your hands all over your body. Massage the oil into your belly, your breasts or chest in smooth round strokes. If you are a woman, cradle your breasts in your hands and let yourself feel your love for them, whatever size and shape they are. Lightly stimulate your nipples. Alternate nipple stimulation with full breast or chest massage.

Run your hands down your body to your genital area. For any gendered body, there are numerous ways to pleasure your own genitals. There are strokes that can bring energy to your genital area, gentle squeezing, stroking, or patting. You can rub your hands together and place them over your womb, ovaries, scrotum, penis, or vaginal opening, bringing warmth and energy to these areas. Gentle, slow strokes can begin to build energy, and faster ones can heighten it. You might want to simply bring yourself to orgasm, or you might want to play with bringing yourself up to a seven or eight on your personal pleasure scale, and then, using slower strokes, relax the energy and then build again. You can also alternate genital stroking with touch on other parts of your body, spreading out the erotic energy and delighting your whole body with pleasurable sensation. You may choose to heighten the pleasure several times before orgasming, or you may choose not to orgasm at all and just breathe the erotic energy through your body so you can channel it into other activities throughout your day.

Both Gabrielle and Michelle described beautiful self-pleasuring experiences with rose. Gabrielle said, "I masturbated with oils infused with rose in a room fragranced with potpourri. I was relaxed, whole, and happy, transported . . . and so turned on with desire. I felt supported and

Tender Titillation Tea

INGREDIENTS

1 tablespoon dried rose petals

1 tablespoon dried oat tops

1 tablespoon dried damiana leaves

2 tablespoons dried hawthorn flowers

Honey, to taste

PREPARATION

1 Boil 1½ cups of water, then place the herbs in a cup and pour the just-boiled water over them.

2 Cover and let the herbs steep for 15 minutes. Strain.

3 Add honey to taste. I definitely recommend adding some. This tea is delicious when sweetened!

HERBAL TIPS

✦ This is a wonderful blend to make in larger batches and store in a jar. (You can do this with any of the dried tea blends in the book—just use the ratio in the recipe to put together a large batch of the mixed herbs.) It can be made by the pot to share with friends.

✦ Though it seems like a lot of herbs for one cup of tea, I find the ratio of 5 tablespoons of herbs to 1½ cups of water makes a really delightful blend.

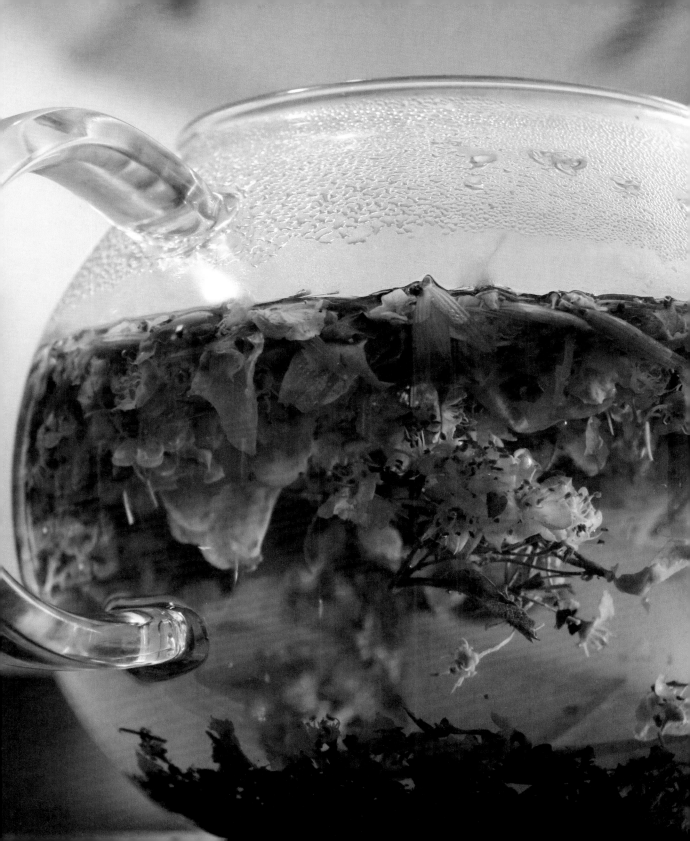

nurtured being surrounded by such overwhelming beauty, an exotic connection. True beauty really is when you can appreciate yourself. Rose surrounded me in love."

Michelle had this experience:

The awakening I had recently with rose was with myself. Robert and I have been working through conflicts and power struggles. We had a morning where I desired lovemaking, but we just weren't connecting. I told him I needed some time to myself for pleasuring. The next 30 minutes were groundbreaking for me. I used rose water and some rose oil and proceeded to pleasure myself using the erotic map concept. I also got inspired in the moment to envision myself as a goddess, aided by rose, sensual, vulnerable, open, receiving. I envisioned being deeply held and penetrated with male energy. Funny, it wasn't a fantasy about a particular man, just very intense, strong, male presence, penetration, support and being held, supported, protected. I actually imagined myself being split open at one point, figuratively of course, like a seed cracking open with new growth, or a bud expanding into a blossom. I was able to build slowly to an amazing G-spot orgasm, and ejaculate, and have a deeply male/female spiritual experience—but I was all alone. It was empowering and unique for me. I'd masturbated plenty, but never with this type of deep spiritual experience. That rose, what an ally!

I love that these women were willing to share these experiences. Gabrielle has not had a sexual partner for many, many years since her husband passed away, yet she expressed the depth of pleasure she was able to experience on her own. Michelle's experience points to the fact that even when we do have a partner, sometimes our sexual connection does not flow. It is wonderful to know

we can take care of our own pleasure needs. This can reduce the pressure to find a partner and reduce the pressure on our partner to fully meet our sexual needs.

Still, let's face it, there is frustration and longing that accompanies not having a romantic or sexual partner. This was present for Rachel many times during our year-long exploration. Having just ended a multiyear relationship, she would show up to video calls with tears and rawness about the ache she felt for a lover in her life, and how being in a group focused on aphrodisiacs and pleasure was extremely challenging because it highlighted that longing for her. I have felt that ache, that longing, too. It is not comfortable. Sometimes it feels like loneliness or sadness, and other times it feels like just way too much sexual energy running through my body and a kind of desperation to share it.

There can be a desire to suppress these kinds of feelings. We may be practiced at ignoring them and distracting ourselves with other experiences or numbing ourselves with alcohol, television, junk food, or drugs. However, there is tremendous value in allowing ourselves to feel them. As we feel them fully, we move through them and allow them to shift and dissipate. This keeps them from becoming stuck in our bodies and leading to illness or coming out in ways that damage our current relationships. Just as we can expand our capacity to feel joy and pleasure, we can expand our capacity to be with ourselves in the midst of challenging emotions. A Seda Blanca Bath (page 61) or an AshwaMacaMocha Shake (page 64) or some Soft Landing Tea (page 229) can help. Also, physically wrapping myself in soft blankets, or lying on a warm stone in the sunshine or on the sand at the beach while the waves wash onto the

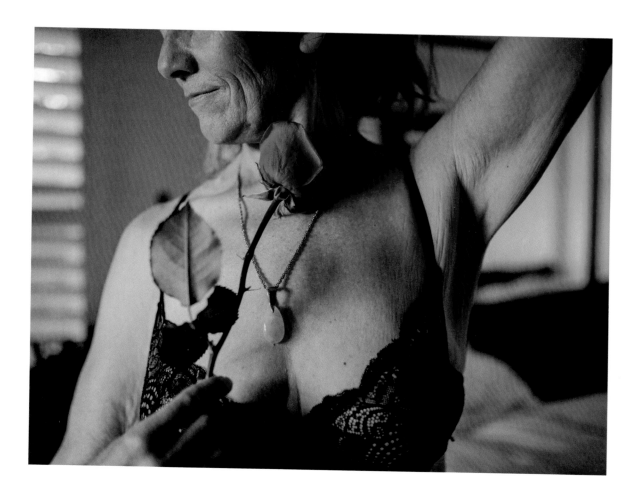

shore, or sitting with my back up against a tree are all things that help me to be present with difficult emotions. Deep breathing and calming music help too.

These same strategies can also work well if challenging emotions come up during our self-pleasuring. Our bodies can store trauma and unprocessed emotions in our muscles and organs. Sometimes massaging or stroking will release feelings from old wounds or experiences.

Our bodies may feel more willing to release these emotions when our partner is not present and we are less self-conscious. Knowing this is a possibility can help us be present with whatever arises. Our presence is the best gift we can give ourselves in this situation. Breathing and feeling and breathing and feeling. The good news is that as the trauma is released, it opens the way for more and deeper experiences of pleasure.

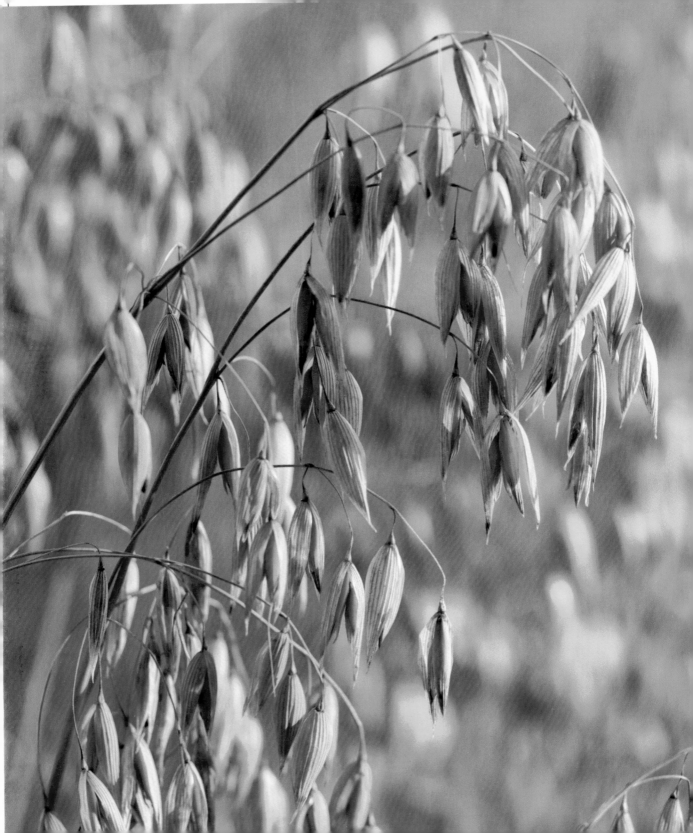

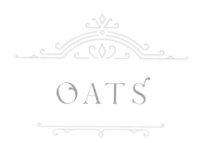

OATS

Avena sativa

My daily Golden Oat Infusion (page 37) has always felt like a sweet, calming gift for my nervous system and a nourishing source of vitamins and minerals (especially calcium) for my whole body. This book project led me to discover that oats have been called a modern-day love potion and to realize the aphrodisiac effects of oats. At one point, I found myself giving a talk on aphrodisiac herbs and suddenly realized that perhaps that daily quart of infusion is part of what led to me giving such a talk!

How Do Oats Work in Our Bodies?

Oats have amazing relaxing, soothing, and calming properties. They work as a nervous system tonic by coating and protecting our nerve endings and helping repair damage to the myelin sheath that covers nerve fibers.[1] This helps reduce stress and irritability so we receive more pleasure from touch.

Oats are also incredibly nourishing and restorative. They are packed with vitamins and minerals and are especially rich in magnesium and calcium.[2] They also can help stabilize our blood sugar levels and nourish our hormonal systems, which helps decrease mood swings.[3] Because they are high in silica, they are also nourishing for our skin, bones, hair, and nails.[4]

Oats also have a unique set of antioxidants known as avenanthramides. These compounds have been shown to have a myriad of powerful protective and nourishing qualities, including suppressing the release of histamine; restoring the skin's natural barrier; reducing inflammation; protecting DNA of skin cells against environmental insults, including UV radiation; and protecting the cardiovascular and neurological systems. Some have even called oats an "elixir of youth" because of all the protective and nourishing qualities of the avenanthramides.[5]

Sexually speaking, oats are nourishing for our endocrine system,[6] the collection of glands that produce hormones that regulate metabolism, growth and development, tissue function, sexual function, reproduction, sleep, and mood. They are a tonic for our ovaries and uterus and nourish our reproductive organs to restore and heal them or to provide optimum nourishment for them if they are already healthy.[7] The demulcent or lubricating aspect of oats also helps promote vaginal lubrication.[8]

When used regularly, oats also nourish and tonify our hearts and blood vessels.[9] They improve blood flow, which can help with erectile dysfunction.[10] Oats also liberate testosterone and improve sperm motility.[11]

A Bit about Oat Plants

There is simple beauty in a field of oat plants—their golden color, their delicate stems bent with the weight of dangling oat tops.

Oats are generally grown in temperate areas and can thrive in most any well-drained soil.

Herbal Shorthand

APHRODISIAC ACTIONS: *cardiotonic, demulcent, endocrine system tonic, energy building, nervine, nutritive, restorative*

OTHER ACTIONS: *diuretic, antispasmodic*

ENERGETICS: *warming, moistening*   TASTES: *sweet*

CONSTITUENTS: *avenanthramides (a unique set of antioxidants), high in vitamins and minerals like calcium, magnesium, silica, potassium, B and E vitamins*

DOSAGE SUGGESTIONS: *Oats are a nourishing herb and can be consumed as you would any healthy food. I recommend 1 quart of Golden Oat Infusion daily. Oat top tincture can be used as needed throughout the day to soothe nerves and calm anxiety.*

How to Use Oats

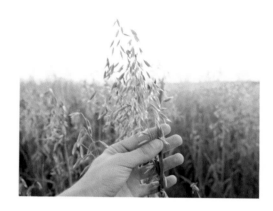

PARTS USED: *Oatstraw and oat tops*

Daily Golden Oat Infusion (page 37)—*for maximum nourishing and tonic effects*

Oatstraw or oat top tea (1 tablespoon of herb in 1 cup of boiled water, steeped for 20 minutes)—for settling and soothing your nerves in order to relax

Soothe Tincture (page 203)—*20 to 125 drops per day—nourishing and relaxing for nervous system*

Seda Blanca Bath (page 61)—*soothing and skin nourishing*

Oatstraw bath or sitz bath—to relax and soften tissues (add as much as a gallon of infusion to your bath water)

Oatstraw foot bath—to soothe and pamper your feet

Mineral Rinse (page 94)—*to nourish your hair and scalp*

Add oats to facial scrubs for gentle cleansing.

Participant Experiences

We found that Golden Oat Infusions brought a soothing, nurturing, grounding, and restorative energy to our lives, a sense of calm resilience. Artemis found that Golden Oat Infusions really grounded her in self-love. She felt "a sense of calm, steady flexibility beneath a feeling of alive and surging passion." She also noticed an increase in vaginal lubrication. Cassie and I also echoed the effect of increased vaginal lubrication.

For Joe, the Golden Oat Infusions led to his most profound healing experience over the course of the project. He'd been experiencing ejaculations that were so strong they were painful, but the oats really smoothed them out, making them more fluid and pain free. This shift allowed him to really sink in and enjoy sexual connection much more.

Another way we really enjoyed engaging with oats was as a Seda Blanca Bath. Michelle and Robert really enjoyed shared Seda Blanca Baths, squeezing the milky oat bags onto each other's skin and massaging each other with them. Lisa enjoyed a luxurious self-pleasuring Seda Blanca Bath.

PARTNER PAMPERING

Practicing exquisite self-care opens a doorway to being able to give to our partners with no strings attached. It allows us to come to our partner filled up and overflowing with positive energy. We can give the overflow to our partner and still be filled up ourselves.

I offer you the poem on page 119 to give you a feeling for the kind of energy you can bring to your partner.

Partner pampering is a delightful and healthy relationship practice, and as I said above it can feel as wonderful to be the giver as it does to be the receiver. You may also find yourself challenged by assuming one or the other of those roles, but there is great value in stretching and trying both out. Bodyworker and intimacy coach Betty Martin has developed a tool called "The Wheel of Consent." It is a wonderful tool for exploring the different roles we can take within the realm of consensual touch and exploring and expanding our comfort with the different forms.

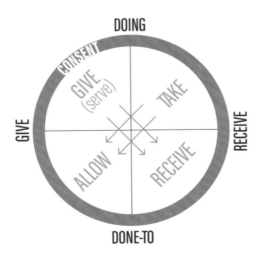

Betty's work highlights some aspects of consensual touch that are critical to be clear about as you embark on a pampering session with your partner. Her wheel breaks up the possibilities for consensual touch into four quadrants that are formed by the intersections of the continuums of giving to receiving and "doing" to "being done to." When we are pampering, it may seem obvious that one of us is giving and the other receiving. One of us is being done to and the other is doing. The brilliance and subtlety of Betty's work comes as you explore the four quadrants of the wheel. Let's do this by looking at how these concepts can play out during a massage.

If you are the person giving the massage, you will be in the quadrant where doing and giving intersect. You are touching your partner's body for their pleasure. Your partner is in the quadrant where receiving and being done to intersect. (They are receiving touch for their own pleasure.) In order to stay within the realm of consent, it is important to practice both attunement and communication. If you are in the role of giver, tune in to your partner's cues (attunement). Even if you are still enjoying massaging your partner's breasts, they may be ready for you to move on. They may let you know with subtle shifting of their position or a light touch on your hand. If you are unsure, ask (communicate). It is a good practice to check in with your partner from time to time about things like the pressure and speed of your touch and about where they would like to be touched. As the receiver, allow yourself to ask for what you want, for something to continue longer or for something to stop or change. Pampering sessions are great opportunities to build your communication skills as a couple and learn more about each other's bodies and preferences,

Just for now, without
asking how, let yourself
sink into stillness. Just
for now, lay down the
weight you so patiently
bear upon your shoulders.
Feel the earth receive
you, and the infinite
expanse of sky grow even
wider as your awareness
reaches up to meet it.

Just for now, allow a wave
of breath to enliven your
experience. Breathe out
whatever blocks you from
the truth. Just for now, be
boundless, free, awakened
energy tingling in your
hands and feet. Drink in
the possibility of being
who and what you really are—
so fully alive that when you
open your eyes the world
looks different, newly born
and vibrant, just for now.

— Danna Faulds, from her book *Prayers to the Infinite*

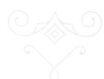

especially if we enter into them with curiosity, openness, and playfulness.

To understand a little more about Betty's wheel, let's go back to that moment when you were still enjoying massaging your partner's breasts, but your partner was ready for you to move on. If you continued to touch her breasts, you would be outside the circle of consent, and would be risking losing your partner's trust. Notice that it is possible to touch your partner's breasts for your enjoyment within the circle of consent, but it requires a different agreement with your partner. They would need to have agreed to be in the quadrant where giving and being done intersect. (They are allowing their body to be touched for your pleasure.) You would then be in the quadrant where doing and receiving intersect. (You are touching their body for your pleasure.) As long as you make clear agreements about who the touch is for, this can all happen within the circle of consent and trust will remain intact. Notice that this second example where the touch is for the doer's pleasure is outside of the realm of both massage and pampering. It is worthwhile to spend some time with Betty's wheel and get your mind around these quadrants. You can find her generous supply of free information at bettymartin.org.

Setting an intention to purely give to your partner for their nourishment and pleasure is a profound gift. In preparation for the pampering session, think about what you want to offer. Perhaps one or more of the spa treatments from your herbal spa experience, a massage, or just holding and hair stroking. Not sure what they would like? Ask. It is wonderful to surprise each other once you know each other's preferences, but if you are

unsure, the pampering will still feel wonderful, even if it is not a surprise. If your partner knows what is coming they can anticipate it, and this can build and extend the pleasure.

Once you know what will happen during the pampering session, you will want to set aside plenty of uninterrupted time and also set up a beautiful space. If you can, include elements you know will delight your partner. What scents do they enjoy? What kind of music do they like? Do they have a favorite set of sheets you can put on the bed? Any of these kinds of special touches can help your partner feel seen and cherished.

One beautiful example of partner pampering came up in February of our Aphrodisiac Circle year together. We were experimenting with oats. Artemis was drinking a Golden Oat Infusion every day and said, "like the grass it grows from, I feel steady, flexible, beautiful, and more attentive and attuned to the nuance of my femininity. I noticed myself slowly rubbing my belly this month, an object I've detested most of my life, except when it was growing life within it. I invited my lovers to rub and caress it, and both of them were drawn to do so, on their own, in long, round strokes. I could feel their adoration rise up through me, loving the soft belly of me, nourishing my sensuality in a way that was different, purer. I have never let people touch my belly, so this was a gift from her [the oats], I am sure."

Setting an intention to purely give to your partner for their nourishment and pleasure is a profound gift.

Personalized Pampering

1   Bring yourself present and into your sensual body using breath, sensory meditation, or another practice you prefer.

2   Close your eyes and imagine yourself being pampered in the most sensual, nourishing way possible. What do you imagine? Let yourself linger over the details of what is happening, who is with you, where you are, and what is around you. Are you getting a full-body massage? Relaxing in a scented salt bath? Are you outside or inside? What are the elements that make this pampering scene extra special for you? Feeling the sun on your skin? The bouquet of wildflowers? The sensual music? The chocolate truffles?

3   Open your eyes and write down (or draw, or . . .) the elements you discovered that particularly delight you.

4   Create a self-pleasuring time for yourself where you bring in some (or all) of the elements you imagined or ask for what you want. Is there someone in your life you could ask to pamper you in these ways? Ask. If you find someone who is willing, set up a time and surrender into being pampered.

5   Is there someone in your life who you would enjoy pampering? Ask them to do this exercise and let you know what elements particularly delight them. Have fun creating a pampering experience for them.

Exotic versus Dooryard Herbs and Sustainable Wildcrafting

When we are pampering ourselves or one another, or even just engaging in sensual or sexual exploration, we may be particularly drawn to exotic herbs—herbs with unfamiliar names that grow in faraway or very specific places, or that are in very limited supply. There is no end to the exotic sounding herbal elixirs marketed as aphrodisiacs—from chuchuhuasi bark to New Zealand deer antler velvet powder to *Cordyceps* mushroom extracts. Depending on where we live there will always be dooryard and exotic herbs available.

Dooryard herbs are the ones that grow right outside our door, those that are easy to cultivate in a garden in our area or that grow abundantly and naturally where we live. These herbs may seem less exciting because we are familiar with them. The truth is that some of our most common weeds, like dandelion, are some of the most potent healing plants on the planet. Often the herbs growing right around us are the best match for our bodies too. We are both living and growing in the same ecosystem. In the Aphrodisiac Circle, people had profound experiences with roses, oats, and hawthorn—three plants that grow well in our area of the world. Roses were especially impactful as people got out and harvested the petals themselves.

Still it is fun to play with exotic herbs as well. There is a place for both dooryard and exotic herbs in our experimentation. Just experiment consciously. Perhaps call on exotic herbs now and then for fun, or for a specific purpose for a specific time period. Consider the impact of having the herbs shipped to you from afar, and always, always check your sources. Make sure the herbs you are getting are being cultivated and harvested in a sustainable way and without the use of fertilizers or pesticides. Note that wild herbs growing in their natural habitat will often be far more potent than cultivated varieties. If you are getting herbs that have been wildcrafted—harvested from the wild—be sure those gathering them are not overharvesting and devastating local plant populations.

If you are gathering plants yourself, do so in a sustainable way. Gather just the plant parts you need (if you are harvesting roses, you need only the flowers, not the whole plant. Take a basket and gather the petals). Also take only the amount you need. Consider what you are going to be making with the plant and what quantity you will need before you head out to wildcraft. Don't take all the plants, flowers, leaves, or roots from a particular plant or stand of plants. Leave enough of the plant intact so that it can continue to grow. Leave some flowers for the bees. If you do so consciously, your wildcrafting can actually be part of tending the plants in a particular area and you can leave the stand healthier for your efforts.

The plants gift us with their flowers, leaves, and roots for nourishment and healing. Caring for the plants that we gather is part of honoring them for the gifts they give. As you bring the plants into your life, please be in this kind of reciprocal relationship with them, caring for them and honoring them even as you accept their gifts.

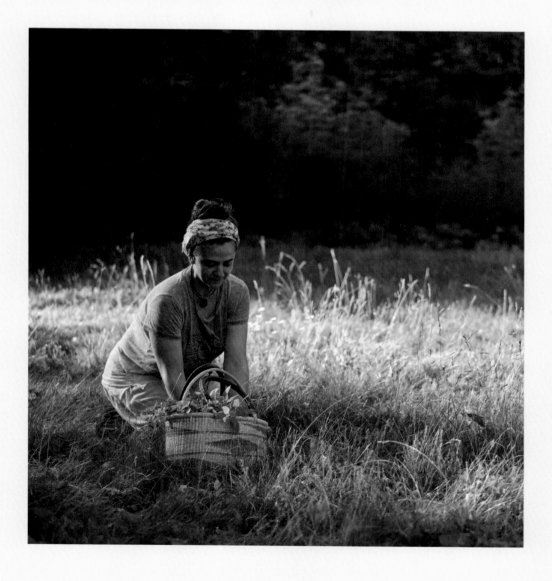

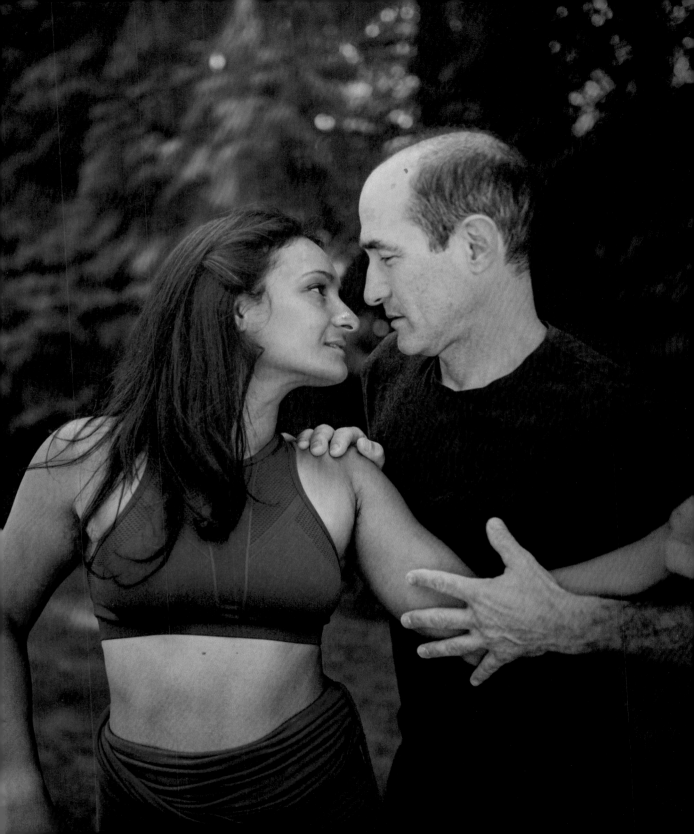

FIVE

DANCE

OF

RELATIONSHIP

eading Artemis's description of her lovers caressing and cherishing her belly inspires relaxation in my own body. I feel myself breathing more deeply, my muscles relaxing. It speaks to the joy and beauty of being in an intimate relationship, the things that draw us in and keep us connected over time—the elements that make all the challenges of relating worthwhile. Anyone who has been in relationship knows that each one comes with its share of challenges. Stepping into relationship with another is truly an act of courage, requiring vulnerability and deep trust.

It requires a level of trust in our partner, but also a depth of trust in ourselves. In order to be in a healthy relationship with another person, we must trust ourselves to look out for ourselves, taking responsibility for our own happiness and well-being.

We've already learned some effective methods of building our level of trust in ourselves. Herbally, we can call on the grounding, nourishing powers of maca and ashwagandha by drinking an Ashwa-MacaMocha Shake (page 64), then taking time for deep breathing, doing a sensory meditation to drop into our bodies, and allowing answers to arise from that place will build our capacity to listen deeply to ourselves. When we follow through on the ideas or answers that arise, we begin to see the results of opening up to our own deep wisdom. As we begin to trust and honor ourselves more, we will naturally begin taking better care of ourselves, gifting ourselves with nourishment and pampering. As we do so, we will be giving more from a place of already being filled up ourselves and our motivation to continue taking care of ourselves will increase, creating a beautiful feedback loop.

One of the biggest challenges in a relationship is staying connected to ourselves while relating with another. I like to think of the interplay involved in healthy relating as a partner dance, because dance requires each of us to be present in our own bodies while also co-creating with another. This, to me, is at the heart of healthy relating. When we are dancing or relating, we are continually reading each other's cues, verbal or nonverbal, risking making requests or invitations to each other, saying yes or saying no, and then taking action based on the answers we get. Sometimes we misunderstand each other and step on each other's toes. Sometimes we are amazed at how beautiful and smooth the dance goes and we don't really even know all the reasons why, only that we want more of that feeling. Rather than looking to the person we were dancing with to provide that feeling, we can learn tools (like the Relating Meditation on the next page) and develop practices that empower us to generate that feeling in dances (relationships) throughout our lives.

THE UNFOLDING OF INTIMATE RELATIONSHIP

Humans are social beings. We need each other, and it is through connection and cooperation that we thrive. From the moment we are born we are dependent on others, and cultivating healthy relationships throughout our lives is not only important for our happiness and well-being but for our very survival. We interact and relate with one another in different ways in different times in our lives. Staying present and connected with ourselves and the energy between us will serve us well, no matter what level of connection is present. We may be single for a time, interacting with others who are mostly acquaintances. We may relate more deeply with some close friends. We likely have family ties that lead to all sorts of relating adventures. And then there is that impulse to move into more intimate levels of relating.

More intimate levels of relating begin with attraction and flirtation. During this part of the relationship dance, we are getting to know each other, feeling the energy between us, and noticing how we feel within ourselves when we are relating with this other human. Flirtation can be fun and energizing for both parties. In healthy, authentic relating, either party is free to choose not to take the relationship anywhere beyond that. If we are relating in a healthy way, flirtation is not an invitation to sex, it is simply joyful play.

Relating Meditation Exercise

A wonderful couple who are friends of mine shared with me something they call a relating meditation. I think it is a beautiful tool for learning to stay connected with yourself while relating with another and for practicing once you've learned it. This is my own version of their work.

1   Find a partner to practice with, and decide who will speak first.

2   Sit facing one another with your eyes closed, and breathe deeply, focusing on your breath. Feel it moving in and out of your body. Take 10 deep breaths this way, tuning in to yourself.

3   After your 10th breath, open your eyes and look into the eyes of your partner. Take five more deep breaths, just being present with one another and breathing.

4   After the fifth breath, the person speaking first says, "Sitting here looking at you, I'm noticing _____." Fill in the blank with a body sensation (e.g., a tingling in your toes, a warmth in your belly, a tightness in your shoulder).

5   The other person speaks, saying, "Sitting here looking at you, I'm noticing _____." Then they fill the blank with a sensation they are noticing in their own body.

6   Go back and forth like this several times. Notice how it feels to be present with another while staying tuned in to your own body sensations enough to identify them and speak them.

SECOND ROUND:
Relating While Being Present with Yourself and Present in Space

1   Take turns again with one person saying, "Sitting here looking at you, I'm noticing _____." This time, fill in the blank with a body sensation and one thing you are noticing in your environment (e.g., a slight breeze on your left cheek, the sunlight streaming in through a window, the beauty of a sculpture behind you).

THIRD ROUND:
Making Requests

1   This is a round for practicing making requests and receiving an authentic response. You need not fulfill the requests that come up during the exercise. Again, take turns in this round, repeating this series as many times as you like.

2   You say, "Sitting here looking at you, I'm noticing _____."
Fill in the blank with a body sensation and a noticing from the environment, and then add a request that bubbles up from this present moment. (This request can be anything. "Smile with me. Let me rub your shoulder. Come run around the room with me . . ." Allow yourself to be enthusiastic, even childlike, in your request.)

3   Allow your partner to feel your enthusiasm for the idea, truly trusting them to take care of themselves when they answer.

4   Your partner, after listening to the cues from their body (as we learned in Chapter 3), will then answer with a yes or a no.

5   Whichever answer they give, say thank you. Their no is as precious as their yes since you truly only want to do the thing with someone who is a full yes. Their no can actually help you trust their yes's much more fully as you learn to trust that this is someone who will take care of themselves.

There is a lot going on in this last round. It's an opportunity to practice being fully present in the moment and allowing a simple request to bubble up from the energy generated between the two of you. It is an opportunity to practice speaking what is alive for you in the moment without attachment to it happening. It is an opportunity to practice feeling into and speaking your authentic yes and your authentic no and to have either answer greeted with enthusiasm and respect. It is an opportunity to practice receiving your partner's yes or no with respect and enthusiasm. At its heart, this is about clear boundaries. It is about being clear about your own boundaries (feeling and speaking your authentic yes or no) and about honoring and respecting the boundaries of others. This is essential skill building for truly healthy relating.

This relating meditation is a simple but powerful practice that can help transform some of our less healthy, more habitual ways of relating. Please do call on the grounding powers of the herbs as you dive into this practice. An AshwaMacaMocha Shake (page 64) will serve you well. As you practice it regularly, notice what starts to change in your relationships. Bring expression to your observations—noting them in your journal or by dancing or drawing or singing them.

In my own experience, I've noticed myself holding back from flirtatious play because of fear of misunderstandings about what the flirtation means and what the other person will assume will come next. Realizing that even after flirting, I can still say no to requests for deeper levels of emotional or physical connection helped free up that playful energy in my life.

If either party feels a desire for a deeper level of emotional or physical intimacy, conversation involving clear requests and mutual consent is an essential next step. These conversations require us to be vulnerable, let ourselves be seen in our desire, and risk that desire not being returned. The truth is that sometimes attraction will be mutual, and other times it will be one-sided. Anyone who has experienced the sublime joy of mutual attraction knows why we risk stepping into this place of extreme vulnerability. When it is not mutual, however, we find ourselves in a challenging situation.

Let's take a deep breath here. And another one. One-sided attraction is actually fairly common, so let's ask ourselves, "How can we navigate this situation well?" The relating meditation exercise has prepared us for this by getting us used to offering and receiving yes's and no's with equal gratitude. Still, let's acknowledge no's are tricky—to receive and also to give. Receiving a no to a vulnerable request may bring up feelings of disappointment, rejection, or shame. Giving a no requires us to witness another moving through these feelings. Either experience is profoundly challenging, so let us hold ourselves and each other in loving tenderness in these moments, acknowledging the vulnerability and risk it took to express the attraction and desire, honoring and celebrating the joyful feeling of it, and then

letting it go, and trusting that each of us will find ways to care for ourselves and move through our feelings.

Building our skill at holding ourselves through difficult emotions and allowing others to move through their own difficult emotions is what truly allows us to honor our own and each other's truths. It is an essential skill to build in order to develop the emotional resilience necessary to navigate relationship at all levels. I consider hawthorn to be a primary herb for this as it nourishes and protects our hearts both physically and emotionally. Tulsi is another powerful ally. As an adaptogen it helps us handle stress with greater ease. It can also help to clear our minds and hearts so we can more easily see the truth of a situation. I find its scent to also be both soothing and uplifting. After navigating a situation involving one-sided attraction, I would likely make myself a cup of Sweet Restoration Tea (page 135) and sink into a Seda Blanca Bath (page 61), breathing deeply and acknowledging the feelings that come up. Moving through them often requires nothing more than this—giving myself some loving attention as I acknowledge and feel them.

There are also emotions to be fully acknowledged and felt when the attraction is mutual and you choose to take a relationship to the next level of intimacy. You may have that joyous, uplifting experience of falling in love. The energy in this phase of a relationship can be quite intoxicating. We feel attractive and happy, like all is right with the world. Our partners seem fascinating and we notice all the things they do right and tend to overlook any of their less-than-perfect traits. There is often a lot of sexual heat present early in relationships. We can't get enough of each other's

Example Conversation

These conversations can be really simple, but there is a lot going on underneath the words.

SIMPLE CONVERSATION:

"Hey, I really enjoyed our dance earlier. I'd love to get to know you better. Would you like to go for a walk with me?"

"Oh, that's really sweet of you to ask. I enjoyed our dance too, but I'm not interested in anything more with you right now."

"Okay, thanks."

The two part and each take care of themselves in the midst of whatever emotions surfaced during the conversation.

WHAT'S GOING ON UNDERNEATH THE EXCHANGE:

Speaker 1: This person has really worked up their courage to be vulnerable and ask for what they want.

Speaker 2: After breathing and checking in with themselves, this person realizes they are a no to this request and they need to find a way to let the other person know with tenderness and kindness but also clarity and firmness.

Speaker 1: This person now must be with whatever emotions are coming up for them and find gratitude for receiving the other person's truth.

bodies. Each touch or kiss sends electric energy through us. This energy has been called "new-relationship energy" because it doesn't last. During this time our judgment can be clouded, so make sure you take some time to ground yourself so you are thinking clearly about whether you want to take this relationship into a place of deep intimacy. Call on grounding and centering herbs like ashwagandha and maca during this time.

If the relationship continues to delight and nourish you and you decide to go into even deeper levels of emotional and/or physical intimacy, then please revel in this energy while it is present.

Cherry Kiss Julep *Hanna Nicole*

INGREDIENTS

½ cup diced rhubarb

½ cup tart cherries
(frozen or fresh)

2 cups coconut water

⅓ cup honey

¼ cup powdered kava root

Pinch of nutmeg

2 egg whites

Juice of one large lemon,
or ¼ cup lemon juice

1 thin lemon slice for garnish
(optional)

HERBAL TIPS

✦ Kava drinks are best
consumed with intention
at a time when you are
ready to drop into your
erotic energy and certainly
not just before getting in a
car to drive. Kava can slow
your reaction time too
much for that.

PREPARATION

1 Place rhubarb, cherries, 1 cup of the coconut water, and honey into a small soup pot on low to medium heat for a couple of minutes, until the fruit begins to bubble.

2 Turn heat to low and simmer for 20 minutes (if it begins to stick to the bottom of the pan, add a tablespoon of water at a time until it loosens again).

3 While that is cooking, place the powdered kava inside a muslin bag.

4 Pour the rest of the coconut water into a bowl, and place the bag of kava into the water.

5 Massage the kava bag with your hand for 10 minutes, until the coconut water is milky and infused.

6 Pour the infused coconut water into a small jar, and place it in the fridge for now.

7 When the fruit is done cooking down, remove it from the heat, and strain the fruit syrup into another small jar. (Compost the fruit.) Place the fruit syrup into the refrigerator until it is cool.

8 While the fruit syrup is cooling, set out a large mason jar and fill it with ice cubes.

9 Separate eggs, saving the whites. Add a pinch of nutmeg to the egg whites.

10 Whisk the whites until stiff, and set aside.

11 Pour the lemon juice, chilled syrup, and kava coconut water over the ice.

12 Shake vigorously.

13 Pour the mixture out evenly between two small glasses.

14 Using a spoon, scoop the egg whites evenly between the two glasses to create a nice, even ½-inch layer over the drink.

15 If you want to add a touch more presentation, place a thin slice of lemon on the glass rim.

16 Enjoy your reveling!

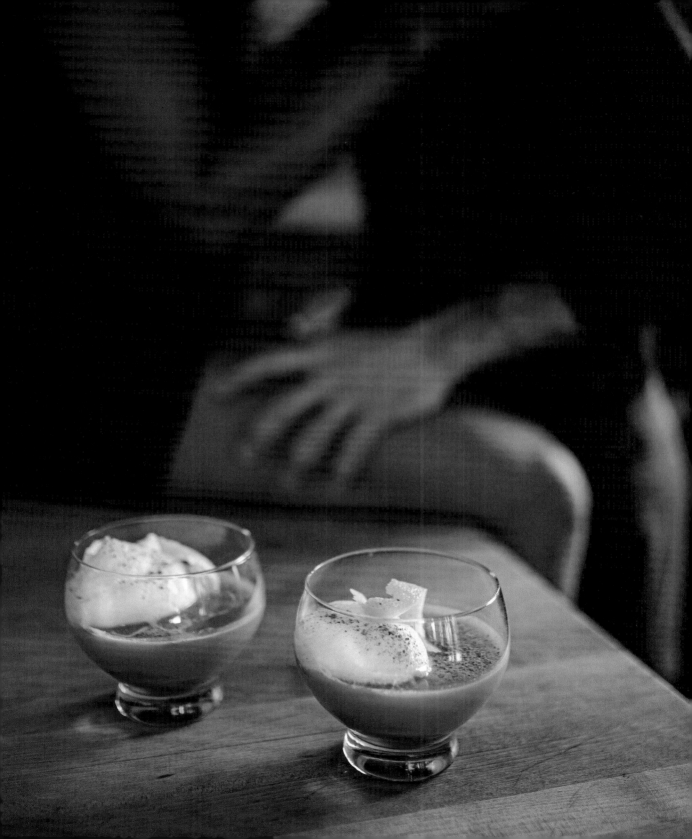

New relationship energy is one of the most joyful, beautiful gifts of being alive. Kava can help you to revel. It will also take you out of your mind and into your body, so be sure you've done that thinking work before you engage with it. Robert and Michelle noticed that kava heightened whatever emotions they were experiencing, so enjoying it while you are feeling the new-relationship high really could be wonderful. You can revel with a Cherry Kiss Julep (page 132).

DEEPENING INTO LONG-TERM RELATIONSHIPS

As we continue to spend time together, this new-relationship energy will slowly fade and our relationship will enter into new territory. We may begin to notice some of the less-than-perfect traits about our partner, and conflicts may emerge. We may decide to end the relationship at this point. Sometimes this is absolutely the right choice, and sometimes as we work through the issues that come up between us, we actually find ourselves experiencing even deeper levels of connection.

We definitely have a cultural myth that leads us to believe that if the person we are in a relationship with is really right for us, then we should just live happily ever after. This is unfortunate because it can lead us to a continual stream of heartbreaks, rather than allowing us to deepen into longer-term relationships. Part of what happens in longer-term relationships is that all the places that we need to heal can get illuminated. This doesn't usually happen gently, but more often through conflict with our partner. Navigating these conflicts and learning and growing through them requires lots of emotional maturity and resilience. The rewards are greater freedom and ease in your own life and much deeper intimacy with your partner.

To reap these rewards, you will need some powerful tools. Let me share with you some of my favorites. First let's look at emotional resilience. How do we build that in ourselves? Emotional resilience requires curiosity and a willingness to learn and grow. When you find yourself upset because of something that happened in your relationship, before reacting, take some time with yourself. I love this Viktor Frankl quote, "Between stimulus and response there is a space. In that space is our power to choose our response. In our response lies our growth and our freedom." Pausing and taking advantage of that space between stimulus and response is the first powerful tool for your toolkit. Take time and space to get clear in yourself before responding to your partner. You may need to discharge some of your angry or upset energy. Take a run, go for a swim, or dance like crazy in your living room.

You may also want to take one of those Seda Blanca Baths (page 61) or settle in with a cup of Sweet Restoration Tea (page 135) and nourish yourself as you acknowledge and give attention to whatever emotions are there for you to feel. For me, this tea blend is deeply calming. The hawthorn nourishes me and wraps my heart in loving protection, and the tulsi soothes my being on a deep level while helping build resilience. The combination is powerful as you take time to nourish and hold yourself while feeling and moving through difficult emotions. This nourishing and holding is a second powerful tool for developing emotional resilience.

Sweet Restoration Tea

INGREDIENTS

2 tablespoons dried
hawthorn berries

1 tablespoon dried tulsi leaves

½ teaspoon honey

HERBAL TIPS

✦ This recipe is a combination
of a decoction and an
infusion. Decoctions are made
by simmering plant material
in water for a period of time
(usually at least 20 minutes)
and infusions are made by
letting plant material steep in
just-boiled water for a period
of time.

✦ Decoctions are used for
harder plant material like
dried berries, roots, and bark.
Infusions are used more often
for delicate plant material
like leaves or flowers.

PREPARATION

1 Put the hawthorn berries and 1½ cups of water into a
saucepan and cover with a lid.

2 Bring the water to boil. Reduce the heat to a simmer.

3 Simmer for 20 minutes.

4 Put the tulsi in a teacup, and pour the berries and water
over top.

5 Steep for 5 minutes.

6 Strain.

7 Stir in honey and enjoy!

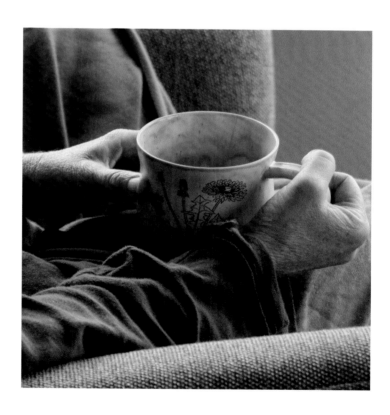

You may also need to allow yourself to express your emotions, crying or moaning or yelling or maybe punching a punching bag or your pillow. Finding some ways to release emotional energy without directing it at your partner is yet another tool for building emotional resilience. As you feel your emotions fully and move that emotional energy out of your body, the intensity of the feelings will dissipate and shift. Grounding and Moving Tea (page 137) can help ground you and allow you to express emotions like anger and sadness so you can move them through your body.

A fourth powerful tool for building emotional resilience is cultivating friendships in your life with people who can help you when you get into challenging emotional situations. We don't have to do this alone! Seek out people who can hear your side of the story and hold space for your pain without feeding your anger at your partner and perhaps even help you to see their perspective. Become a person like this for others in your life. Getting empathy and perspective can help you discern what you need to tell your partner and also allow you to show up with an open mind so you can hear your partner's perspective.

Building emotional resilience is a primary key to being willing to risk entering into the vulnerable space of intimate relationships. Knowing that we can feel and move through difficult emotions without having them incapacitate us allows us to be more willing to enter into vulnerable situations, like asking for that first date, requesting some pampering, or bringing up a secret desire. Without emotional resilience, we will fall into self-protective behaviors that most often isolate us from others. We may decide to put our sexuality and sensuality on a shelf, dressing in dumpy clothes or overeating so we don't feel attractive.

While protecting us from some level of heartbreak, these behaviors also cut us off from our vitality, our creativity, and our source energy and can lead to depression and other illnesses.

Moving through the difficult emotions may in itself allow for tranquil connection with your partner once more, but you may still need to work through the source of the conflict. Some of my favorite tools for navigating conflict include open communication, deep listening, self-reflection, and presence.

It is important to be able to speak our own truth and equally important to listen with an open mind to the truth of our partners. When we are present with each other in this way, listening deeply and communicating vulnerably, we can begin to hear each other's perspectives. As we listen to each other and reflect each other's truth, much of the charge of a conflict situation dissipates. Sometimes just hearing each other is enough to resolve the conflict.

Other times, we may find that our partner's perspective inspires us to self-reflect. Maybe we see something we would like to apologize for or a change we would like to make in our behavior. One person taking responsibility and apologizing can lead to the other being willing to do the same. Joe noticed that hawthorn was a good ally for him for this aspect of relating. He expressed that it opens him up, allows him to stay focused, be an active listener, and come from heart-open space, giving him more compassion for Cassie. A hawthorn tea or infusion or some Autumn Blush Cordial (page 39) could be good choices.

Another possible herbal ally here is kava. I will often make a cup of chai with kava creamer when John and I want to have a heart-connected conversation.

Grounding and Moving Tea

INGREDIENTS

1 tablespoon dried eleuthero root

1 tablespoon fresh ginger root

1 teaspoon dried schisandra berries

HERBAL TIPS

✦ This recipe is another example
of a decoction—simmering
hard plant material in water
for 20 minutes to extract
constituents into the water.

PREPARATION

1 Place the ingredients and 2 cups water in a small saucepan.

2 Bring the water to boil.

3 Turn the heat to low and simmer for 20 minutes.

4 Strain and drink slowly, letting the eleuthero ground you
while the ginger and schisandra get your energy moving so you
can release it.

5 Run or dance—move your body—to release the energy. Allow
yourself to release with sound as well.

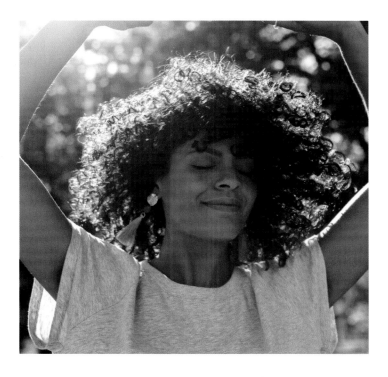

Kava Coconut Creamer

Hanna Nicole

INGREDIENTS

¼ cup powdered kava root

1 can full-fat coconut milk

HERBAL TIPS

✦ This creamer makes a great addition to Warm Nights Chai (page 171). You can let the chai simmer as you knead the kava into the coconut milk. You can also add it to a tea of your choice.

PREPARATION

1 Place ¼ cup of kava powder into a muslin bag.

2 Place the bag in a large bowl along with 1 can of coconut milk plus ½ can of water.

3 Knead the bag for 20 minutes or more, kneading your intention into the milk as it turns cloudy with kava goodness.

4 Compost the kava powder and clean the bag.

5 Pour yourself a cup of chai and stir in 1 to 2 tablespoons of the kava creamer.

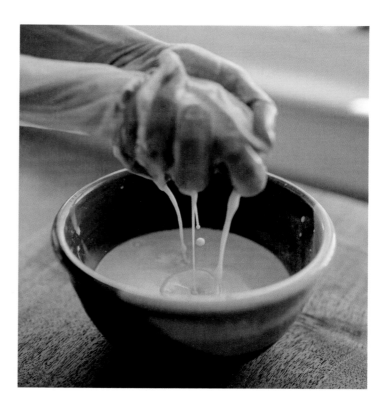

Conflict Resolution Conversation

Since this is not a kind of communication we practice much in our culture, let me give you some steps for creating a successful conflict resolution conversation. This format is based on Imago Dialogue work developed by Dr. Harville Hendrix and Dr. Helen Hunt and the Nonviolent Communication work of Marshall Rosenberg. Setting up regular times for these kinds of conversations is a powerful choice for successful long-term relationship.

1 Set aside time for a conversation. Give yourselves at least an hour in a private space where you will not be interrupted. Sit down with some Five Springs Tea (page 73) for courage or kava chai for heart-connected conversation.

2 Begin by offering each other appreciations—take turns and be sure to really take in what your partner is offering. (Example: Look each other in the eyes and say something like, "I really appreciate that delicious dinner you made for us last night" or "I appreciate you for sitting down with me for this conversation and really working with me to get through this challenging time." If you are receiving, let their gratitude sink in and thank them for it. Then offer an appreciation in return.)

3 Decide who will share first. That person will then speak for two or three minutes, sharing their perspective on the situation while the other person quietly listens.

4 Have the other person reflect back what they heard and then ask, "Am I getting you?"

5 Clear up any miscommunications and then continue with the first person sharing their perspective, pausing every couple of minutes for reflection and clearing of miscommunication.

6 When the first person feels complete (aim for about 15 minutes of sharing, and be as clear and succinct as possible) the listener says, "You make sense to me, based on what I know about you, I can really see how you saw things that way," and offers specifics. This is a powerful step. Even if you don't agree with the way your partner sees things, acknowledging their truth as a valid perspective is healing.

7 The listener then empathizes by guessing at what their partner might be feeling, and then the speaker gets to offer their own understanding of what they are feeling.

8 Switch roles, following these same steps and allowing the other person to share their perspective.

9　This work is actually often the bulk of what needs to happen for conflicts to be resolved. Once each person's perspective has been heard and validated and their feelings acknowledged, it becomes much easier to take the final steps.

10　Identify needs and come up with some possible solutions to meet those needs.

11　Choose a solution to try out, and set a time period to come back and revisit the solution and make adjustments if necessary.

12　End by appreciating each other for engaging in this process.

By the time we get into a long-term relationship, we have likely had many experiences in our lives, some of which have left us with residual trauma. Often, when we get really good at self-reflection, we will find that the conflict at hand does not really have much at all to do with what has just happened with our partner. Rather, their behavior, or the situation in general, has triggered an old wound from childhood or a past relationship. Instead of looking at that wound, we humans are brilliant at self-protection strategies that often look like shaming or blaming our partner for our own upset.

As we practice the emotional resilience tools above and gain more emotional maturity, we can learn to notice when we are triggered into these old wounds and we can make different choices. We can take each other's words less personally, and use the conflict as an opportunity to heal, learn, and grow. This can mean reflecting deeply to discover the source of our pain. When we find the source, we can begin to do the work to heal the old wounds. This is vulnerable work that takes tremendous courage, and you may very well want to employ the help of a counselor or coach to help you through it.

One practice that has helped me personally is to ground myself in the most powerful, grown-up version of myself that I can access. For me, this is the powerful priestess part of myself. Once I am firmly in touch with this, I can, through meditation, invite the little girl or younger version of myself to surface and be held by this powerful part of me. I can make space for her experience and feelings, holding her in the way I wish she could have been held when the wound occurred.

Though challenging, recognizing and healing these old wounds is freeing and has the potential of positively transforming all of the relationships in your life. After nearly 25 years together, John and I agree that this healing is one of the most valuable gifts of a long-term relationship. Along with it comes an incredible deepening of intimacy.

None of this is easy. This kind of relating requires whole new ways of thinking, skill building, and lots of practice. Some of my favorite books and resources for cultivating this depth of relating include Imago therapy, *Undefended Love* by Jett Psaris and Marlena S. Lyons, *Nonviolent Communication* by Marshall Rosenberg, *Self-Compassion* by Kristin Neff, and *Passionate Marriage* by David Schnarch, Ph.D. Alison Armstrong's work on gender differences is also one of my key resources for healthy relating.

Here is a poem to remember as you navigate your relationship:

Dear Human: You've got it all wrong. You didn't come here to master unconditional love. That is where you came from and where you'll return. You came here to learn personal love. Messy love. Sweaty love. Crazy love. Broken love. Whole love. Infused with divinity. Lived through the grace of stumbling. Demonstrated through the beauty of messing up. Often. You didn't come here to be perfect. You already are. You came here to be gorgeously human. Flawed and fabulous. And then to rise again into remembering. But unconditional love? Stop telling that story. Love, in truth, doesn't need ANY other adjectives. It doesn't require modifiers. It doesn't require the condition of perfection. It only asks that you show up. And do your best. That you stay present and feel fully. That you shine and fly and laugh and cry and hurt and heal and fall and get back up and play and work and live and die as YOU. It's enough. It's Plenty.

—Courtney Walsh

CULTIVATING EROS IN RELATIONSHIP

The kind of relationship work described above leads to more understanding of ourselves and of one another, more trust and safety, and a much deeper level of intimacy. Does that translate into a healthy and vibrant sex life? Not necessarily. Often in long-term relationships we develop a comfort with one another that decreases the polarity and dynamic tension that leads to hot sex. We can no longer rely on intoxicating, new-relationship energy to carry us into the bedroom, but we can learn to cultivate eros in our long-term relationships while also deepening into new realms of sexual pleasure.

We have already explored some of the keys to cultivating eros in a relationship. Slowing down, creating time and space for intimacy in your busy schedule, learning about your body and your partner's body, and pampering yourself and your partner are all ways of doing this. Another key is really valuing and nourishing your connection with your partner. Set aside time in your life to do things you love to do together—take walks on the beach, go out dancing or to a concert to listen to music, or take each other out to dinner. Identify the things you both love to do, and look for opportunities to do them. Sometimes it's fun to surprise each other. Set aside a date night and have one person in the couple make the plans while the other gets to be surprised.

Going out together is wonderful, but sometimes our schedules get so full that cramming in a date night just adds more stress. Luckily, we can continue to cultivate connection even in the midst of our busy day-to-day lives. Pausing for a kiss before heading off to work, celebrating a moment of beauty together (a sunset or blooming flowers), giving each other compliments, or offering appreciation all take very little time, but really do nourish our connection with each other. It may seem challenging and awkward at first, but the more you practice, the more it will become habitual and fun to notice and voice things you appreciate about your partner. Even if you are in agreement about whose turn it is to do the dishes, it makes a difference when you say thank you when the kitchen is all cleaned up. Or what about that moment when you were way too exhausted to deal with your teen's stress or upset and your partner stepped in and was able to hear them and diffuse the energy? Let them know how grateful you were and what a difference it made for you in your life. Appreciations build positive energy between you, and positive energy is a foundation for intimate connection.

This foundation of connection and positive energy allows us to step into an intimate space feeling safe and open. As we are present with one another in this safe space, we can open to the possibility of being vulnerable with each other. Try lying side by side and gazing into one another's eyes. Feel what is there for you and between you and your partner. This presence, this connection, is the heart of lovemaking and deep intimacy. So often we enter into lovemaking with an agenda of bringing one another to orgasm. What would it feel like if we changed our intention to feeling connected? Perhaps we would spend a half hour or longer just gazing into each other's eyes or merging our energies by holding one another in the Yab-Yum position (see photos on page 143), or in a close embrace. What emerges as you are fully present with one another? Be curious. Maybe you are drawn to kiss, or maybe tears begin to flow

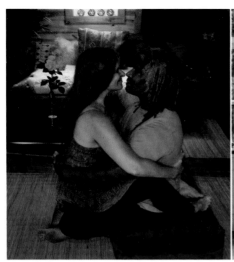
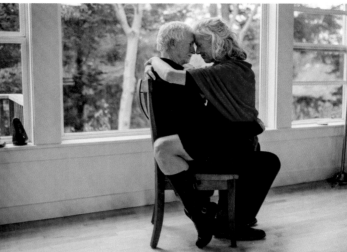

as emotion bubbles to the surface in that safe, intimate space. Allow whatever emerges, continuing to be present with one another. Follow your impulses, feeling what emerges as you do. Move slowly, appreciating each other's bodies, the exquisite sensations of touch, the release that comes from being held in your sadness, and the joy of connection.

Damiana Chocolate Love Liqueur (page 144) is a wonderful aphrodisiac to employ when you have dropped into this place of deep safety with another. I find that damiana quickly drops me down into my body and out of my head. For me, it is not an herb to call on when I want to be able to think clearly, but rather when I am feeling completely safe and excited to enter into deep, physical connection. Artemis calls damiana the engorger and speaks of feeling expansion in the energetic realms in her sacrum. She said, "She is a powerful ally, yet a friend that I will discerningly invite into my life. . . . For those wild nights where sleep escapes me from dusk to dawn, where I can play among the nightfall in a lover's arms, fully

surrendered to the wantings of my body. Where trust runs deep enough with the other, that she can join me and have her way, and I won't be left regretful in the morning." Several of us in the Aphrodisiac Circle agreed that this is an herb to call on when we want to deepen our physical connection within an already established loving, trusting relationship.

Sometimes this dance of intimacy will take you to orgasmic states, and sometimes you may find yourself experiencing sensations you have not experienced before, like a kind of floating together in a bubble of love, or perhaps riding waves of ecstatic energy up into peaks and down into valleys and back up again. Diana Richardson's book *Slow Sex* is a phenomenal resource for this sort of intimate relating. Knowing that there are a wide range of experiences possible, and not seeking to get to one particular state, can help remove pressure from sexual interactions and free up erotic energy in a relationship. If my partner proposes sex and I feel like that means I have to work myself up to orgasm or bring him to

Damiana Chocolate Love Liqueur

Diana DeLuca

INGREDIENTS

1 ounce dried damiana leaves

2 cups vodka or brandy

1 cup honey

Dash of vanilla extract

Rose water, to taste

½ cup chocolate syrup (you can use the Chocolate Body Drizzle recipe on page 157)

2-3 drops almond extract

HERBAL TIPS

✦ The alcohol and water each extract different constituents from the plant material, so in this recipe you are getting the benefits of both.

PREPARATION

1 Soak the damiana leaves in the vodka or brandy for 5 days in a jar on your kitchen counter.

2 Strain, reserving the liquid in a bottle and the leaves in a separate jar.

3 Soak the alcohol-drenched leaves in 1½ cups of water for 3 days.

4 Strain and reserve the liquid. (Compost the leaves.)

5 Gently warm the water extract over low heat, and dissolve the honey in it.

6 Remove the pan from the heat, then add the alcohol extract and stir well.

7 Pour the liquid into a clean bottle, and add a dash of vanilla and a touch of rose water for flavor.

8 Let it mellow for one month or longer; it gets smoother with age.

9 To each cup of damiana liqueur, add ½ cup of chocolate syrup, 2 to 3 drops of almond extract, and a touch more rose water.

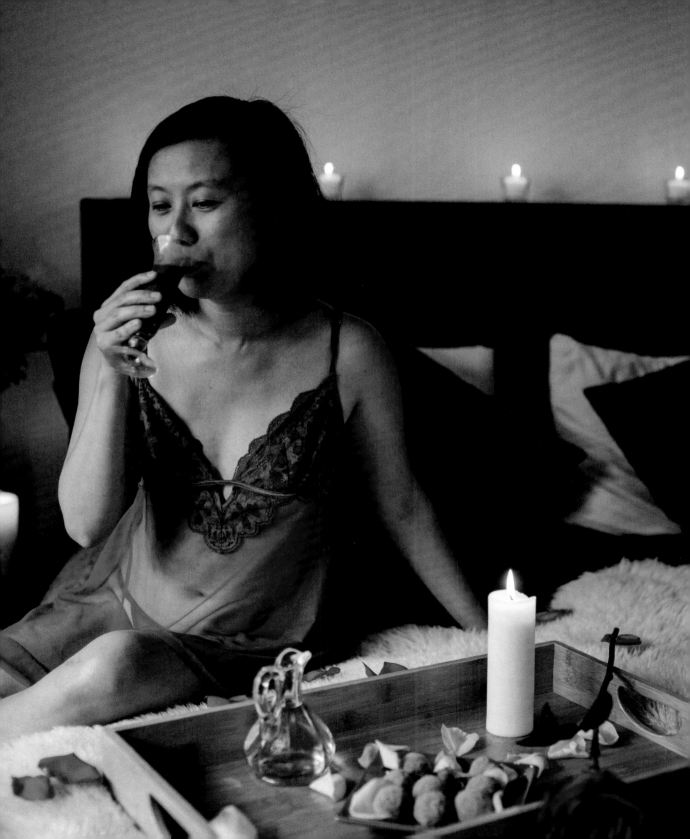

one, I can easily feel too tired to engage. If I know our intention is connection and that my prowess as a lover is not being judged by whether either of us come to orgasm, then I can engage more easily, bringing myself just how I am and being open to what emerges. This gift of releasing orgasm as the ultimate goal of lovemaking or as a measure of your skills as lovers is one of the most beautiful and powerful gifts you can give to each other.

But what if you're angry with your partner at the time you have set aside for intimate connection? Cultivating eros in our relationships can help to reduce relationship conflict as people who are sexually satisfied are naturally less aggressive, but still, there are bound to be times when we are upset with each other. So, feel into it. Sometimes physical connection can help diffuse anger between you. Or perhaps intimate connection time today will look like taking a step toward conflict resolution—sitting and listening to one another, hearing each other's perspectives. Sometimes the work of resolving conflict can lead to vulnerability in our interactions with each other, which creates an opening for deep, intimate physical connection. Vulnerability can actually be an aphrodisiac. If the anger is too intense in the moment, it really might be best to just take space (remember how pausing and taking space was one of those tools for emotional resilience?), setting up a later time to come together and hear each other and setting up another time for physical connection.

Sometimes in relationships sex becomes a manipulative tool, with people withholding or offering it to get what they want. Part of cultivating eros is not allowing that to happen in your relationship. Keep it clean. Engage in sex when you both want to for the purpose of connecting deeply with one another. Period.

All of this is truly such a dance. From the moment we are born, we are in relationship with other humans. We start learning about relating right away, and we develop skills and strategies to get our needs met, some healthy, some not. We create stories about how things are, and we act out of our personal view of reality. Sometimes our interactions with others help us revise our story or learn a new skill or a healthier strategy. Sometimes the dance of relationship goes too fast, and we are not able to employ all the healthy skills and strategies we have, and we step on each other's toes or lose connection with one another for a time. Things won't always go perfectly, but if we stay grounded in love and compassion for ourselves and our partners and keep being willing to learn and grow, we will find that our relationships gain resilience, begin to stand the test of time, and we are able to deepen into the kind of intimacy we truly crave.

We can help cultivate eros along the way by noticing things that help us feel more connected or turned on and then consciously doing more of them. I'll leave you with this story from Simon about ginger. During our month of experimenting with ginger, he started enjoying coffee brewed with ginger. He would brew it and then take time at the table with Rebecca while enjoying it. This was during the holidays when he had some days off of work. The ginger coffee provided a touch point of connection for them that they both noticed and enjoyed. Cultivating eros can be that simple.

BEING IN RELATIONSHIP WITH PLANTS

If any one of the recipes in this book has a positive impact on your journey toward sexual fulfillment and vital living, you will begin to develop a relationship with the plants that are used in that recipe. You may choose to make the recipe multiple times or you may be inspired to try another recipe using that same plant. Each time we make and use an herbal preparation, we are developing our relationship with the plants. We are taking them into our bodies and benefiting from their healing, nourishing, or enlivening qualities. This naturally leads to feelings of gratitude for what they are offering to you in your life.

Plants are living beings with whom we share this planet. When we get in touch with their beneficial

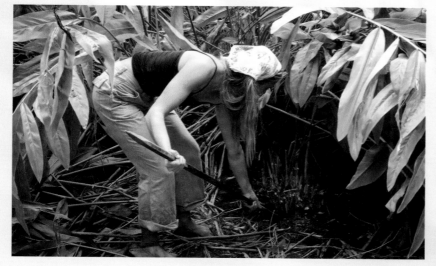

qualities, we may be inspired to get to know more about them. We may want to see if we can grow them in our garden or if they grow wild somewhere near us so we can go and harvest them ourselves. We might discover what kind of soil they like and whether they like to grow in the sun or in the shade and how much water they prefer. These are ways we are deepening our relationship with the plants.

As we come to really enjoy the benefits these plants bring to our lives, it is natural to find ourselves wanting to care for them—to create their ideal growing conditions in our garden or protect the wild places we have found to harvest them. We will want to learn how to harvest them in ways that allow them to keep growing and reproducing so we can harvest them again and again. We will give thanks for the gifts they give. Just like our human relationships, our relationships with the plants that we use for our preparations are reciprocal. As we use them, we are inspired to get to know more about them and to honor and take care of them. In return they thrive and continue to provide benefits for us, which inspires us to keep caring for them and so on.

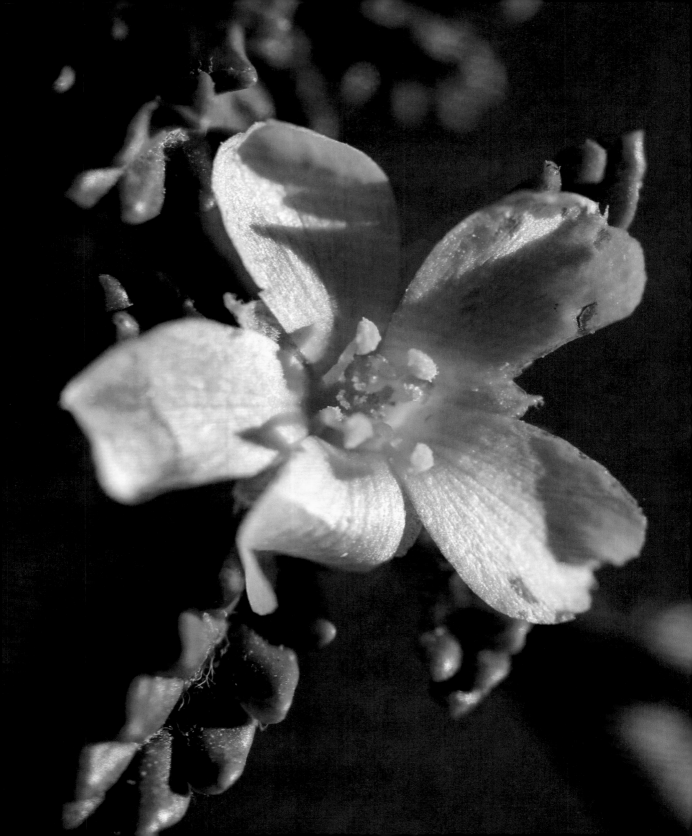

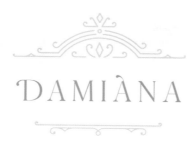

DAMIÀNA

Turnera diffusa, syn. *T. aphrodisiaca*

I fell in love with damiana the first time I drank a cup of Tender Titillation Tea (page 110). Each time I have engaged with damiana, it has quickly relaxed my mind and brought me into arousal and sensation. I call on damiana when I am with a partner I love and trust and want to surrender into a place of deep fulfillment.

How Does Damiana Work in Our Bodies?

Damiana can help bring more oxygen to the genital area,[1] help strengthen our reproductive systems,[2] and help regulate the pituitary gland and therefore our hormones, including increasing testosterone.[3] When used over time as a tonic, it can help restore and improve sexual vitality and fitness.[4]

Damiana is deeply restorative and energizing, partly due to its high phosphorous content, which can lead to better physical endurance and orgasmic ability.[5] As part of various formulas, damiana has demonstrated its ability to enhance female sexual function in human studies.[6] In her book *Down There*, Susun Weed said, "a cup of damiana leaf infusion or teaspoon of tincture improves her interest and his staying power."[7]

Damiana is wonderful for our nervous systems. It is relaxing, can help restore exhausted nerves, and relieve depression.[8] It has demonstrated anxiety reducing and antidepressant effects and an ability to positively modulate behavior.[9] Damiana is a useful aid for people who have a reduced libido due to depression, anxiety, aging, or reduced thyroid function.[10] Brigitte Mars suggests damiana to treat performance anxiety in adults and self-consciousness about puberty in teens.[11]

Several flavonoids have been studied specifically within damiana, namely acacetin, acacetin 7-methyl ether, and vetulin. These compounds have shown very promising research about being MAO inhibitors.[12] MAO inhibitors prevent the breakdown of serotonin and dopamine in the brain, thus enhancing the feel-good effects from these neurochemicals within the body. Another bioactive compound found in damiana, apigenin, is a mild sedative and has been found to greatly reduce anxiety and relieve pain.[13] By enhancing mood and decreasing stress and pain, these compounds found in damiana contribute to its powerful effects.

A Bit about Damiana Plants

Damiana is a small aromatic shrub with beautiful yellow flowers. It loves wild, dry, sunny places and is especially fond of rocky hillsides. Native to the northwest desert region of Mexico, it also grows in Texas, Southern California, and Central America.

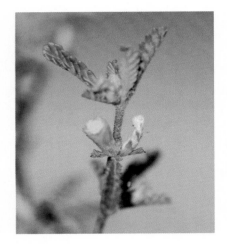

Herbal Shorthand

APHRODISIAC ACTIONS: *antidepressant, aromatic, energizing, hormone balancing, nervine, restorative*

OTHER ACTIONS: *astringent, diuretic, emmenagogue (stimulates menstrual flow)*

ENERGETICS: *warm, dry*   TASTES: *bitter, pungent*

NOTABLE APHRODISIAC CONSTITUENTS: *apigenin, flavonoids, volatile oils*

DOSAGE SUGGESTIONS: *Damiana is a medicinal-level herb and should be consumed occasionally for a specific purpose. (This could look like an infusion added to a bath or a liqueur or tea before making love.) For strengthening and anti-anxiety effects try 15 drops of tincture three times per day or a cup or two of tea (2 teaspoons of leaves per cup of water steeped for 20 minutes) per day for a limited period of time.*

SPECIAL CONSIDERATIONS: *Avoid taking damiana during pregnancy or nursing, if you have anemia, a urinary tract infection, or hypertension.*

Use with caution if you are diabetic as it can drop your blood sugar level.

Long-term use may interfere with the body's assimilation of iron.

Large doses can be laxative and may cause insomnia and headaches.

How to Use Damiana

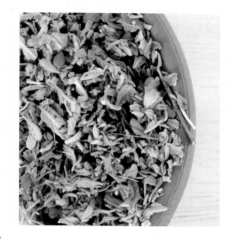

PARTS USED: *Leaves*

For tonic or healing effects of damiana, take a regular, consistent dose over a period of several weeks. (See dosage suggestions provided earlier.) Listen to your body to know if you are at a place in your sexual journey where this tonic or medicinal dose would truly be helpful for you.

A simple cup of damiana tea can have a mild euphoric effect, which can be stimulating for intimacy. If you choose to try damiana as a tea, know that it is bitter and is tastier when mixed with other herbs. I love it with oat tops, hawthorn, rose petals, and a little honey.

The leaves can also be smoked or used as incense to achieve a mild euphoric effect.

Damiana liqueur is a traditional herbal preparation where the leaves are steeped in rum and honey with spices like vanilla, galangal, cinnamon, and pimento berries for two weeks.

Participant Experiences

Damiana had pronounced, immediate effects for us. It brought us into slightly altered state experiences that had an embodied, primal quality to them, definitely moving us out of our normal thinking state. Sarah noticed that it slowed down her thinking and speech and slightly blurred her vision. Lisa described a sort of floating experience that led to great lovemaking. We definitely felt increased sexual energy, which was wonderful when we were with a loving partner and induced longing for touch when we were not. Christina noticed a profound connection with nature when she could be outside but found that damiana increased her mind chatter when she took it just before trying to sleep.

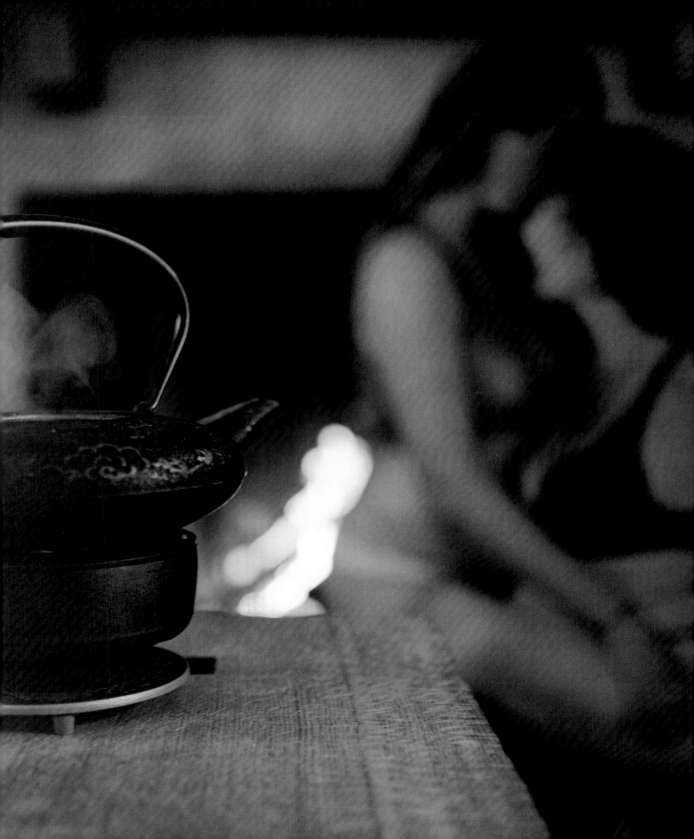

SIX

STOKING

YOUR

FIRE

FOR

SEXUAL

FULFILLMENT

Imagine you live in a culture that has prioritized pleasure and healthy sexuality. As you walk down the street with others who are feeling sexually fulfilled, what do you notice?

Close your eyes and really imagine before you read on.

I feel a relaxation in the muscles in my body, a sense of ease and joy. People are walking with their shoulders back, heads up, and with some extra spring in their step. I see smiles on their faces. People are making eye contact with one another while enjoying the world around them—the feel of the air on their skin, the rustle of tree leaves, the song of birds. I notice acts of patience and generosity—someone helping an elderly person cross the street, a man taking time to talk with a child who accidentally bumped into him.

I believe that sexual fulfillment brings out the best in people. When we feel sexually fulfilled, we are more at ease in the world, happier, more confident, and less prone to violence.

We are sexual beings, and yet for many, the idea of feeling truly sexually fulfilled seems impossible. Many of us live within cultures of sexual repression and exploitation that tie sexual expression with shame or profit. We may feel guilty for having sexual desires at all. Even if we do welcome our desire, we may painfully feel the lack of a partner to explore with or perhaps we are so busy just trying to make ends meet or raise our children that time to explore sexually feels like a distant luxury. Maybe we have a partner, but with the busyness of life or as a result of weathering the conflicts of relationship, the fire has just gone out between us.

So, how can we stoke our fires? What steps can we take toward healthy sexual expression and leading lives where feeling sexually fulfilled is a common state of being? For me, sexual fulfillment is a state of being that arises when we are no longer ashamed of our sexuality, are confident in our knowledge about our bodies and what brings us pleasure, and are consciously cultivating the kinds of experiences that fulfill our desires. Everything we have been exploring in this book so far can be part of cultivating this kind of fulfillment as we apply it directly to our sexuality. Our next steps toward fulfillment are going to be different for each of us. Let's begin by imagining . . .

Imagining and Manifesting Sexual Fulfillment

Part I

1 Take a few minutes right now to breathe deeply and bring yourself into that sensual, embodied space.

2 Imagine yourself moving through your life feeling sexually fulfilled. Allow thoughts and images to rise up into your consciousness. In your imagined sexually fulfilled life, do you have one sexual partner or many or are you most fulfilled by your own self-pleasuring? Have you created a beautiful space for sexual expression and carved out time in your schedule for physical connection? How does your body feel physically? Emotionally? Give yourself permission to dream and to really feel into and enjoy that dream.

3 Write or draw or dance your dream.

4 Hold this dream in your heart as a guiding intention, being curious about where it will lead you.

Part II

1   Look back over your expressions from Chapter 3, getting in touch with your own journey of sexual empowerment. Where are you in that journey right now?

2   Breathe deeply and bring yourself into that sensual embodied place again.

3   Let a next step bubble up for you.

4   Write it down and commit to doing this one thing. That is how manifestation happens. One step at a time. Feel free to call on schisandra for courage. Sometimes these steps are not easy. Call on close friends for support as well. You don't have to do it alone.

5   With each step toward your dream, new opportunities will emerge. Let yourself be open to the surprises that life brings your way. Ideas may emerge for a next step or you may find your dream changing over time. Perhaps you will start to see things you could not have even imagined before. Keep dreaming, identifying and taking steps, enjoying and celebrating each moment of fulfillment you find along the way.

FOSTERING EXCITEMENT AND SEXUAL CHARGE

Part of moving toward a sexually fulfilled life is learning to foster excitement and sexual charge. Though what brings sexual excitement to each of us is unique, there are some underlying, universal truths about human sexuality and arousal as well.

One of my teachers, Pamela Madsen, said during a workshop that eros thrives on space and obstacles. That sentence stuck with me and I have found it to be true. There is a part of our psyche that thrives on longing for something or someone that we cannot have. It can feel torturous to be separated from someone you love, and yet the separation does also serve to increase our interest and desire. When we do finally come together, the sexual energy is hot and intense.

Knowing this truth can help us enjoy the times when obstacles keep us separated from someone we are attracted to or whom we love. The key here is to build our tolerance for feeling longing. Emotions like longing can be so uncomfortable for people that we choose to numb ourselves with alcohol, food, or television. What if, instead, we fantasize about the time when we will be with our love? We can prepare a beautiful space or a new aphrodisiac concoction for our time together. Flirting (even if only by text or phone if you are far from one another) can build the sexual energy even more. Feel and enjoy that energy moving in your body. Instead of numbing it, let it light you up.

Here are some aphrodisiac concoctions you might prepare in anticipation of the fulfillment of your desires.

Chocolate Body Drizzle

INGREDIENTS

½ cup water

½ cup cocoa powder

⅓ cup honey

1 teaspoon vanilla extract

Pinch of salt

¼ cup full-fat coconut milk

PREPARATION

1 Combine the ingredients except the coconut milk in a saucepan.

2 Bring the mixture to a boil and simmer, whisking constantly for 5 minutes.

3 Remove the saucepan from the heat.

4 Stir in the coconut milk.

5 Store in the refrigerator for up to 2 weeks.

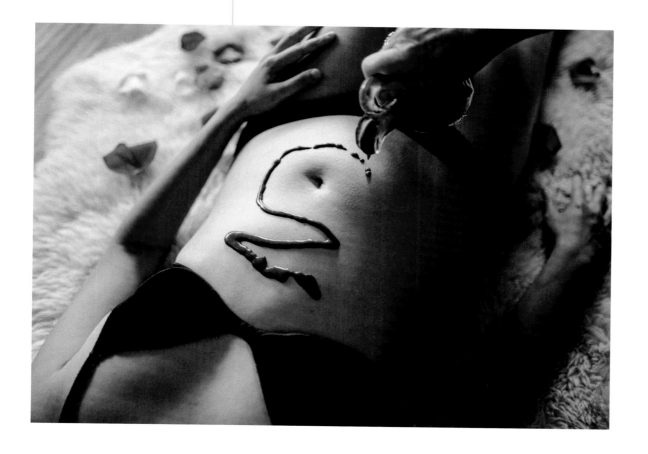

Love's Nectar

This is a beautiful rose syrup that is lovely for body drizzling as well.

INGREDIENTS

2 cups fresh (1 cup dried) rose petals

1 cup honey

HERBAL TIPS

✦ This recipe combines a honey and water infusion to get the benefits of both in a tasty, sexy treat.

✦ Mixing a few tablespoons of this syrup with fizzy water makes a refreshing, delicious beverage.

✦ You can also drizzle this syrup over other tasty desserts like the Eros Cream or the Maple Oat Squares in Chapter 12.

PREPARATION

1 Prepare a Rose Honey (page 14).

2 Bring 1 cup of water to a boil in a saucepan. Remove it from the heat.

3 Add 1 cup fresh or ½ cup dried rose petals to the water, then cover and steep for 1 hour.

4 Strain, reserving the water and composting the rose petals.

5 Strain the petals from the honey (or leave them in if you like to have petals in your syrup).

6 Stir the rose honey into the warm rose-infused water.

7 Store the syrup in a jar with a lid in the refrigerator for up to one month.

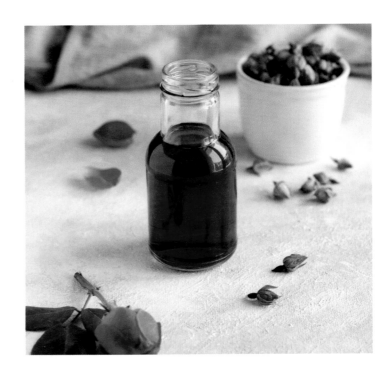

In order for longing and anticipation to be positive forces in our lives, fulfillment is an important component—getting to actually drizzle that chocolate sauce or rose syrup over your partner's body and experience licking it off. Learning to allow longing to lead to anticipation has allowed me to welcome the times when John and I are apart as moments when the sexual energy between us naturally increases. Reunions become sweet and delicious. Taking space can be a way of cultivating eros in long-term relationships, but in any length relationship, frustration will ensue if desires go unmet for too long. So I would modify my instructor's statement to be *eros feeds on space and obstacles with just the right amount of fulfillment.*

When anticipated and prepared for, moments of fulfillment after separation may lead to new experiences that are outside the realm of our everyday lovemaking. (Like licking chocolate body drizzle from your lover's breasts.) Experiences like these can be particularly "fire stoking." Humans are inherently curious and thrive on new and different experiences. Allowing yourself to play and gently push the edges of your comfort zone can be very exciting. As partners, we can encourage each other as we begin to acknowledge our desires. Play with letting your partner seduce you into something new or with seducing your partner into new experiences. As you do so, gift each other with the power to stop the play at any moment if the leap out of comfort becomes too large for any reason. The more we move in and out of our comfort zone, the easier it becomes and the more possibilities for sexual play can emerge.

Our sexual, animal nature also thrives on polarity, the coming together of differing energies. In Chapter 3, we gave ourselves permission to claim our gender preferences, sexual identities, and our desires. As we get clear about and cultivate our own unique sexual energy, we will likely find ourselves attracted to partners who have done the same and whose energy is very different from our own. The exciting, dynamic tension created in the interplay of these different energies is part of what stokes our sexual fires.

Intercourse is the merging of penetrating (masculine) and welcoming or enfolding (feminine) energies. We can build the dynamic tension between these polarities and increase the sexual charge by cultivating healthy masculine and feminine energies within ourselves. Living within a patriarchal culture makes this challenging. Both masculine and feminine energies have become unhealthy within this system. In patriarchal culture, men are in power over women, and masculine forms of power are venerated. This imbalance has led to the repression of feminine energy and feminine forms of power. We have come to think of masculine energy as strong and feminine energy as weak, but in truth, both are equally powerful. The merging of healthy masculine and feminine energies generates source energy for creation.

So, how can we cultivate healthy masculine and/or feminine energies within ourselves? Alison Armstrong's work on this topic has been revolutionary for me. She has interviewed thousands of men in order to develop her understanding of masculine energies and has devoted her life energy to understanding both men and women and helping us all learn how we can be healthy and strong and partner in mutually beneficial ways. One of the things she said about how to cultivate feminine energy that stuck with me is to "do less in more time." Feminine energy

Sharing Your Secret Desires

This opportunity is written as a partner exercise, but can be equally powerful when explored solo, giving yourself the gift of naming your secret desires, sitting with the truth of them with acceptance, tenderness, and gratitude, and gifting yourself with self-pleasuring fulfillment time. You may also choose to disclose secret desires with a close friend as an exercise in claiming them even if you don't practice the fulfillment part with each other.

This is an exercise that can help you move out of habitual lovemaking patterns and into fulfillment of deep desires.

1   Ask your partner if they are willing to engage in an activity to learn more about each other's sexual desires. If they are willing . . .

2   Set up a two-hour block of time to spend with each other where you will not be inter-rupted. Bring a notepad and a pen or pencil.

3   Settle into a comfortable space with your partner, look into each other's eyes, and take a few deep breaths together.

4   Set an intention to spend the next 15 minutes writing a list of sensual or sexual desires to share with each other. Agree also that when you share them you will meet each other's shares with openness and curiosity, responding with the words "Thank you for sharing that with me," and that once you have shared your lists, each of you will choose one desire from the other's list to fulfill together.

5   Set up desire fulfillment time(s) in your calendar right now—one two-hour block for each of you within the next week. (You can adjust the amount of time later if this is too much or too little.) You can choose to fulfill each other's desires on the same date or set back-to-back dates so you have time to revel in each experience without having to immediately switch roles.

6   Spend 15 minutes making your lists of desires. Include a variety of desires from a 20-minute foot massage to 20 minutes of G-spot stimulation to exploring anal stim-ulation or penetration. Include some that you feel your partner will most certainly be willing to fulfill and some that you feel would only be fulfilled in your wildest dreams. Be as specific and descriptive as possible so you have the greatest chance of your desire being fully met.

7   When the time for list sharing comes, settle back in together, look again into each other's eyes, and take a few deep breaths together.

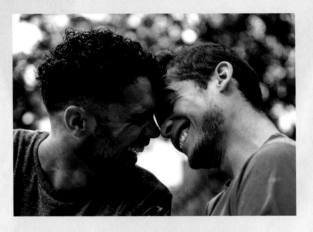

8   Re-presence your agreement to greet each other's desires with openness and curiosity, responding with, "Thank you for sharing that with me." (This allows you to be certain your desires will not be met with shock, shaming, or ridicule.)

9   Check in with each other to see if there are other agreements you could make that would help either of you feel more comfortable sharing your lists. If so, make those agreements as well.

10 Take turns with each partner sharing one desire from their list and then responding to a desire from the other. Continue until you have each shared as much of your list as you are willing to share. (I encourage you to share the whole thing.)

11 In a moment you will be exchanging lists and choosing which desire you would like to fulfill with your partner. Before you do so, take a moment to consciously release any attachment about which desire will be met. No matter which one your partner chooses, their doing so is an expression of their care for you and their willingness to be vulnerable, connect, and give you pleasure.

12 Exchange lists. Give yourselves five minutes to read over each other's lists and choose a desire to fulfill for one another during the time you have set aside.

13 Come back together and tell each other which desire you are going to fulfill.

14 Use the time in between to prepare and enjoy the anticipation.

15 When you have taken turns fulfilling on your desires, come together again to share your experiences. Start by appreciating each other for taking this step together. Share about how it felt to have your desire fulfilled and to fulfill your partner's desire—in your body, your mind, and emotionally. Meet each other's sharing with gratitude, saying something like, "Thank you for being so open with me. I really appreciate your vulnerability."

16 Consider setting up another time to fulfill on another of your partner's desires.

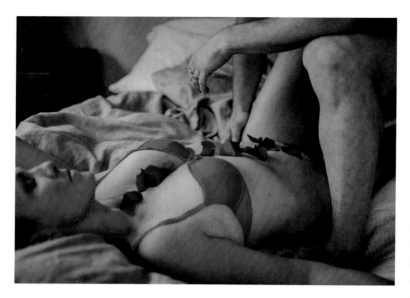

energies of dominance and submission within sexuality. This movie does a brilliant job of weaving the two explorations together and highlighting how the energies of dominance and submission can also foster excitement and sexual charge. People enjoy controlling and being controlled by each other, lovingly challenging and surrendering to one another, exploring fantasy and desire together. Both energies require strength, clarity, and vulnerability. The vulnerability leads to deep connection, and through this loving connection, we can allow ourselves to experience the joy of fully satisfying the desires of our partner, of having our own desires fully satisfied, the joy of full surrender, and the exquisite pleasure of moving beyond our comfort zone into new experiences and explorations. These explorations can range into the areas of kink but can also simply be about one person allowing and providing fulfillment while the other directs the course of the lovemaking. When explored among consenting adults, these energies provide another source of dynamic tension and stoke the fire of sexual fulfillment in surprising and exciting ways.

is more about being than doing. We can cultivate feminine energy by keeping ourselves nourished and filled up. This allows us to be our best selves, and that is our greatest contribution to those we love. Masculine energy is more about doing, so we can cultivate masculine energy by claiming our unique gifts and doing work in alignment with those gifts.

As we explored in Chapter 3, we can cultivate masculine and feminine energies within ourselves, regardless of our gender. We can embody masculine or feminine energies at different times even within the same lovemaking session. One of the challenges of this time in history is to cultivate healthy forms of these energies and equalize their power. As we do so, we stoke the fires of deep sexual fulfillment and also generate powerful co-creative energy to help us through the myriad of challenges facing us today.

I loved the movie *Professor Marston and the Wonder Women* as an exploration of powerful masculine and feminine energies and also of the

SEDUCTION

Cultivating these energies of polarity can be part of seduction, part of helping us transition from daily life activities into lovemaking. As we cultivate our own unique energy, be it masculine, feminine, dominant, submissive, or some combination of all of them, we become comfortable in our own skin. We gain confidence, and confidence is an important foundation underlying successful seduction. Part of being truly seductive is being ourselves, knowing what turns us on, and daring to stand in it. Wearing clothes that make you feel beautiful or sexy, taking time to style your hair and/or put on your makeup or jewelry, maybe adding some cologne or perfume.

We might do all of these things with the hope of being able to convince someone who has communicated that they are not interested in having sex with us to engage anyway. We might wonder if there are herbal aphrodisiac concoctions that can help us with that, like modern-day love potions. Well, what I can tell you is that herbs do not work that way. If someone is not giving you clear indications about feeling attracted to you, please respect their no. Seduction and herbal aphrodisiacs are not about coercing or pressuring someone into doing something they do not want to do. Experiencing sexual advances or seductive energy from an unwelcome source can feel very uncomfortable and sometimes downright scary.

Joe shared this experience with one-sided attraction:

While I believe it's true that women are the recipient of most unwanted advances, most of the men I know have had their share of unwanted advances too. One of my worst experiences was downright scary. I was in college, and a young woman was very into me . . . too into me, if you know what I mean. After several unsuccessful advances, one dark night she came to my house during a rainstorm, wearing only short-shorts and a sopping-wet white T-shirt. When I opened the door, she practically forced herself into my home and then she forced herself onto me. I was caught

by surprise and didn't have enough self-confidence to say no. We slept together. Afterward, I felt awkward, shame and guilt. The next morning, I told her as kindly as I could that I only wanted a friendship. She snapped, and for the rest of the year, she spread nasty lies about me to anyone who would listen. Eventually she found a new boyfriend who happened to be a gun-loving macho ex-Marine. But instead of letting things go, she called me up and said, "I told my new boyfriend that you are trying to steal me away from him. I hope he kicks your ass, or even better, I hope he hunts you down!" I was scared to death!

If someone says no, respect it, and go your way. Though it may hurt in the moment as you feel the rejection, pursuing someone who does not want to be pursued is unhealthy for both parties. Instead, move on, trusting that you will find others who are attracted to your unique energy and who will ultimately be a better fit for you.

When mutual attraction is present and both people are clear that they want to engage in deeper levels of intimacy, seduction is simply a playful way of encouraging another to let go and engage in connection with you. It is about being confident in yourself and fully present with your lover so that they can feel safe, connected, and aroused. It is about going slow, teasing them with the look in your eyes, or a gentle caress of their arm, a light kiss on their neck. It is about knowing your partner and what helps them relax and transition into a state of arousal. Perhaps you have set up a space with soft music playing and some Warm Caress Massage Oil (page 164) by the bedside. Perhaps there's a feather there too or one of their favorite sex toys to begin to stimulate their imagination about what is to come.

The intention behind your actions is important. Yes, you are coming to your partner with

Warm Caress Massage Oil Recipe

Rosalee de la Forêt

INGREDIENTS

¼ cup grated or finely minced fresh ginger (30 grams)

½ cup jojoba or almond oil

10 to 15 drops lavender (*Lavandula angustifolia*) essential oil

PREPARATION

1 Add the freshly grated ginger to a small jar. Pour the oil over the ginger and stir to combine. Let this sit for 12 to 24 hours.

2 Strain the ginger from the oil, reserving the oil and composting the ginger.

3 Add the lavender essential oil and stir.

4 The water in the fresh ginger will cause this mixture to eventually spoil, so for best results, store the massage oil in the fridge and use within 1 to 2 weeks.

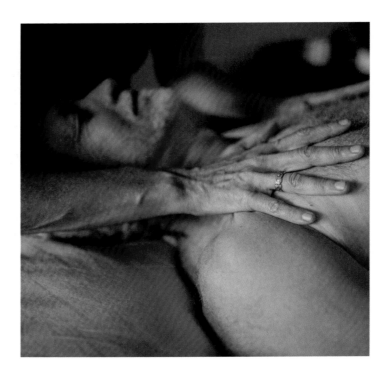

your own turn-on, and you are being vulnerable in sharing your desire to engage sexually, but if you are focused on your own sexual pleasure or your own orgasm as your goal, your seduction will be less effective. I invite you to come back to the intention of presence and connection. As you are present in the moment and build connection with your partner, you will find yourself creating a safe and playful space where you can lovingly coax or seduce them into new explorations that may surpass any goal you originally set for your time together.

HEALTHY SEXUAL INTERACTION

Time together with bodies entwined, exploring touch and pleasure is truly precious time, and our lovemaking can look different every time we engage. Sometimes we may be super hot for each other and quickly tear the clothes from our bodies and lose ourselves in passionate kissing, stroking, and penetration. Other times we may want to explore an erotic edge like anal play, wearing sexy lingerie, or being tied up. Maybe we've just taken a tantra workshop and are excited to try out a new breathing technique. Or perhaps we are feeling tender and raw after an argument or other emotional experience and we just want to feel held and loved.

All kinds of possibilities exist within the realm of healthy sexual interaction and at the heart of them all is mutual consent. As long as all of those involved in the interaction are participating with full consent and are free to change their minds at any point, experimentation and play are beautiful gifts we can give to each other. Differences in age and power must be taken into consideration here. Even if there is verbal consent, if one party is clearly in a position of power over the other (e.g., adult/child or boss/employee or teacher/student) true consent and therefore healthy sexual interaction is not really possible.

Betty Martin's Wheel of Consent highlights the fact that there are a myriad of exciting possibilities for us within the realm of mutual consent, and it is beneficial to enter into sexual activity with a great deal of consciousness. In Chapter 4, we explored the idea of pampering each other and touch clearly being for one partner or the other. During lovemaking there is a dance of pleasurable touch that happens. But what about those moments when you are not fully enjoying the touch you are receiving? Do you just grit your teeth and endure because you don't want to hurt your partner's feelings or because you think they are enjoying it? Sometimes it is pleasurable to allow our bodies to be touched primarily for our partner's turn-on, but the tragedy comes when we are enduring and our partner believes they are touching us for our pleasure. Neither one of us is truly enjoying what is happening. Try playing Betty's Three-Minute Game (page 166) to get a deeper understanding of this. Open communication during or after sex can help us learn to touch and be touched with more consciousness and greatly increase our pleasure.

Betty Martin's Three-Minute Game

This simple game from Betty's website can help you understand this idea more fully. You'll find more details on her site at bettymartin.org if you want to really dive into this. Here's how to play:

1   Sit with a partner. Take turns making the following offers to each other and following through with touch. Betty recommends going slow and starting with neutral (non-sexy) body parts like the back of a hand.

    Offer #1: How would you like me to touch you for three minutes? (Please scratch my back, kiss my neck, bite my toes, hold me, etc.)

    Offer #2: How would you like to touch me for three minutes? (May I feel your arms, explore your back, play with your hair, etc. Do not offer to "give" anything, like a massage. This is for your pleasure.)

2   When you make the offer, you are giving a gift. Negotiate as needed. Never give more than you are happy to give.

Each of the four rounds of the game creates a different role for you. Either you are doing or they are doing, and either it is for you or it is for them. Those two factors combine in four ways: you are doing and it's for you (Take), you are doing and it's for them (Serve), they are doing and it's for you (Accept), and they are doing and it's for them (Allow). Consent (your agreement) creates the quadrants. Without agreement about who it is for, the quadrants do not exist. Each quadrant is enjoyable and challenging in different ways, each will access a different aspect of yourself and your sexuality, and each has the potential to teach you something new.

MASTERING OPEN COMMUNICATION TO INCREASE PLEASURE

Learning to communicate openly about our experiences of sex and pleasure is incredibly fire stoking as it leads us to increasingly engage in physical experiences that heighten our mutual pleasure. Yet there are multiple challenges to successful communication. One challenge I've noticed is that during sex, I have largely dropped out of a mental, thinking space into my body. Forming coherent thoughts and finding and speaking words can be difficult. If we do find words, communicating them with consciousness and compassion can pose another level of challenge, yet compassionate communication is particularly important during sex. It is important because when we are connecting sexually, we are open and vulnerable, so it can be particularly challenging to hear feedback. So what do we do?

I have several suggestions that can help make open communication more successful. First, talk about the idea of communicating openly with your partner when you are not engaged in a sexual interaction. Create an agreement that you would like to try this so you can both increase your pleasure. Also, I recommend making a recovery plan. What will you do if it doesn't go well? Find ways to give each other space to make mistakes, like agreeing to take an hour break from each other after a difficult interaction where you each do some self-care and then coming back together to talk through what happened without blaming or shaming.

We are always communicating during sex, even if not with words. If we are attuned to one another, we will notice all kinds of ways that our bodies are communicating with us about what is happening, like increased vaginal moisture or penises becoming erect, or increased or decreased heat in the body. We can also communicate positive feedback vocally without words, using moans, sighs, or other sounds. All of these kinds of communication are valuable as we seek to give ourselves and our partners the most pleasure possible. If we need to let our partner know that something they are doing is not feeling good, we can do so gently by simply shifting our body position or asking for a change that would make something feel better. You can say, "Mmmmm.

Slower please" or "I'd love a little more pressure." These kinds of suggestions are much easier to hear than "Ugh, I don't like that," when we are open, raw, and vulnerable.

Taking time after sex to tell each other what you liked and to share ideas for future lovemaking sessions is a great practice as well. Feedback can be much easier to hear when we are not actively engaged in lovemaking. Gifting each other with appreciations for what we liked and enjoyed before making requests or suggestions for changes is important as well. As we practice giving and receiving feedback it gets easier and we begin to build our emotional resilience and trust. We begin to understand that feedback is a gift that helps us become a better lover rather than an indication that we are bad or wrong and will never satisfy our partner the way they want us to. We can relax and let go of the fear that if we do not perform perfectly, our partner will stop loving us or stop wanting to interact with us sexually, and we can open to the possibility of increasing our skills.

KEEPING IT HOT

Besides struggling with open communication, couples can also come to a place in their sexual interactions where sex becomes primarily about satisfying a biological need and is reduced to bringing each other to quick orgasm or ejaculation. If this is so for you, you are missing out. There is greater depth of intimacy and connection possible and it can make a powerful, positive difference in your life. One way to change this habit is to drop the goal of orgasm entirely and instead be present with body sensations as they arise. Let's call on rose to help us with this. Remember that first exploration with the rose petal way back in the Introduction when I invited you to brush a rose petal across your lips? Well, rose petals brushed across nipples or over pussy lips or penis heads also feel exquisite. Set up a lovemaking session just to feel those sensations. Agree in advance that the session will not lead to intercourse.

Play with holding space for each other's pleasure. How can you help each other feel safe enough to fully open to your desires? Remember that pleasure map we made of our bodies in Chapter 3? What were the strokes that helped your partner relax and open? As we help each other feel safe and give ourselves and our lovers permission to explore our desires with open curiosity, we begin to unlock our true potential for intimate, pleasurable connection.

Perhaps during one lovemaking session, your partner will focus completely on you and your pleasure, allowing you to fully surrender into your sensations. Perhaps you will feel inspired to offer the same to them. You can also trade sessions where the person receiving gets to ask for whatever they want. These trades are exquisite lovemaking sessions in and of themselves and they can also help us learn about ourselves and each other. This learning can then be brought into a dance of lovemaking. In a single session, we can take turns creating space for our own and our partner's pleasure. We can ask for what we want and encourage our partner to give us feedback about their desires. We can give exquisite sensation and surrender to it. We can even both completely surrender to the pleasure we are mutually creating and experiencing.

We can consciously set ourselves up for experiences like this. At one point during our study, Lisa and her husband were traveling to Seattle to see a show. Knowing they would have a night in a hotel together, Lisa packed her sexy lingerie as well as a bottle of rose massage oil, schisandra berry honey, and some rose syrup. Before the show, she set these items on the bedside table and put on her lingerie under her dress, building the anticipation for the night to come. When they returned to the hotel room, they took turns licking the schisandra honey from each other's fingers, licking rose syrup from each other's bodies, and massaging each other with the oil. It was a night of reveling in delicious sensation and their connection with one another.

Having a backpack packed with supplies for comfortable outdoor sex (a cozy, soft blanket, some massage oil, some Damiana Chocolate Love Liqueur . . .) is another example of setting yourself up for these kinds of experiences. This is so beautiful for summer lovemaking.

In the winter, you may want to call on ginger to keep your fire stoked. In the winter, Christina added dried ginger to her tea and other hot drinks and found she was less huddled against the cold and more bubbly and flirtatious. She described feeling warmed up in her sexual self in a whole and integrated way. Lisa and her husband shared a bath using ginger bath salts and it led to a hot, somewhat fierce, lovemaking session. "When we emerged from the bath, we could feel the heat from the ginger coursing through our bodies and fueling our desire for one another. Our kissing was passionate. My husband's cock felt amazing pounding hard and fast in my pussy."

Some Like It Hot

A stimulating bath salt blend.

INGREDIENTS

1 cup dead sea salt

¾ cup Epsom salts

¼ cup baking soda

¼ cup ginger powder

⅛ cup dried peppermint leaves

PREPARATION

1 Mix ingredients together.

2 Put 1 cup into a mesh bag and add the bag to the bath.

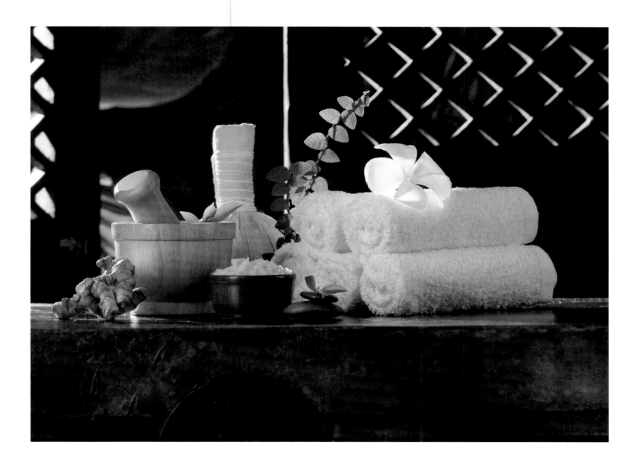

OTHER HERBS FOR KEEPING YOUR FIRE STOKED

Ashwagandha: Robert found this herb raised his overall energy level, helping him feel stronger and last longer during sex.

Cacao: James found that daily consumption of cacao led to him feeling more available, expansive, and aroused, and his sexual experiences "had a more connected and authentic feel . . . [and his] orgasms were more embodied, pleasurable . . . longer and more deeply fulfilling."

Schisandra berries: Rachel found that eating a few schisandra berries each day helped her feel stronger and more energetic, which led to her feeling more open to connection. Christina found the effects of schisandra berry consumption to be even more pronounced. She said, "despite having a month of being unexpectedly slammed at work, a few days around ovulation, I felt like I want sex NOW even though I also felt tired and exhausted. It was unexpected to have some energy for self-pleasure in the midst of living so much in my masculine and being tired from working so hard."

Fenugreek: Lisa found that the warming herbs in Warm Nights Chai (page 171) helped heat things up while also increasing her nipple sensitivity.

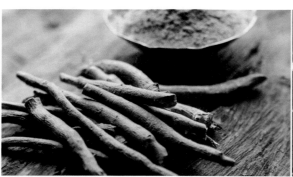

Ashwagandha

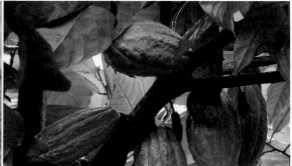

Cacao

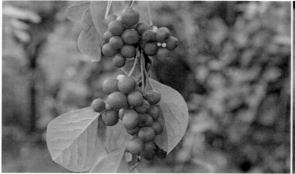

Schisandra berries

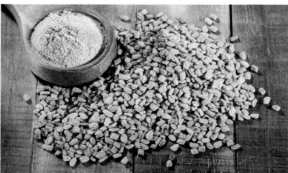

Fenugreek

Warm Nights Chai

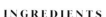

INGREDIENTS

1 heaping teaspoon fenugreek seeds

1 cinnamon stick

1 heaping teaspoon fresh
ginger, grated

¼ whole nutmeg, chopped

1 teaspoon cardamom
pods (crushed)

¼ teaspoon whole cloves

¼ teaspoon black peppercorns

2 whole star anise pods

1 teaspoon whole allspice

½ teaspoon whole fennel

½ teaspoon whole coriander

4 tongues (slices) astragalus, or 1
tablespoon cut and sifted astragalus

1 tablespoon dried burdock root

1 tablespoon dried dandelion root

Cream (or coconut milk), to taste

Honey, to taste

Rose water, to taste (optional)

PREPARATION

1 Combine all the herbs and spices in a saucepan with 4 cups
of water.

2 Bring the mixture to a boil, and reduce the heat to a simmer.

3 Allow it to simmer for at least 20 minutes.

4 Strain and pour the chai into cups. (Compost the herbs
and spices.)

5 Add cream (or Kava Coconut Creamer, page 154), honey,
and/or rose water to taste.

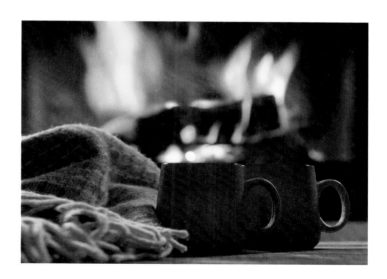

HERBAL TIPS

✦ This recipe is another example of a decoction—simmering harder plant material in water for a period of
time to extract constituents. I enjoy simmering this chai for even longer than 20 minutes, sometimes for
a full hour, and I often let the herbs rest in the water after it is done simmering for several hours before
finally straining it to drink.

EROTIC CONNECTION WITH NATURE

The herbs are here supporting us, and so is the natural world as a whole. Our sexual nature is our wild, animal nature. When we are turned on sexually, we are fully embodied, present in the moment and trusting our animal instincts. All of nature supports this aspect of ourselves, and being out in nature and in our sensual selves can be another beautiful way of stoking our fire.

Robert and Michelle found this to be true as they harvested rose petals together. . . . Come with them out to the Kah Tai Lagoon. The sun is shining and warm on their skin. The sky is blue, and the birds are singing. It's June and the world is vibrant with spring greenery around the water of the lagoon as they walk the dirt path to the rose bushes. Already their senses are piqued; now add the smell of the rose blossoms in the rising heat and the silky feel of the petals on their fingers. If you let yourself, you can be completely seduced by the beauty and sensuality of the natural world.

Joe and Cassie remembered being seduced by nature in this way on a trip to Ireland to visit a site with a ring of old growth hawthorn trees. Joe writes, "There we were, all alone with a grove of sacred hawthorn trees at early dawn. As the sun began to rise, we suddenly and unexpectedly felt the urge to make love underneath one of the beautiful trees. And so we did! Maybe it was because we were in Ireland, or maybe it was

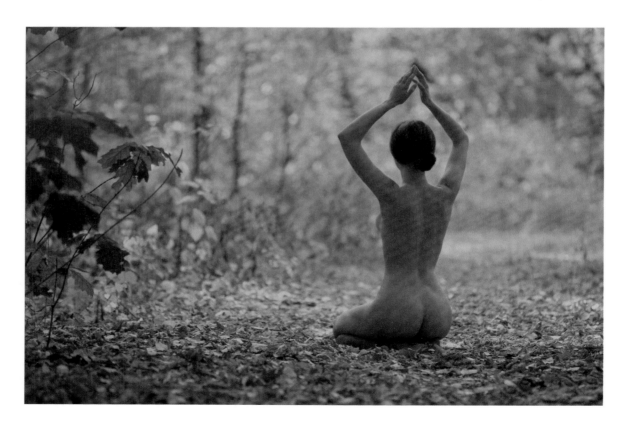

because we knew these trees were considered sacred by the locals, or maybe it was the genuine magic of these sacred hawthorn trees, but our experience making love in the misty dawn was unique in its pleasure and delight. We felt a sense of playful danger, like these old trees were watching. I imagined that they were cheering us on, as if they were relishing in the delight of our lovemaking as much as we were. I've never quite experienced a sense of magic like that before."

Excerpts from "Biosexual"

. . . a flower is really nothing more
than spread open botanical labia,
love-lips smiling at the world.
A flower is a sexual invitation
luring insect pollination . . .

. . . soft green moss
on the velvet loveseat of a fallen tree trunk
seduces my skin with the promise of sweet sensation.
Delicate blue and purple wild flowers entice me
like little fairy poems printed on flower vellum,
and in the center of each one,
five tiny secret hearts,
like a cluster of elfin candy valentines
within the flower vulva,
protected by the luscious flower lips . . .

Dona Nieto (La Tigresa)
from *Naked Sacred Earth Poems*

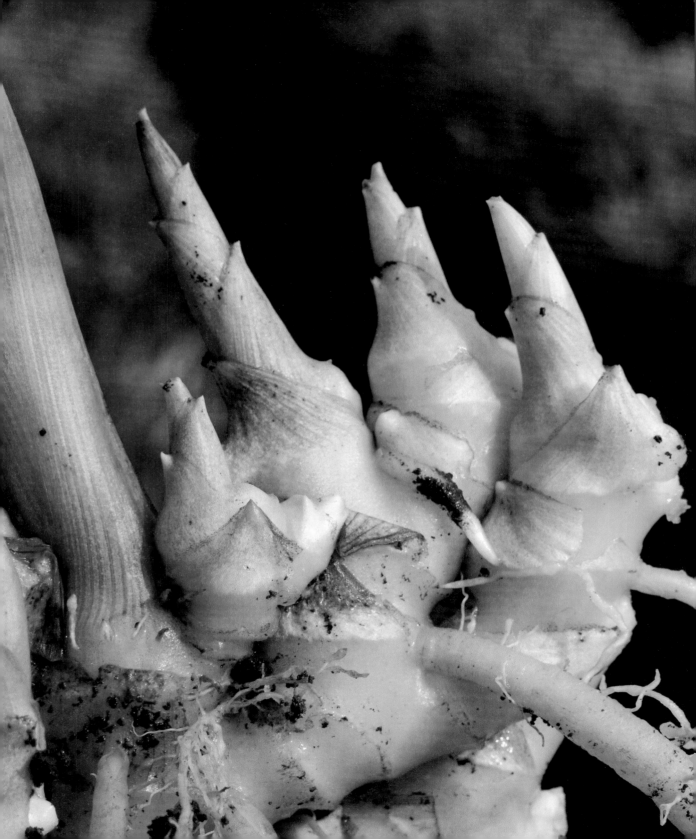

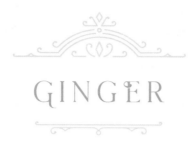

GINGER

Zingiber officinale

Mmmmm. Can you smell it? I've got ginger tea simmering on the stove. Just the smell warms me up. I keep a ginger chai brewing on the stove all winter long. Ginger is a wonderful aphrodisiac ally during the cooler months. It can help generate internal body heat that allows us to relax and open even as the snow falls outside. Drinking my tea, I feel a fire glowing in my belly and energy coursing through my veins. When I'm warmed up like this, I feel open and ready for intimacy!

As it warms us, ginger can stimulate our ambition, our personal power, and our sexual centers.

How Does Ginger Work in Our Bodies?

Ginger works as a circulatory system tonic. It dilates our blood vessels and increases circulation.[1] This increased circulation is what warms our bodies. Shogaols, one of several types of polyphenols in ginger, have been shown to protect and regulate the cardiovascular system and decrease blood pressure.[2]

Ginger helps to remove atherosclerotic plaque from blood vessels throughout the body,[3] which in turn brings more blood flow and energy to the pelvic region and invigorates our reproductive system. Rosemary Gladstar names it as a primary herb for the reproductive system.[4] As regular use helps remove plaque from penile blood vessels, ginger can help treat low libido and low sperm quality and motility.[5] Ginger may also improve female fertility.[6]

Ginger is also a wonderful remedy for painful menstrual cramping and delayed menstruation as it can help release blockages in the pelvic region and get the blood flowing.[7] It is also a helpful remedy to reduce heavy menstrual bleeding.[8] Ginger is a common and well-studied remedy for nausea and morning sickness.[9]

Ginger has broad anti-inflammatory and antioxidant effects that help to prevent and treat the degenerative diseases of aging, such as dementia, metabolic syndrome, and cardiovascular disease.[10]

Ginger is a very effective anti-inflammatory for the brain and helps us form new neurological connections.[11] These new connections may open us up to deeper connection to ourselves, our desires, and our partners.

A Bit about Ginger Plants

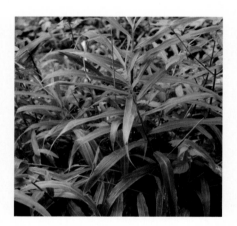

The ginger root we buy at the store is actually a rhizome, technically a part of the plant stem that grows horizontally just underground. Culinary ginger plants grow two to four feet tall and have long narrow leaves, and the flowers are cream or yellowish with purple lips that grow in a conelike formation. There are also ornamental varieties (1,300 different species) of ginger with much showier flowers. Ginger has a long record of use in Southeast Asia and grows best where it is hot and humid and the soil is rich with nutrients.

Herbal Shorthand

APHRODISIAC ACTIONS: *aromatic, cardiotonic, circulatory stimulant*

OTHER ACTIONS: *analgesic, anti-inflammatory, antimicrobial, antioxidant, antispasmodic, carminative, diffusive, stimulating diaphoretic, rubefacient (skin irritant), stimulating expectorant, vermifuge (destroys parasitic worms)*

ENERGETICS: *warming, drying*   TASTES: *pungent*

NOTABLE APHRODISIAC CONSTITUENTS: *many powerful polyphenols including gingerols and shogaols, volatile oil*

DOSAGE SUGGESTIONS: *Ginger is a strong herb, so you need only use a small amount to notice its effects (e.g., about 1 tablespoon grated ginger to flavor a dish for four).*

SPECIAL CONSIDERATIONS: *Ginger is very warming and drying, so avoid large doses if you have acne or eczema.*

Discontinue use if you get heartburn.

It is important to consult your doctor about your use of ginger if you are taking blood-thinning medication.

How to Use Ginger

PARTS USED: *rhizome*

Ginger is a wonderful herb to include in your cooking—adding it to everything from stir-fries to soups to certain baked goods.

Ginger tea is a warming treat, and it is also a primary ingredient in chai blends and is wonderful in other tea blends as well. Because of the ways it works with our circulatory system, it helps deliver the benefits of other tea herbs through our bodies. You will get the most benefit from ginger tea by preparing it as a decoction—simmering it for 20 minutes—rather than simply steeping it in hot water.

Ginger honey and syrup are delicious, warming treats.

Powdered ginger can be added to a foot bath to warm up our feet or mixed with salts for a warming bath salt blend.

Ginger can also be infused in oils to be used for a warming massage.

Participant Experiences

We experimented with ginger in the winter and really appreciated its warming and enlivening qualities, which kept us more relaxed and open during this cold time of year. Christina noticed it helped create a "warm, steady hearth fire of erotic energy rather than a burst of heat that quickly burns out." Both Christina and Artemis reflected a sense of heightened personal power, increased ambition, and willingness to take action. Ginger can get too hot. Sarah was just starting a new relationship and found the heat of ginger to be too much when combined with the new-relationship heat. Artemis is also in a time where her sexual energy is high, and she described ginger as "ridiculously warming." Christina also noted the need to moderate her intake and balance it with more cooling herbs.

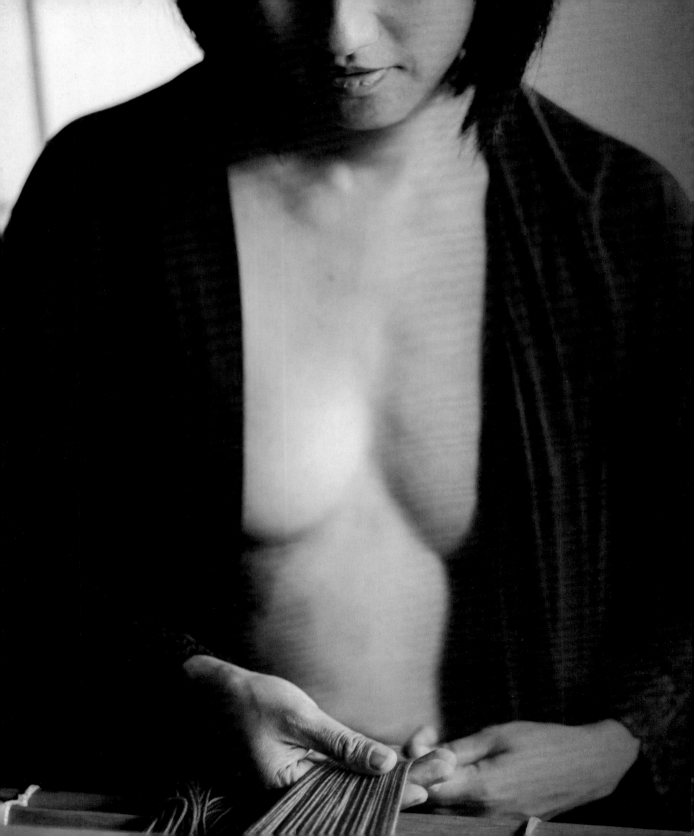

SEVEN

CHANNELING EROTIC ENERGY

INTO

VITALITY

AND

CREATIVITY

Sometimes the first thing I do when I wake up in the morning is say the "Total Permission" poem (from Chapter 3) to myself as I run my hands over my body. This is a beautiful way of bringing myself out of dream space and into my body; gently waking my arms, my legs, my hands and feet, my belly, breasts, and vulva and to bathe in self-love. "I give myself total permission . . . to listen to my desires . . . to turn myself on, to bathe in love . . . I say yes to sensuality . . . to my soul's purpose . . . to sexuality . . . I say yes to life!" Waking myself up in this way begins to fuel that flow of erotic energy from the very beginning of my day.

I love how, in this poem, Sitka puts saying yes to her soul's purpose right between saying yes to sensuality and sexuality. In my mind, that is right where it belongs because sensuality and sexuality provide that flow of erotic source energy that can fuel your life's work, your soul's purpose, your creativity.

In the opening essay of her book *Ecosexuality*, Lindsay Hagamen refers to erotic energy as a "renewable resource that energizes our communities." I love that! I love the idea of love and eros replacing fear and greed as the primary energy behind our actions.

In her book *Vagina*, Naomi Wolf explains that "the healthy, sexually well-treated vagina in a society that respects women can . . . deliver a strong activation of dopamine to the female reward system as well as surges of oxytocin for connection, and opioids/endorphins that drive the sensations of joy. So the vagina delivers to women the feelings that lead them to want to create, explore, communicate, and transcend." This idea is born out in her research of the lives of women artists and revolutionaries as "luxuriant stretches of creative and intellectual expansion in their work" are linked to "a particularly liberating sexual relationship or affair." Her book does a brilliant job of explaining the link between healthy sexuality and creativity for women, and Mantak Chia's work highlights this truth for men as well. In a video talk, he said when he channels his orgasmic energy, instead of ejaculating, he has so much energy he can't sleep. So instead he writes books. He's written 40 books!

Each of us has so much to offer. Each of us has a set of unique gifts and talents that we bring to this world. We live in a time when we are facing incredible challenges. A global pandemic is reshaping our lives, social justice issues are becoming even more illuminated, and climate change is threatening our very existence. It is becoming increasingly clear that we need to get really creative if we are going to be able to survive as a species and even more creative if we want to truly realize the full potential for health and vibrancy that is possible on this beautiful earth. In working through Julia Cameron's *The Artist's Way*, I began to realize that my creativity is a precious resource. This is true for every one of us. Cultivating our gifts and our creativity and being conscious of how we choose to express and direct them is, in my mind, an important and essential responsibility of being human on this earth in this time.

Through some personal growth work with my friend Tanya Brakeman's Revel program, I defined my purpose on this earth as this: "I am a promise that humans will come into healthy, ecstatic relationship with ourselves, each other, this beautiful earth, and all of life." This is what drives me to create, and it is a touchpoint that I come back to when I am choosing how to dedicate my creative energy. It is the primary motivating force behind this book, my work at LearningHerbs, and each interaction I have with people. Have you defined your own life's purpose? There is an opportunity to do so on the next page.

One of my favorite ways of expressing my purpose is through my writing. I love playing with words, finding ways to express my ideas and share what I've learned. For me, writing is pure joy, and still it requires energy, dedication, and time. As I've gained comfort with erotic energy being present in my body, I've found it easily and naturally translates into creativity. The tricks to being able to channel erotic energy into your work are learning to consciously create an erotic flow of energy in your life and gaining comfort with its presence in your body when you don't release it through orgasm. Not only can this bring creative juice to your own work, it can amplify the energy of love and eros as an energizing force in our communities and the world at large.

Defining Your Life Purpose

1 Take a few deep breaths and bring yourself into a sensual, embodied place.

2 Read this quote from Tanya, creator of Revel, about the process and value of identifying your life's purpose:

> *In creating my life's purpose, the aim by which I hold myself true, I am inviting my own sense of loving authority to align my energies from intrinsic inspiration. A sense of life purpose isn't about the prize at the end of the journey. By articulating my life's purpose as a principles- and values-based aim, a clear statement of my purpose, I have found the rewards in my everyday movements. As I engage in projects large or small, the rewards are in becoming aware of and accepting my own humanity as I struggle to discipline my own life force, an erotic and naturally self-interested venture, and that I can greet the selfless and selfish parts of myself with equal respect. That I can take my messy and unformed arousals and be formed by my natural self-discipline, letting that devoted discipline organize my passions and energies to serve a bigger purpose than simply my passing whims.*
>
> *Having an aim, a spelled-out life's purpose, gives me the opportunity to experience my human arousal, embrace the discipline of honest connection, and turn my egoic self over to my purpose, in service and surrender.*

3 Take a few deep breaths down into your belly, letting her words settle into your body.

4 Ask yourself, "What do I love to do? What lights me up? What is it I will stand for, no matter what others think of me, no matter how impossible it seems?" Let answers emerge into your conscious mind. This is less about creating a life purpose for yourself and more about identifying the life purpose that already underlies all you do.

5 Take time in your particular style (e.g., writing, speaking, dancing, etc.) to bring expression to the ideas about your own life purpose that rise up within you.

Don't worry if a clear purpose does not emerge the first time you engage with this exercise. More ideas will likely surface in the days and weeks ahead. Come back to this exercise regularly for a while until something settles out for you.

You may also be in a time in your life when you are so busy making ends meet that thinking in this big-picture sort of way just doesn't resonate. Give yourself permission to come back to this exercise (or any other exercise in this book) when you feel resonance with it.

Becoming clear about your purpose can help center you and create motivation and vibrancy in your life. If you are struggling to articulate your purpose and want to dive more deeply into this idea, I suggest looking into a program like Tanya's that can take you more deeply into this kind of personal exploration.

KEEPING A SLOW SIMMER OF EROTIC ENERGY ALL DAY

Beginning your day with the "Total Permission" poem or some other simple self-loving ritual can ignite your erotic energy, and with some creativity, you can keep that energy simmering all day, so that it can fuel whatever you are up to in your life. When you choose your outfit for the day, choose something that makes you feel beautiful or handsome or sexy. More and more, my wardrobe is becoming comfortable, beautifully feminine, form-fitting dance clothes. I love how dressing this way leads me to feel joyful and confident and happy. If you really want to up the erotic energy, try wearing loose pants or a skirt and going without underwear for a day. You will be in touch with your genital region all day long.

As you continue with your day, remember to weave in pleasure. Have you set yourself up with spaces in your house and yard that encourage love and eros to flourish? Take time to enjoy

them. What about those simple rituals you created for yourself back in Chapter 1? Remember to slow down, bring your full attention to what you are doing, and take time to notice and revel in sensation. When you get in the shower, take a moment to really notice the delicious feel of the water on your skin. Notice the feeling of the water soaking your hair and running down over your shoulders and back. Enjoy the slippery feel of the soap bubbles on your skin, the shampoo in your hair. Appreciate being wrapped in warmth by the water.

In addition to being present and reveling in physical sensations, anticipation can be a wonderful tool for keeping the erotic energy simmering. If you've set aside time for sex with your partner, especially if you are going to try something new together, the anticipation can be an aphrodisiac, keeping a stirring of erotic energy alive to be tapped into any time during the day. Anticipating an upcoming date can work in a similar way. You can also build erotic anticipation by setting up time in your week or month for partner dancing or signing yourself up for a cuddle party or a tantra workshop. Imagine what it will feel like in your body to be interacting in a sensual or sexual way. Allow the excitement to build as the anticipated event grows nearer, feeling the flutter of your heart that means you are alive and stretching and risking, the tingle in your genitals, perhaps the damp, slippery juiciness of your pussy or the energetic surges in your pelvic floor. Noticing and enjoying these kinds of body sensations in the present moment is what creates the erotic simmer.

When the anticipated event arrives, allow yourself to fully revel in the pleasurable sensations. In the days and weeks afterward, allow yourself to replay the pleasurable events in your mind now and then, feeling again the excitement of the moments spent in pleasure. Notice and enjoy the body sensations that arise. In this way, the memories become another avenue to continue the simmering of erotic energy in your life. Put another pleasure date on your calendar so you can begin anticipating again.

As you walk through the world anticipating and remembering your pleasure, allow your joy to bubble over. Smile at people you pass on the street. Give compliments freely. Notice opportunities to do random acts of kindness. Buy a bouquet of flowers for the young, harried mom trying to shop while juggling two children. Feel your own beauty, and perhaps even allow yourself to flirt some. Regena Thomashauer describes flirtation as "enthusiastic self-love . . . overflowing to others." It is a source of empowerment that "leaves the giver refreshed and the receiver

OPPORTUNITY FOR CULTIVATING EROTIC ENERGY FLOW
Designing Personal Simple Rituals

1   Brew yourself some of that chai or another cup of tea, and find a cozy place to sit and contemplate.

2   Look back at your list of sensual delights from Chapter 1, and brainstorm some simple rituals that you can add to your life on a regular basis or some experiences you want to set up for yourself that will start to build a level of erotic anticipation.

3   Bring your own creative expression to your ideas, writing, drawing, or dancing them.

4   Pick one ritual or experience and take a step toward bringing it into reality right now, today.

Each step toward bringing more vibrancy, pleasure, and joy to your life will build upon the last, and before long, you will be filled to overflowing.

enhanced." Knowing your own beauty and seeing and recognizing the beauty in others lifts everyone up and contributes to the flow of erotic life energy.

Some of my other favorite ways of keeping this simmer going for myself include being naked outside, whether sitting in hot springs or hot tubs, skinny dipping in the ocean, or sunbathing. I love the way the natural world physically stimulates my senses and the tingling excitement of daring to go without clothes. Reading books about sexuality can also contribute to the erotic flow. From Regena Thomashauer's book *Pussy: A Reclamation*, I adopted her suggestion of frequent pussy gazing. I bought a special little hand mirror that I keep in my purse so I can sneak a peek now and then throughout the day. Another of my favorite ways of cultivating erotic life energy is the practice of kundalini yoga. This form of yoga involves lots of breath work and movement, meditation and chanting, all of which serve to enliven my life-force energy in profound ways.

And let's not forget to involve the herbs in our simmering rituals. Remember those herbal honeys we made in Chapter 1? Spread some rose or hawthorn berry honey on your toast in the morning, or even better, lick some off your finger now and then throughout the day. In our family, we love to have an airpot of chai on the counter throughout the fall and winter. The warming herbs can help increase your circulation, keeping your energy moving and helping you feel vibrant and open (see the Warm Nights Chai recipe, page 187). Plus, the delicious smells of the various chai herbs provide an opportunity to sink into pleasurable sensation and to have an aphrodisiac experience just by brewing the tea.

To wrap up this section, I want to share with you the artist's prayer that I wrote for myself as I was working through *The Artist's Way* book. I have it on my wall by my bed so I can read it when I go to sleep at night or wake in the morning. It is my way of reminding myself of this interweaving of spirituality, sensuality, and creativity that is at the center of my life.

Dear Goddess,
Fill me with your strength and beauty
So that my life is always
A true expression of the Divine Feminine.
Guide me to rich, deep, connected experiences
That leave me gasping in awe and wonder
As I delight in this sensual life
Drinking in body sensations
And fully feeling my emotions.
May my life be a
Creative gift to the universe.
May I weave beauty as I dance my truth
Living always
For the highest possible good.

GAINING COMFORT WITH EROTIC ENERGY IN YOUR BODY

Erotic energy is powerful energy and cultivating it can lead to feelings of longing for sexual connection with another. You may feel like the energy is too much for your body to hold and like you need to discharge it through sex. The first step to changing this patterned response is setting an intention to do so. (This can be as simple as, "I intend to channel my erotic energy into _____." Fill in the blank with your current creative project.)

Now, allow yourself to feel the energy in your body. Is it focused in your pelvis or somewhere else, or is it moving through your whole body? Just allow it to be, say yes to it and be curious about it. What does it feel like? Is there a tingling sensation? A feeling of pressure or fullness? A buzzing sensation? Notice how your acceptance and curiosity increases your ability to be with it and hold yourself while it is present within you. Speak your intention aloud or in your head to anchor it.

The herbs can help you to ground this energy so that it becomes a stable force that can fuel you throughout your day. Both maca and ashwagandha are particularly grounding herbs, so the AshwaMacaMocha Shake from Chapter 3 is wonderful to keep on hand for moments when you want to stabilize the erotic energy moving through you. If you are cultivating this flow in your life on a daily basis, this drink may become a daily tonic. During the month we were exper-imenting with maca, Cassie was working long, stressful hours and drinking a meal-replacement smoothie with maca as a main ingredient. Despite the long hours, she noticed she felt turned on and energetic. At the time, she was frustrated that she didn't have more time for intimate connection with Joe during the month, but in reflecting, she realized that the sexual energy was helpful in getting through the work she had to do. (Pssst . . . when she did find some time for intimate exploration, she also noticed heightened sensitivity and pleasure.)

A bath can be another way to stabilize and ground the energy. I find that immersing myself in warm water is centering. Creating a Mineral Soak by adding some salts and clay to the bath can enhance that effect.

Our breath is also a powerful tool to integrate into our practices. Breath can help move energy through our bodies and ground it as well. I am going to share a couple of breath work practices for you to try. Please know that working with the breath is also a way of clearing blocked energy in your body. If doing any of these practices creates an emotional response in your body and you find yourself crying or shaking or having some other physical response, please hold yourself tenderly, knowing that stuck energy is being released through the physical experience. Healing is happening. As the energy is released, the physical sensations will pass. You may feel tired after the release. I recommend doing something that feels nourishing for yourself like a warm bath, a nap, or a walk in the woods. Each release will ultimately lead to feelings of greater freedom, ease, and clarity in your life.

Mineral Soak

INGREDIENTS

1 cup Epsom salts

1 cup magnesium flakes

½ cup French green clay

¼ cup baking soda

PREPARATION

1 Measure ingredients directly into the bath. (Mixing and storing does not work for this blend.)

2 Relax into your bath, and enjoy your soak.

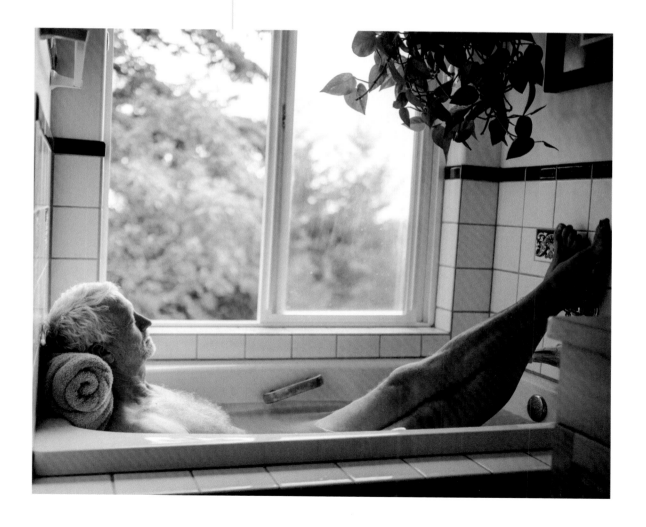

BREATH PRACTICE #1

Jamie Renee Lashbrook, a friend and breathwork practitioner, says:

"When we engage in the breath with intention, we are accessing the inherent erotic energy that is constantly birthing life all around us. Love is literally in the air. This ambrosia mixes with the oxygen in our blood and can reach into all of the places that forgot how to receive pleasure. Breath is life. Life blossoms from the erotic."

She offers this practice:

You can take a seated or lying-down posture. Place one hand on your pelvic bowl and one hand on your heart. Begin breathing in for a long count of four through your mouth. Visualize this ambrosia rising from the earth through your pelvis up your spine to your crown. Hold for a count of two. Exhale through the mouth, bringing that ambrosia down your front body for another count of four. Let it circle around your breasts, spiral around your navel, and back through your pelvic bowl. You are creating a circle of pleasure around you from earth to sky and back. Do this for 10 to 20 minutes. Breathing through the mouth—can you taste the life in each breath?

You can quicken this cycle by reducing the count to two and eliminating any pause between the inhale and exhale. This will accelerate your response systems. Please tune in to the aforementioned body sensations that may indicate that an emotional release is occurring for you. If this happens, take time to allow the release to complete itself and be sure to find a way to nourish and nurture yourself afterwards.

Complete this practice with three audible exhales while envisioning roots growing down from your base into the earth beneath you. Sit in stillness for a moment, envisioning the fruition of your creative work or asking how this energy wants to be channeled if you do not have a particular project in mind.

BREATH PRACTICE #2

1 Find a comfortable place to lie down.

2 Settle in, and bring your attention to your breathing.

3 Begin to breathe in through your nose and out through your mouth.

4 Increase the force and speed of your breathing, making your exhale audible.

5 Keep the inhale and exhale roughly the same duration.

6 Notice how this breathing builds and expands the energy within you. You can vary the force and speed to move and build the energy as you like.

7 Breathe this way for at least 10 cycles.

8 When you feel ready, raise your head and feet off the floor and clench all the muscles in your body as tightly as you can.

9 Hold for 20 seconds and then release, allowing your head and feet to rest again on the floor, and feeling the energy circulate and settle in your body.

10 Lie still, envisioning the fruition of your creative work or asking how this energy wants to be channeled if you do not have a particular project in mind.

BREATH PRACTICE #3

If you would like to add movement to your breathing practice, try this exercise:

Begin standing up, and breathe deeply in and out. As you do so, begin to bend and then straighten your knees, creating a gentle up and down bouncing through your body. Allow your arms, hands, and head to move freely as you do, and if sound wants to emerge through your mouth, allow that as well. Continue bouncing and shaking in this way for a full minute or two.

Find a comfortable seated position in a chair or perhaps cross-legged on a pillow or meditation cushion. It is helpful for your spine to be straight. Feel the effects of the bouncing and sounding. I am always amazed at how still and calm I feel as I sit after this shaking. Notice how the erotic energy has been distributed through your whole body with the bouncing. You have charged your being and are poised to create. When you are ready, begin your creative work.

As you engage with your creative endeavor, a cup of this herbal tea blend can help the energy flow into your work.

Day Bright Tea

INGREDIENTS

1 tablespoon dried nettle leaves

1 ½ teaspoons dried ginkgo leaves

1 teaspoon dried peppermint leaves

½ teaspoon cinnamon chips

1 ½ teaspoons fresh grated ginger

PREPARATION

1 Mix the herbs together in a pint jar.

2 Fill the jar with boiling water, cover, and steep for at least 45 minutes.

3 Strain and enjoy. (Compost the herbs.)

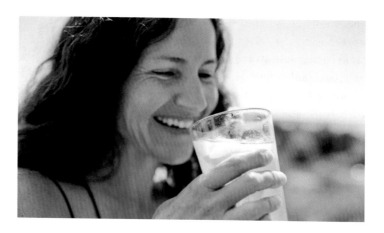

BUILDING CREATIVE ENERGY BY PLAYING WITH THE EDGE

As you increase your capacity to channel erotic energy through these kinds of practices, it will become exciting to play with building it so that you have more of it to draw on as fuel for all that you do in the world. We've explored many ways to cultivate sensual, turned-on energy in your life. Now, let's look at consciously building sexual energy for the purpose of channeling it. This kind of building can be done by playing with the edge of your peak excitement, either by yourself or with a partner. As you come to the edge of orgasm and then back off from it, sexual/creative energy begins to build. Each time you come close to orgasm without going over, more energy is created. Moving this energy throughout our bodies with our breath increases our vitality, and this energy can then be channeled into creative projects.

We started exploring the idea of building erotic energy back in Chapter 4 when we were exploring the possibilities of pampering increasing our capacity for pleasure. Let's go a little more deeply into it now. Get out your rose massage oil and your herbal lube and let's explore how we can build sexual energy in our bodies. Mapping our arousal onto a number scale of 1 to 10 can help us here. If you are practicing some of the ways to keep erotic energy in your daily life, perhaps you are operating most often at a 2 or 3 on this scale, feeling vibrant and resourced.

Erotic massage is a wonderful way to start practicing building sexual pleasure without "going over" and having an orgasm. We associate massage with relaxation and pleasure. Adding the erotic element adds the dimension of building sexual pleasure without the expectation of "going over" into orgasm. As you set up the space for the massage, you will find yourself moving up—maybe to a 3 or 4 on your pleasure scale. Put a beautiful spread on the bed or table and set that massage oil and lube nearby. Get out your favorite sex toy(s). Add some soft music and candlelight and some herbal incense or air freshener. Delight all of your senses.

You can massage yourself or your partner or allow yourself to receive a massage from your partner. If offering partner massage, I like to begin with my partner on his belly so I can oil up his back, gently starting to wake up and stimulate his whole body. Using long, sensual strokes, rub the oil into his back, buttocks, and legs. Offer some focused massage to relieve muscle tension and heighten relaxation. You can also gently rock your partner's body side to side and offer some percussive massage to increase the flow of energy and wake the body up. Be in communication with your partner, asking what pressure feels just right. Keep your touch pleasurable, adding in some erotic elements. A little breath in the ear or blowing down the back, a slight pass of the hand down toward the genitals. Continue this sensual, teasing massage style when your partner rolls over. Give ample time to the legs and arms, belly and chest, occasionally brushing across the erogenous zones, the nipples, vulva, or cock.

Breast and nipple massage can really start to build the energy on your pleasure scale. Take your time here. Cup and hold the breasts or massage the area around your partner's nipples. Use gentle strokes, and maybe some nipple kisses. Sometimes nipple massage can send erotic energy right through your genitals as well. Are you up to a 5 or 6 now?

Bring your attention down to the genitals. You may want to switch to using your herbal lube at this point in the massage. There are some strokes that can be used to wake up the genital area, bringing energy there, like gentle pressure on the mons pubis just above the vulva, under the pubic hair, or a gentle squeezing of the outer labia toward one another. Move your hands up and down the outer labia, awakening the whole vulvar area. For men, gentle squeezing up and down the whole shaft of the penis can serve this purpose as well.

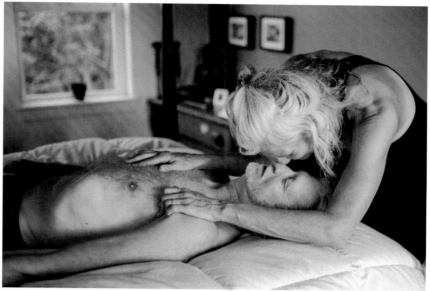

Other strokes are perfect for really building sexual energy, like circular strokes around the clitoris or a gentle rubbing of the clitoris itself. One of my favorite strokes for building sexual energy in a man is to wrap my hands around his cock with my thumbs in front so that they are stimulating that particularly sensitive spot near the tip of his cock. Using plenty of lube, move your hands up and down the shaft. Play with raising the sexual energy to an 8 or 9 on your scale, and then change to slower strokes or just gentle holding. Use your breathing to circulate the energy in your body. Massage strokes down the legs or up toward the belly can also help to distribute the energy. After a few minutes, transition back to strokes that build the sexual energy again. You can take yourselves to higher and higher levels of pleasure this way. Edge play like this can be easier if you start in the self-pleasure realm because you can really feel when you are near the going over point and know when to switch to calming strokes. With partner massage, this takes being really tuned in to each other or really clear communication.

Building your vocabulary of massage strokes can help you to expand this practice. There are classes and workshops offered to help you learn and also some wonderful classic videos available on the subject. *Fire in the Valley: Female Genital Massage* with Annie Sprinkle and *Fire on the Mountain: Male Genital Massage* with Joseph Kramer, Ph.D., are excellent, classic resources that offer many ideas for strokes with clear video instructions for performing them. As you practice them, you will be able to call up different strokes at different times in your lovemaking or self-pleasuring.

You may set out to build sexual energy to channel into projects through erotic massage, or you may choose during a lovemaking session not to "go over" into orgasm, but rather to breathe the energy through your body and ground it so it will be available to you as source energy. Practice and playfulness are the keys here. Enjoying the exploration, whether you end up in orgasm or not. Just swimming in the pleasure and loving yourself and your partner is source energy.

CHANNELING FULFILLED SEXUAL ENERGY

Periods of time when we are in particularly sexually fulfilling relationships can be exceptionally creative times as well. This is borne out by Naomi Wolf's observation about heightened creativity being linked to periods of sexual fulfillment for women artists and revolutionaries throughout the course of history. In our Aphrodisiac Circle, Michelle, who was in a particularly expansive time in regard to her sexuality, wrote about channeling erotic energy into her Soul Motion dance apprenticeship and series. She is in a fulfilling sexual relationship with her partner and also has a very fulfilling self-pleasuring practice, which she says is "an amazing generator of erotic energy and self-confidence . . . especially if I do it at a time when I am feeling the need for sensual, erotic energy and a partner may not be physically or emotionally available." She finds that this practice leads to her dance project being "a reflection of 'me' and my unique experience in the world—as a woman, biologist, naturalist, adventurer, and dancer."

Several men I have spoken with have shared with me the value of learning to separate their orgasm from ejaculation when wanting to channel their erotic energy. Ejaculation can leave men feeling exhausted rather than energized, but orgasming without ejaculation is what left Mantak Chia with the energy to write all those books. His books *Taoist Secrets of Love: Cultivating Male Sexual Energy* and *The Multi-Orgasmic Man* are great resources for learning to do this while still feeling sexually fulfilled. Robert, from the Aphrodisiac Circle, has had good success with this practice and said that the orgasmic sensation is different without ejaculation, and in his opinion it is better. It's not as intense and extends for a longer period of time. It allows men to have multiple orgasms within the same lovemaking session and also to generate creative energy for their work.

Though none of the men I have spoken with thought of turning to herbs as allies when they were learning these skills, both Robert and herbalist jim mcdonald have voiced agreement for my intuition that ashwagandha could be really helpful. As an adaptogen, it can help support in times of change. It also helps with strength and stamina, which are helpful in the learning process. Finally, jim observes that it can help with presence, which he finds is key. He also noted that kava can be helpful in supporting presence, so these two herbs could be helpful to experiment with as you engage in this learning.

For people of any gender, new-relationship energy or venturing into new territory sexually can be particularly energizing. Lisa has noticed that starting new relationships with her polyamorous partners leads to surges of self-confidence and creativity that gets channeled into her work.

Interacting with a new person leads to new insights and new ways of looking at the world. Trying something new sexually, like anytime we shake up our routines and risk doing things differently, leads to expanded neural networks and hence, new and creative ideas. When fresh insights and exciting explorations become part of our lives, it is natural that we experience creative energy and expansion.

Fulfilled sexuality also leads to production of neurotransmitters and hormones in our bodies that increase our creative potential. In her book *Vagina*, Naomi Wolf explains that dopamine, serotonin, oxytocin, phenylethylamine, and over 20 different endorphins are released in the body in association with sexual pleasure and orgasm. These chemicals are responsible for generating feelings of bliss, confidence, contentment, passion, attention, and focus. These feelings provide a beautiful foundation for creative expression and the confidence necessary to put your ideas out into the world.

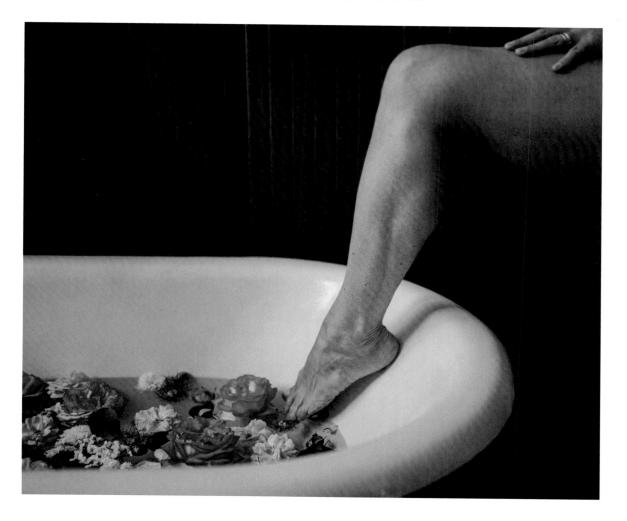

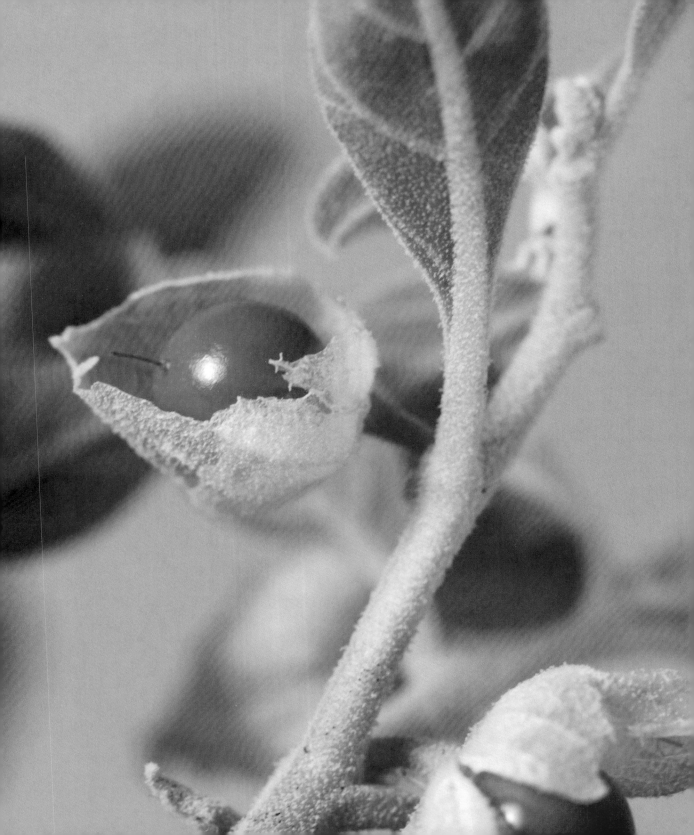

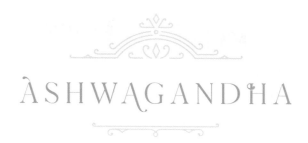

ÀSHWAGANDHA

Withania somnifera

Ashwagandha is a powerful root medicine that both energizes us and increases our stamina, heightening sexual interest and performance. This root is calming, grounding, and deeply rejuvenating. *Ashwagandha* is a Sanskrit word that loosely translates as "the smell of a horse," perhaps referring to the distinct smell of the root, but also alluding to its ability to bestow horse-like strength and endurance.

How Does Ashwagandha Work in Our Bodies?

Ashwagandha nourishes our whole body and promotes an overall sense of well-being. As an adaptogen, it regulates endocrine processes that help us handle stress more easily. It also enhances our immune system and promotes longevity.[1]

Rosemary Gladstar calls ashwagandha a "classic reproductive system tonic," explaining that it "helps restore sexual chi or energy."[2] By decreasing oxidative stress and regulating hormone levels, it can improve sperm count and semen quality for men.[3] For women, it can increase lubrication and improve orgasms.[4] Its blood-thinning properties can help with impotence.[5] It can also help relieve muscle pain and cloudy thinking associated with perimenopause.[6]

Ashwagandha is also a powerful herb for our nervous systems. It contains alkaloids and steroidal lactones known as withanolides that nourish and relax our nerves,[7] helping to relieve anxiety and nervous exhaustion. Triethylene glycol (TEG) is a component in ashwagandha that has been shown to induce sleep and enhance the quality of sleep.[8] Khalsa and

Tierra say that, in their experience, ashwagandha is particularly good at helping reestablish healthy sleep patterns in people with chronic sleep issues.[9]

Ashwagandha also affects our brain, heart, and circulatory system. It is neuroprotective and can increase the availability of dopamine in the brain.[10] One study showed the powerful ability of withanolides to reconstruct neural connections.[11] It also improves cardiovascular function, increasing the size of the heart and improving blood sugar fuel to the heart.[12] Finally, its ability to protect against pulmonary hypertension and relax our blood vessels helps promote an overall feeling of well-being.[13]

A Bit about Ashwagandha Plants

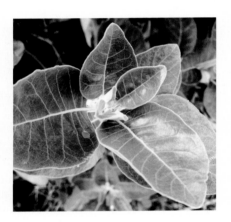

Ashwagandha is a tropical plant native to Africa, India, and Asia. This perennial shrub in the nightshade family actually thrives in arid conditions and in poor quality, alkaline soils. It grows to about three feet tall and produces small, yellow-green, star-shaped flowers and a berry that grows within a papery calyx. The stem and leaves are covered in silver-gray hairs. Though the leaves and berries are sometimes used, people mainly cultivate it for the roots.

Herbal Shorthand

APHRODISIAC ACTIONS: *cardioprotective, adaptogen, energizing, hormone balancing, nervine, neuroprotective, restorative, reproductive system tonic*

OTHER ACTIONS: *anti-inflammatory, antioxidant, antispasmodic, astringent, diuretic, immunomodulator*

ENERGETICS: *warming, moistening*   TASTES: *sweet, bitter*

NOTABLE APHRODISIAC CONSTITUENTS: *35 alkaloids, steroidal lactones (withanolides), amino acids, iron, triethylene glycol (TEG)*

DOSAGE SUGGESTIONS: *Ashwagandha is a tonic herb and so should be taken regularly, in medium dosages, for a specific period of time. A basic tonic dose is 3 to 6 grams of powdered root per day. For more acute situations, use a medicinal dose of up to 15 grams per day.*

SPECIAL CONSIDERATIONS: *Seek professional advice if you are pregnant.*

Do not take this with barbiturates.

People with nightshade sensitivities may not tolerate it.

Do not use this if you have an upper respiratory infection or lots of mucus congestion.

How to Use Ashwagandha

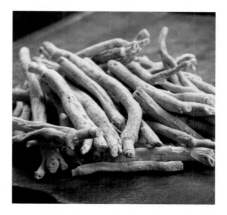

PARTS USED: *root*

USE POWDER IN: *AshwaMacaMocha Shake (page 64)*
*or **Dream Cream (page 234), Date Treats (page 236)** or*
other energy balls

Mix with honey and fruit concentrate and
spread on toast.

Tincture or capsules

Participant Experiences

As a group, we benefited from the deep nourishment offered by ashwagandha. Artemis found it to be calming, helping her to be less reactive to stimulus, fear, and anxiety. Christina was taking the tincture twice a day and found she slept better and felt more grounded. She had more energy for work and enjoyed the regular herbal support in her life. Robert had the strongest reaction of all of us. He noticed a marked energy boost and increased staying power during sex.

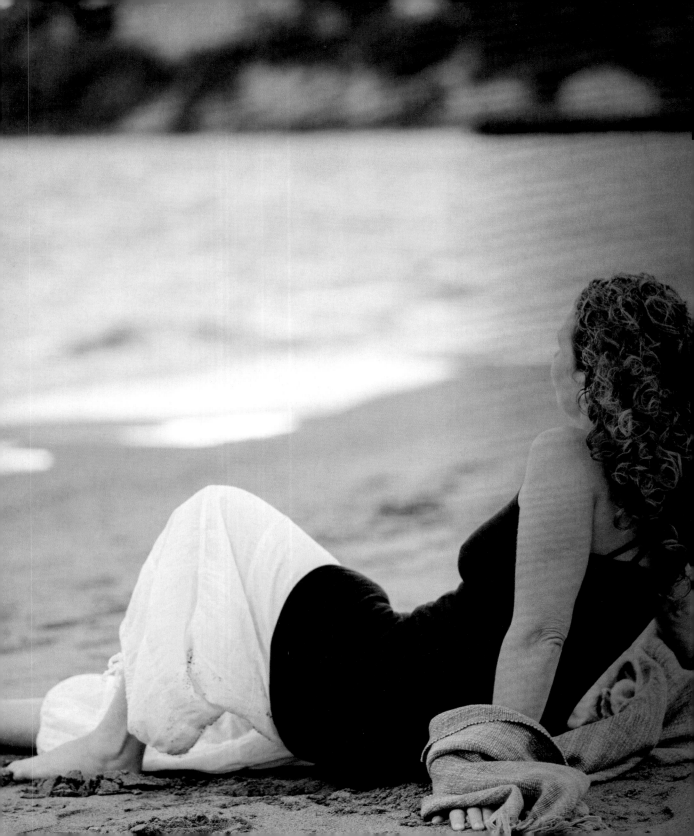

EIGHT

RELAXING

INTO

YOUR

BODY

Come with me down to the beach. Let's go to my favorite one. It's just five minutes from my house by car, but let's walk today. We can take our time, and I'll show you my favorite route, taking advantage of the little public trails that get us off the concrete and among the trees. We'll wind through the neighborhood.

Okay, just down this hill, and you'll be able to see the ocean. There. Beyond those houses. See the water? Just down this way to the bluff top. Look at that skyline. Snow-capped Mount Baker and the Cascades. You're lucky to be here on a clear day so you get this full beauty! Let's go all the way down onto the sand. There's a stairway just ahead. See? These hundred steps down the bluff are an opportunity to slow down. Let's descend slowly so we can really tune in and notice the feelings that arise as we transition from the busy world of everyday life to the quiet world of waves and sand.

Oh, let's take off our shoes so we can feel the sand on our bare feet! Doesn't the sun's warmth feel glorious on your skin? Let's sit over here with our backs against this driftwood log. This is where I come when I need to relax. The sound of the waves washing up on the shore, and the repetitive motion of them, calms my nerves in a way nothing else does.

This is a perfect place to practice our sensory meditation, dropping fully into the sensual experience of being right here, right now. Close your eyes. Feel the sand with your fingers, notice the feel of your body resting on the sand, the places where your back meets the log behind you. Listen to the gentle rhythm of the waves washing in and flowing out, washing in and flowing out. There's a seagull calling overhead, oh, and an eagle too. Breathe deeply of the fresh, salty sea air. Slowly open your eyes, take in the beauty of the ocean, the seabirds, the mountains. Feel how your body relaxes as you stay present and in your senses. This is just the way you want to feel as you make love. Relaxed, present, and tuned in to your sensual nature.

CULTIVATING RELAXATION

Most everyone I know is beyond busy right now in their lives. There always seem to be multiple things vying for our attention. We work long hours and juggle family obligations and social commitments. We have come to equate a busy lifestyle with success. We try to fit sex in between other obligations or at night at the end of a long day when we are beyond tired from all of our doing. Then we wonder why we don't have enthu-

siasm and energy for it. Cultivating relaxation can be a practice that improves our sex life while also transforming our whole life in positive ways.

Sitting outside in nature and practicing a sensory meditation like we just did at the beach is one beautiful way of cultivating relaxation in your life. This can be as simple as finding a small grassy area in a nearby park or sitting with your back against a tree. As natural beings, we are soothed by the sensations that arise as we spend time outside—rich, earthy smells or the scent of flowers, the sounds of birds, the feel of the sun's warmth or the caress of a breeze on your skin.

For a while, I was doing an independent nature studies course with Wilderness Awareness School and they had me go to the same place outside every day for a year. I sat with my back to a cottonwood tree right on the bank of Lake Washington. It was at a park within walking distance of my Seattle home. Years later, I can still easily call up the scent of the cottonwood buds, the sound of the wind in the tree's leaves, the sight of the coots and cormorants on the water. That spot held me through one of the most turbulent times in my life. It was a place where I felt safe and relaxed. Can you find such a place for yourself and visit every day or even once a week?

Our time spent gathering plants can serve in this way as well. Sarah shared about her experience collecting hawthorn flowers from a tree near her home. As she spent time with the tree, picking the abundant, delicate, white flowers, her body began to relax and become increasingly receptive to sensation.

If you do not have an inspiring natural area near your home, you can create a space in your home dedicated to natural beauty. Perhaps a small table or shelf near a window that you can

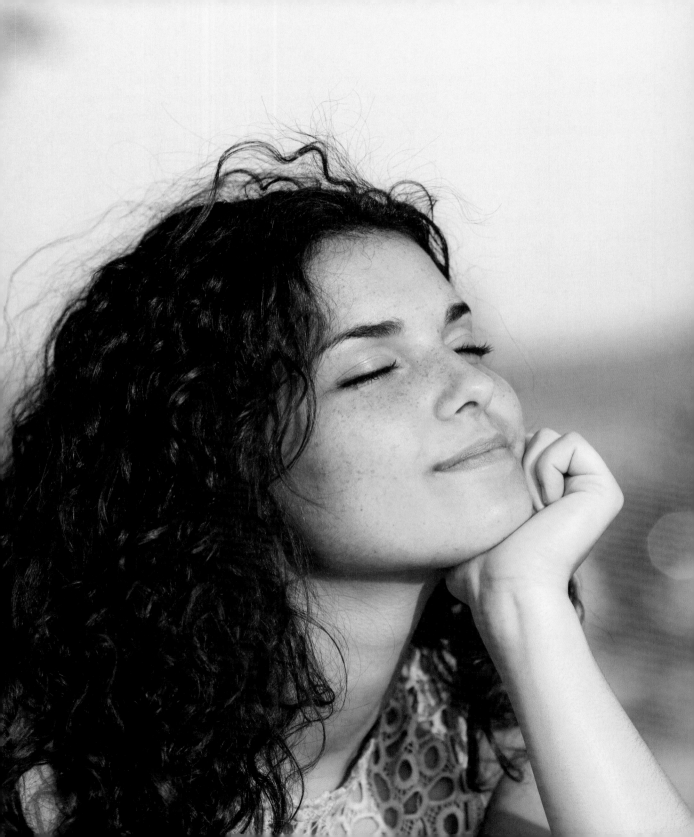

Soothe Tincture

INGREDIENTS

1 cup fresh milky oat tops

1 cup 100-proof vodka

PREPARATION

1 Put the oat tops in a ½-pint jar, loosely packed.

2 Pour vodka over the herbs to fill the jar.

3 Stir and cover. Make sure the alcohol fully covers the oat tops.

4 Let sit on your kitchen counter for 6 weeks, stirring daily for the first week.

5 Strain, reserving the liquid and composting the herbs.

6 Take by the dropperful.

HERBAL TIPS

✦ Tinctures are a great way to access the medicinal qualities of plants because alcohol will naturally extract the more medicinal plant constituents. 100-proof vodka is 50 percent alcohol and 50 percent water, which makes an excellent tincture.

✦ Other alcohols like brandy or tequila have a lower percentage of alcohol but can still be used to extract plant constituents. These are more often used when making tasty drinks like cordials, bitters, or liqueurs.

✦ Herbal tinctures are most potent when made with alcohol, but if you need to avoid alcohol, you can make a glycerin tincture or drink an oat top tea as a relaxing alternative.

✦ Milky oat tincture is one of my favorites for relaxation, but fresh milky oats may be hard to come by. You can also easily purchase a pre-prepared tincture. If you would like to practice making a tincture, but do not have access to oat tops, you can make a soothing tincture with 1 cup finely chopped tulsi leaves instead. Use the same method described for the Soothe Tincture. (If using dried tulsi leaves, use only ½ cup.)

✦ Making just a cup of tincture is a great idea when starting out. Small amounts are best. Then you can try the tincture and see how it works for you. If you love it, you can make a bigger batch next time. Over time, you will come to know which herbal preparations you use and want to make every year, and you can plan your harvesting accordingly.

open when the weather is nice. Place beautiful natural items here—leaves, flowers, rocks, shells, feathers—whatever inspires you. Sit with them daily. Take them in with your eyes, noticing the shapes, textures, and colors. Pick them up and feel the weight of them in your hands. Add to your collection as you find new things, and return some of the older ones back to nature for someone else to find and enjoy.

Make this time with nature cell phone free. Turn it completely off and leave it at home or in another room. We have become very tied to these devices and their continual alerts about incoming messages or news. It is impossible to fully relax and drop into your body with the continual distraction our phones provide. Consider turning yours off for a whole day. Or try just an hour or two. To cultivate relaxation, spend more time with your alerts silenced, without your phone, or with your phone completely off. Leave it behind and go for a walk, practice yoga or meditation, or go to the spa or get a massage.

Getting a massage or going to the spa are wonderful ways of cultivating relaxation in your life. So often we finish one big project only to start right away working on the next. What if you commit to treating yourself to a spa day or massage when you finish a project? Or better yet, what if, as you plan the project, you predict when the busiest, most intense period of work will be and schedule yourself for a massage in the midst of the push time? Setting up your schedule with relaxation as a priority can be truly life changing. You will likely find yourself getting through more work more efficiently and with less stress than ever before.

Making a practice of gratitude can also support this shift. It is perhaps one of the simplest and most effective ways of cultivating relaxation that I know. Any time you catch yourself feeling stressed or anxious, you can simply ask yourself what you are grateful for in that moment. Refocusing your mind on those things will instantly diffuse some of the tension. You can make a practice of speaking or writing your gratitudes from your day before you go to sleep at night or when you first wake up in the morning. I also love to write thank you notes to people for the wonderful things they do for me or how they enhance my life. As we put more and more of our attention on aspects of our lives that we are grateful for, those parts of our lives have a way of naturally expanding.

I often feel extreme gratitude for the herbs and their healing qualities in my life. Of course, herbs can help support our cultivation of relaxation as well. A milky oat tincture (Soothe Tincture, page 203) can be a beneficial ally in this regard. Oats are a nervous system tonic. They are both soothing and restorative. Taking a dropperful of milky oat tincture before your massage or time in nature can heighten the relaxation. Similarly, if you are wanting to engage sexually after a big day of work, taking a dropperful or two of milky oat tincture can do wonders to help you relax. Cassie uses this tincture as a quick remedy on hectic days to bring down stress in the moment and to soothe her jittery nerves before bed at the end of a long workday.

RELAXATION VERSUS NUMBING

Notice that my suggestions for cultivating relaxation did not include settling down in front of a movie, drinking alcohol, or taking drugs. These kinds of activities can be relaxing, but they can also be a form of numbing. If we truly want to live a vital, turned-on life, it is important to be aware of the difference between relaxation and numbing. Relaxation is about settling into your body and senses and resting there. Numbing is about distracting yourself from what you are thinking, feeling, or sensing—escaping your mind, body, and senses.

Drinking a glass of wine at the end of a long day can be relaxing. Continuing to drink, overindulging, is more likely numbing. Start to notice the difference in your own life. When you engage in an activity to relax, ask yourself if you feel more dropped into your body and senses or more distant from them. In my experience, numbing activities provide temporary relief, but ultimately leave me feeling worse. Relaxing activities, in contrast, can help relieve tension in a way that leads me to more freedom and ease. Over time, you may find yourself choosing activities that are relaxing more often than those that are numbing.

Life is not easy. Over the course of a lifetime, we face innumerable challenges. The death of loved ones, natural disasters, loss of a job or our whole livelihood, sickness, pain, or rejection. Each challenge comes with its own set of emotions, thoughts, and physical sensations—some of which feel completely unbearable. Part of the journey of life is bearing the seemingly unbearable. Occasional numbing may be part of what makes this possible, but when you choose numbing more and more often, you cut yourself off from the possibility of vital living and from life itself.

One of the most comforting gifts we can give each other during times of challenge is a hug, and cultivating a culture where everyone has easy access to comforting touch is vitally important to human survival. We can more easily bear difficult feelings and sensations if we know we are not alone. Touch helps us feel our connection to others on a body level, and a hug is simple, full-body touch.

Unfortunately, for many reasons, hugs and loving touch may be hard to come by. With COVID-19 running through the population, social distancing protocols have cut us all off from a multitude of opportunities for loving touch. After doing some deep work on racism with Holistic Resistance, I have come to understand that certain members of our society, especially Black men, are chronically under touched because of the racism in our culture. May this book serve as a prayer that we can find our way to changing this reality.

In the meantime, if you find yourself alone and experiencing difficult emotions, a warm bath or soft blanket can provide soothing sensations similar to a hug. Instead of numbing, try allowing yourself to be wrapped in comfort and warmth as you feel whatever it is you are feeling. When fully felt, emotions tend to dissipate rather quickly, and relaxing into a hug can help you move through challenges much more effectively than numbing and stuffing your emotions.

DROPPING INTO YOUR BODY

As we experience soothing and pleasurable sensations, we begin to enjoy inhabiting our bodies more and more. Unfortunately, many modern professions encourage us to be more in our heads than our bodies. This is true for some because they require mostly brainpower and very little physical movement. For others we need to wear fashionable outfits that are uncomfortable and thus encourage us to distance ourselves from our body sensations. Other jobs lead us to dissociate from our bodies because they require us to do heavy physical or repetitive work that causes us pain. We turn off access to our bodies in order to make it through our day.

Though writing this book requires lots of creative brain power, I have chosen to do my writing on my sheepskin rug in front of the fire in my feminine, comfortable, dance clothes. I take periodic stretch breaks and enjoy moments of just feeling the softness of this sheepskin and find I am aware of the warmth of the fire on my skin even as I write. Perhaps you can find ways to do your work that also allow you to remain connected to pleasurable body sensations. Maybe splurge on a soft, cashmere sweater to wear to work and delight in the feel of it against your skin all day. Or bring some Sweet Heart Tea to your desk. Sarah noticed her nervous system being calmed by this tea and the scent reminded her of being outside in spring with the bees.

There are also activities we can choose outside of work time that drop us into our bodies. My favorite of these is ecstatic dance. I love this form of dance because for me it is pure joy to just let the music move my body. I am not focused on leading or following as I am in partner dance, and since everyone in the room is actively in motion, I do not feel self-conscious about how I am moving. I simply let the music vibrate in my body and move in whatever way I am inspired to move in the moment. This can be a wonderful practice of being actively dropped into your body. In my town there is a morning ecstatic dance every

week. If this is not the case for you or if you feel self-conscious dancing with others, you can just turn on your favorite music in the privacy of your own living room, close your eyes, and allow the music to inspire movement.

I also love swimming in the cold ocean or in mountain lakes, any natural water, really. This brings me out of my mind and fully into my senses in a flash. What are your favorite ways of dropping down into your body?

MOVING THROUGH CHALLENGES OF BEING EMBODIED

I acknowledge that for some people, dropping into your body and being very aware of physical sensations can feel uncomfortable or downright scary. If we are used to numbing and stuffing our emotions, they can lodge in our bodies and manifest as sore muscles or sick stomachs. When we drop into our bodies we will likely feel these unpleasant sensations as well as pleasurable ones more acutely. Rather than avoiding these sensations, I encourage you to breathe into them, sense into what kind of movement might feel good to release the tension you feel. Take some time nourishing yourself with a massage or soak. Massage oil made with kava is fantastic for sore muscles (Sensations Massage Oil, page 224). Often we get angry or frustrated when our bodies are sore or in pain and just push through, continuing to do the activities that brought on the pain in the first place. Being compassionate with our bodies and offering some love and care will bring healing much faster.

Sweet Heart Tea

INGREDIENTS

2 tablespoons dried
hawthorn flowers

Honey, to taste

PREPARATION

1 Place the hawthorn flowers in a teacup.

2 Boil water and pour over the flowers to fill the cup.

3 Cover, and steep for 15 minutes.

4 Strain, composting the flowers.

5 Add honey to taste.

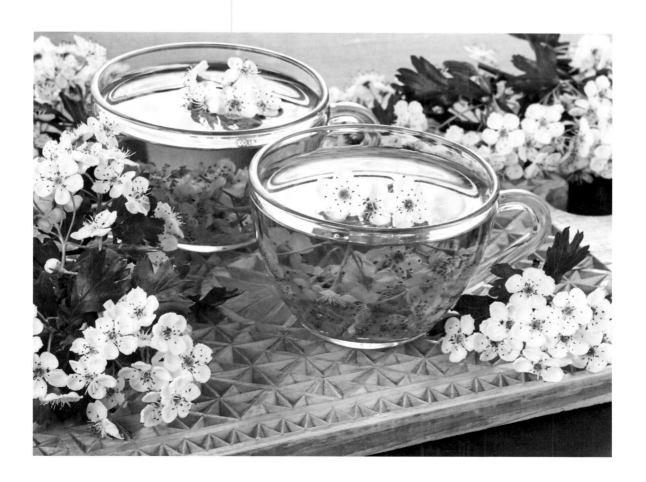

Sensations Massage Oil

Inspired by Rob Montgomery via jim mcdonald

INGREDIENTS

½ cup kava root powder

1 cup almond oil

Essential oils for scent (optional)

PREPARATION

1 Place kava root and almond oil in a pan or jar that fits inside your slow cooker without touching the sides. (I like to use the top pan of my double boiler.) Cover it with a lid.

2 Place a folded dish towel on the bottom of your slow cooker.

3 Place the pan with the oil on top of the towel so that it is not touching the sides or bottom of the slow cooker.

4 Put enough water in the slow cooker to reach ¼ way up the side of the pan.

5 Set the slow cooker to warm, and leave the lid off.

6 Allow the oil to infuse on warm for 5 days, stirring once or twice per day, and refilling water as needed.

7 Strain, reserving liquid and composting herbs.

8 Optional: Add essential oils for scent. I like 3 drops vetiver, 2 drops bergamot, and 1 drop ylang-ylang for this oil.

9 Store in a squeeze-top jar for easy use during massage.

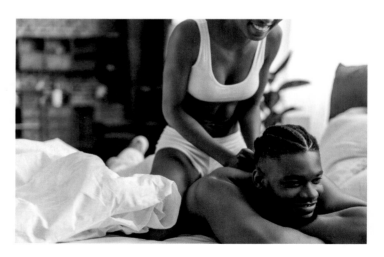

You might also try a practice of lying still and bringing your focus to one body part at a time, breathing slowly and deeply while encouraging that body part to relax. Begin at your toes and work your way up your body, relaxing your feet, ankles, shins, knees, thighs, pelvis, belly, chest, arms, hands and fingers, neck, and finally your head, paying special attention to your jaw or any area where you routinely store tension.

It is also possible you are storing trauma in some areas of your body. You may have trained yourself to dissociate from your body as a way of avoiding reexperiencing past traumatic experiences. Recognizing a pattern of dissociation can be the first step to healing from it. An increasing amount of work is being done in the arena of healing trauma, and I really suggest finding a professional to work with if you are dealing with sexual

OPPORTUNITY FOR CULTIVATING EROTIC ENERGY FLOW

Relaxing into Your Body

1 Find a comfortable position and take a few deep breaths. Use a sensory meditation or other technique to drop yourself into a sensual, embodied place.

2 Imagine yourself moving through a typical day. Are there certain activities that bring you more into your body? Others that distance you from your body?

3 Imagine yourself on a relaxing vacation. What are you doing that helps you to relax? Now, allow yourself to imagine a vacation for yourself that is focused on relaxing, sensual embodiment. What activities would you plan for yourself?

4 Write down (or dance or draw) the ideas that emerged for you.

5 Perhaps you already have activities in your day-to-day life that help you relax into your body. Consider if there are ways you can prioritize them even more.

6 Are there activities that emerged from your dream vacation that you might be able to bring into your daily life? Be creative as you consider this question. Perhaps you can't go to a spa for a sauna and massage on a daily basis, but you could spoil yourself with a warm, relaxing bath, followed by some Love Your Body Lotion.

7 Pick one activity to integrate this week. And one for next week. Allow yourself to make them a regular practice in your life. The more you begin to inhabit your body, the more you will find yourself craving these kinds of activities and the easier it will be to prioritize them.

abuse issues or are healing from other forms of trauma. While herbs can certainly be helpful in these situations, that level of healing is really beyond the scope of this book. If this is the case for you, herbs like hawthorn and oats and tulsi will be a good starting place for you, as will gentle exercises like the sense meditation and relaxing one body part at a time. Always listen to your own body, and choose what feels right to you. Move as slowly as you need to, letting yourself step into inhabiting your body more fully over time.

All of these practices for dropping down into your body can help increase your awareness of pleasurable sensations during sex. They can be helpful for transitioning from the pressures of a busy workday to time in the bedroom with your love. Taking time for a cup of Tender Titillation Tea (page 110) or a few sips of Kava Cordial (page 211) can be a lovely transition ritual, just like those hundred stairs down to the beach. Feel yourself dropping further into your body with each swallow.

GIFTS OF RELAXING INTO OUR BODIES

When we are fully relaxed into our sensual bodies, we are extremely present in the moment. There is no worry about the future or angst about the past. This is the place where full surrender is possible—full surrender into the pleasurable sensation of your lover's touch, into orgasm, love, and connection. These moments of complete surrender are, for me, moments of exquisite pleasure and belonging. It is in these moments that I feel a sense of oneness with the whole swirling

universe. There is serenity here. Peace. Freedom from fear and connection to vast possibility. When we go through life feeling sexually fulfilled, we are consistently in touch with these beautiful feelings and able to handle the stress of daily life with much more ease and grace.

Inhabiting our bodies more fully on a daily basis also gives us access to a trustworthy guidance system that can help us navigate our lives. When faced with a choice, we can breathe down into our bodies and notice what sensations arise as we consider our different options. A tight stomach or a feeling of butterflies there may be a warning to choose differently, as can an elevated heart rate or difficulty breathing. Conversely, a relaxing of tension in our muscles, an ease to our breathing, or a relaxed heart rate can let us know when we are on the right track. When faced with requests from others, it is good to check in with our body's guidance system as well to know if we truly want to answer with a yes or a no. Our brains are good at coming up with reasonable arguments both ways so we are left spinning in confusion and unable to choose. Our bodies often provide much clearer signals if we tune in to them and begin to trust what they are telling us.

Listening to and trusting our bodies can also lead to increased health. When we are present and dropped into our bodies, we will notice pleasurable sensation, but also at times, we may become aware of discomfort and pain. These sensations can be early warning signs that our health is at risk. When we are making choices that allow us to be dropped into our bodies throughout our daily lives, we can catch these early warning signs, get the rest or treatment we need, and avoid having them turn into larger health challenges.

Kava Cordial

INGREDIENTS

½ ounce dried, cut, and sifted kava root

¼ cup dried rose petals

1 tablespoon dried hibiscus flowers

4 cardamom pods, crushed

3 tablespoons honey

1 ½ cups pitted sweet cherries (or enough to fill jar)

Brandy to cover ingredients in pint jar

HERBAL TIPS

✦ Any time you are infusing herbs into liquid, make sure the liquid fully covers the herbs and other ingredients after you stir them. This will keep your preparation from growing mold. The ingredients may float more to the top for the first few days and then sink lower after a week of stirring.

✦ Kava drinks are best consumed with intention at a time when you are ready to drop into your erotic energy and certainly not just before getting in a car to drive. Kava can slow your reaction time too much for that.

PREPARATION

1 Place all the ingredients in a pint jar.

2 Pour the brandy over the herbs to fill the jar.

3 Stir and cover.

4 Let it sit on your kitchen counter for 2 to 4 weeks (to taste), stirring daily for the first week.

5 Strain, reserving the liquid. (Compost the herbs.)

6 Sip straight or add a splash of seltzer water.

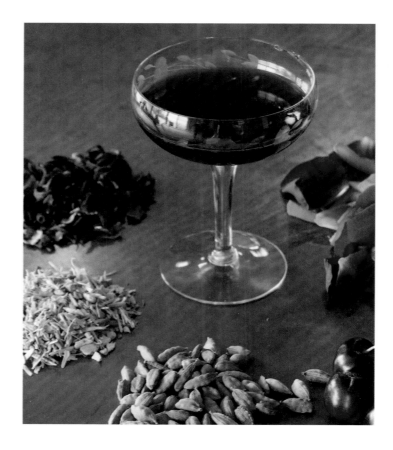

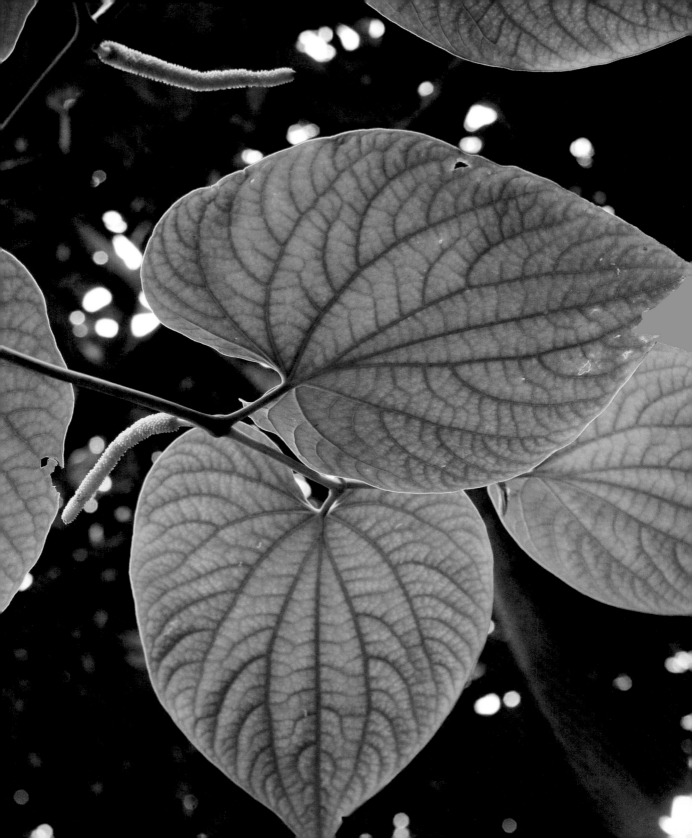

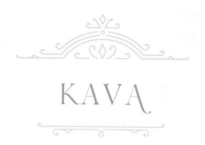

KAVA

Piper methysticum

Kava is a beautiful ally for sexual surrender. Taking it into our bodies is both deeply relaxing and can lead to feelings of euphoria. Approach kava with profound respect. It is a powerful plant ally to be enjoyed with intention and care. Take it into your body and allow it to help you revel and connect.

How Does Kava Work in Our Bodies?

Kava's scientific name translates to "intoxicating pepper," which gives a hint about its effect on our bodies. In my experience, kava's effects are marked and immediate. When chewed it increases the saliva in your mouth and has both a tingling and numbing effect on your tongue. This experience is temporary and normal. I also notice kava's relaxing and euphoric effects within minutes.

Kava is both a relaxing nervine and muscle relaxant, so it helps calm our nervous system and relax any tightness in our muscles at the same time. The kavalactones in kava work on the GABA receptors in our brains to reduce or inhibit anxiety.[1] The specific kavalactone, desmethoxyyangonin, increases dopamine levels in the body,[2] and kavain helps to keep feel-good neurotransmitter serotonin in the body for longer periods of time.[3]

Kava can be great for relieving stress and pain that has settled into our muscles.[4] In small doses, kava can relax our muscles and reduce pain without blocking central nerve signals so our minds remain bright and active and our muscles fully functional.[5]

Herbalist jim mcdonald points out that large doses can "still the mind and make the limbs a bit wobbly."[6]

Kava is being explored as a treatment for generalized anxiety disorder.[7] It also reduces the anxious depression sometimes seen with menopause and can also be helpful with the anxiety that is associated with PMS, so it can help women who find that anxiety negatively affects their libido.[8]

Kava's combined actions of relaxation and euphoria have made it a favorite drink ingredient for social occasions. It also can help relieve tension and prepare the way for conflict resolution and deeper levels of connection.[9] Rosemary Gladstar says, "There can be no hate in the heart when one has kava."[10]

It is also noteworthy that kava's spicy, stimulating qualities increase circulation, warming us and bringing more blood flow to our whole body, including our genitals.

A Bit about Kava Plants

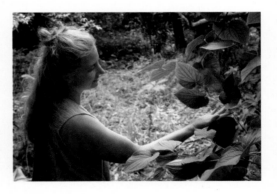

Kava is native to the Pacific Islands and has been used ceremonially there for thousands of years. It likes to grow in tropical areas with lots of humidity and rainfall. Kava is a small shrub or tree with dark green, heart-shaped leaves. It is cultivated for its roots, which are best harvested when the plant is four to five years old.

Herbal Shorthand

APHRODISIAC ACTIONS: *euphoric, muscle relaxant, nervine*

OTHER ACTIONS: *analgesic, anesthetic, antispasmodic, diuretic, sialagogue (stimulates secretion of saliva)*

ENERGETICS: *warming, drying*   TASTES: *acrid, bitter, pungent*

CONSTITUENTS: *kavalactones*

DOSAGE SUGGESTIONS: *Kava has been used traditionally for ceremonies and special gatherings. It is a powerful herb, best consumed consciously and occasionally in small amounts (e.g., a dropperful of tincture or as an addition to a cup of tea).*

SPECIAL CONSIDERATIONS: *High dosages can impair coordination, so don't take kava and then drive or engage in other activities that require quick reflexes.*

Use only the root as a compound found in the stem and leaves can cause liver damage. Also, seek out a noble variety of kava and buy from a source that properly handles the plant from harvest through the final product (to be sure stems and leaves are not included).

Do not use if you have any type of liver disease or if you are taking Parkinson's disease medications.

Do not use kava during pregnancy or when breastfeeding. Do not give it to young children.

Do not mix kava with alcohol, sedatives, tranquilizers, or antidepressants or with pharmaceutical anxiolytics (e.g., benzodiazepines).

Large amounts of kava may cause dry, peeling skin that will clear up when kava consumption is stopped.

Kava is best taken occasionally rather than as a daily supplement.

How to Use Kava

PARTS USED: *root*

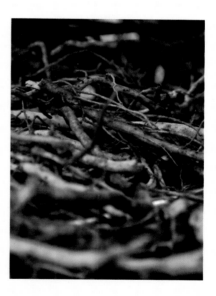

Add to drinks like tea, punch, or fermented soda. To add it, squeeze kava root in a mesh bag to release the constituents into water and add the water to your drink of choice. Kava was traditionally used in fermented form and I found that adding it to my fermented sodas yields good results.

*Kava root massage oil **(Sensations Massage Oil, page 224)** is both warming and muscle relaxing.*

Add decoction or milky kava root water to your bath for muscle relaxing.

Kava tincture has immediate relaxing effects and can be used to induce restful sleep.

Participant Experiences

As a group, we really connected with the powerful potency of this herb, and agreed it is best used on occasion and with intention. I'll often make a batch of kava chai for John and me when we need to resolve something in our relationship and want to be sure we are connected on a heart level. During the Aphrodisiac Circle year, I ordered some fresh kava root from Hawaii and combined it with ceremonial cacao for a beautiful birthday ritual that included heart-connected conversation, sensual dance, and snuggling.

Both Sarah and Christina noted the tingling in their mouths with the use of kava as being erotic and creating a desire for kissing or oral sex. Sarah also noticed increased sensitivity around her breasts, clit, and vagina. For me, kava chai before sex has led to increased sensation deep within my yoni during penetration.

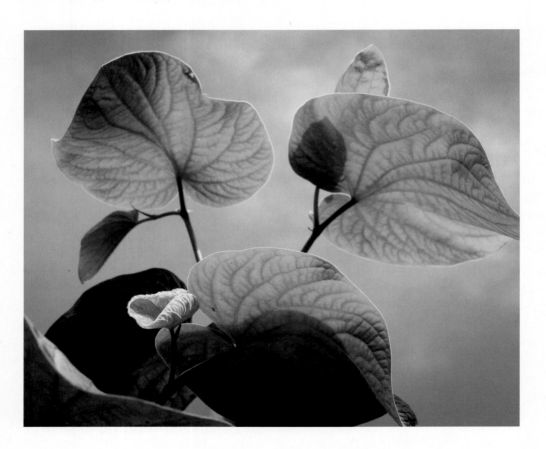

FULL SURRENDER

Complete relaxation and dropping into our bodies may happen easily and naturally, but this state of full surrender will more likely be reached through conscious cultivation, using the ideas presented in this book. We've learned about creating environments where love and eros flourish. These are the kinds of environments where full surrender is possible. There are elements present that speak to all of our senses, encouraging relaxation and arousal. Things that we know impede our arousal have been consciously handled. Our bedroom door is locked, and the kids' needs are being met by others. The room is set up in a way that meets the arousal needs of both partners (e.g., even though roses increase the erotic delight of one of us, the smell is too much for the other, so we have settled on a tulsi room mist, a scent we both enjoy).

In addition, we have created and shared erotic pleasure maps for our bodies and have talked about the kinds of touch that help us to relax and drop into our bodies and the kinds of touch that excite us as we become increasingly aroused. Along the way we've also learned that some kinds of touch can bring us right out of arousal and up into our heads. It is important to notice and communicate about those kinds of touch as well, so that we can avoid jolting each other out of our aroused states, and instead continue to increase arousal and surrender through our touch. We learn through exploring with each other and deepening our capacity to listen to each other's arousal cues. We can help each other by making

sounds or speaking words that communicate the heightening of our pleasure, gently pushing each other away when something does not feel good or by asking for a change in speed or pressure. "Mmmmm. Slower, please . . ."

Being able to communicate our needs and desires to each other requires the kind of deep trust that is built through our conscious dance of relationship. Practicing the relating meditation, offering each other words of appreciation, always increasing your tools for healthy conflict resolution, treating each other with love and respect, taking responsibility for what is yours and making amends when necessary. Risking being vulnerable and transparent, not withholding things from one another. These are the kinds of things that build trust over time. When you are feeling that kind of trust and attunement with your partner, you might pull out your Damiana Chocolate Love Liqueur (page 144) or indulge in a Cosmic Surrender Bath (page 218) before lovemaking. I've found both of these preparations bring me into a deep state of surrender.

Full surrender to the delight of pleasurable sensation is truly a beautiful gift. States of surrender inspire feelings of serenity, love, and connection. These are the states we can reach when we feel deep trust in our partners and we have set ourselves up for maximum pleasure. As we continue to learn and grow and practice things we learn in books like this one, we will naturally deepen into states of greater and greater surrender, and we will get to delight in so much pleasure along the way!

Cosmic Surrender Bath

INGREDIENTS

1 ounce dried damiana leaves

1 cup kava root powder

PREPARATION

1 Place damiana leaves in a quart jar.

2 Pour water over the leaves to fill the jar.

3 Let the leaves steep for at least 4 hours.

4 Strain into a large bowl, reserving the liquid and composting the damiana leaves.

5 Put the kava powder in a muslin bag.

6 Put the bag with the kava into the damiana infusion and knead the bag for 20 minutes or more to release the kava goodness into the infusion.

7 Pour the infusion into your bath, and enjoy relaxing into it.

HERBAL TIPS

✦ Our skin is the largest of our organs, and a bath like this one allows us to take in the effects of the herbs through the full extent of our skin. As you will experience, the result can be quite potent.

✦ Please use this bath with respect and care, entering into it with intention and when you have plenty of time to enjoy the effects and are not in need of swift reaction times.

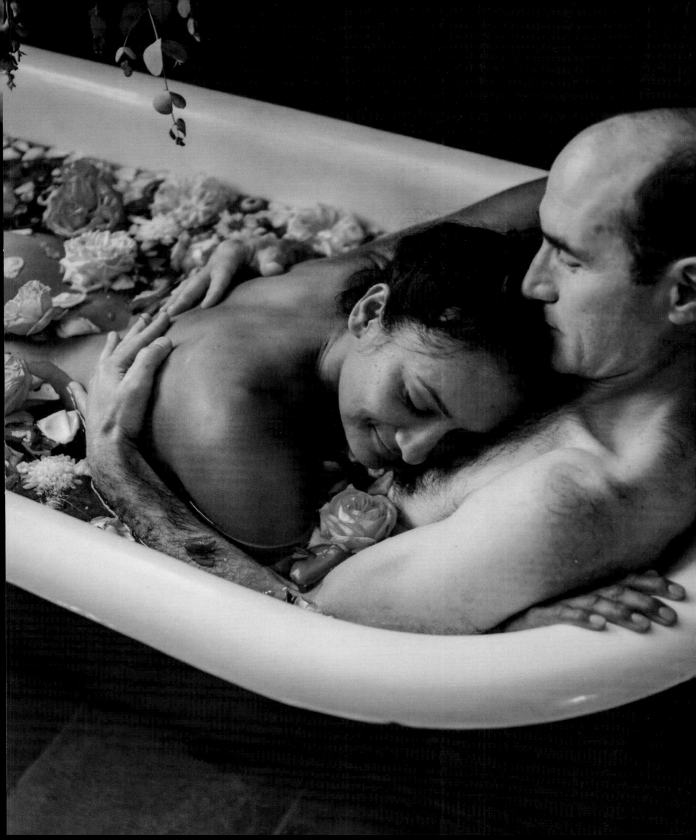

Surrender

She lay herself open
Upon an earthen cradle
beneath the crescent moon,
Each shaping their form
to her body softening,
After years of searching
upright and rigid
for sanctuary and rest.
It was not a light giving,
Of her weight to the forest floor,
It was a heavy thud
releasing years of stories,
Of a mother's expectations to be good,
Of a father's want of her one way,
So he could parade her like a trophy, about.
In the falling,
something opened, she could not shut,
The light wanting in, with piercing points
Needling her pliant,
This time, she allowed it, by her own accord
Not because someone told her to,
Because it sought her.
She invited it in to her,
Not pushing for something,
but releasing
to its unrelenting want to find her.
She let it search her,
absorb her skin,
Open its mouth to taste her,
Gazing eyes upon its beauty for her alone,
Then, taking it inside her she felt all that she needed,
To surrender.

The words flung at her to judge,
The shoulds packed on her back like musts,
The avalanche of deeds she must do,
The body she must sculpt, just so
To be recognized.
And she flung it all in dry stick heaps
to the dark woods beside her,
Compost for the soil of her new rising.
Offering permission from the one who mattered,
The one she answered to, when the moon had fled,
And found other trees to shine on.
She spread outward,
An exquisite sigh,
The ecstatic relief of,
No longer needing to hold on,
For in this releasing she freed herself
Of all that did not belong,
Cocooned matted layers of other's dreams.
The veils unwrapped,
Tumbling her form nakedly seen,
In one single stream of sunlight,
Leaving only the beauty
of her warm essence glistening
On warm mossy rocks.
And here, spent,
she knew herself,
And took her place among all things,
Bathing herself sovereign in a moonlight stream
Like a birthed newborn doe,
skin touching warm air,
For the first time.

— Artemis Mandala

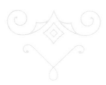

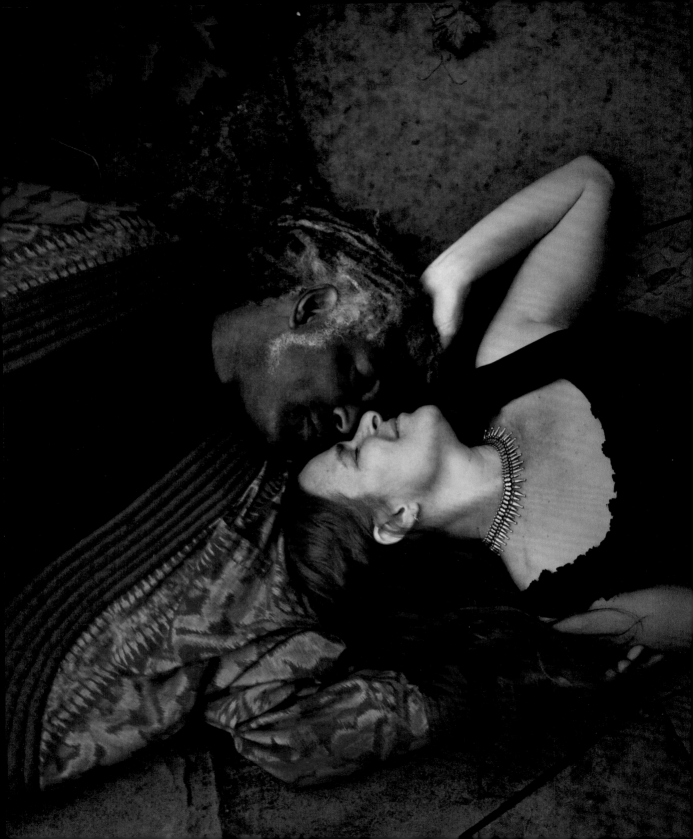

NINE

DEEP NOURISHMENT

Mmmm. Sunlight is streaming through the window as I yawn and stretch myself awake. Usually my alarm goes off at 5 A.M., and it is still dark outside, but it's Saturday and I'm taking a day to deeply nourish myself. I've found that letting myself sleep until my body naturally wakes up is one of the most nourishing things I can do for myself. Quality sleep, and enough of it, is foundational to vital living. I gently and sensually wake myself up with the "Total Permission" poem, running my hands over my body as I say it out loud to myself. I revel for a moment in the delicious sensations of my own touch and the feeling of the soft sheets against my skin, allowing my body to move against the sheets, slow and sexy. It is a delight to be awake once again in a sensual, human body.

Then I reach for my journal. I start each day with three pages of free writing—my morning pages (a practice I learned from *The Artist's Way* book). This practice helps keep me connected with myself and what I think and feel about things that are going on in my life and the world. It also allows me to dump all the circular thoughts that run around in my brain onto paper, freeing up space for more creative thinking later in the day. Sometimes it gives me a chance to think creatively about something by writing about it. Yesterday, I wrote about all the ways I could nourish myself today, so I've had a whole day to delight in the anticipation of my day of nourishment. I end my entry with my affirmations and writing my core life purpose to help ground me in those elements of my life that I want to be at the center of all of my actions.

I slip on my cashmere leggings and sweater, gifts from my sweet husband, and start a fire in the wood stove. I pull the lambskin off the couch and lay it out in front of the fire, creating anticipation for the day to come. I've already got my knitting and my favorite novel and a journal by the fireplace. Once the fire is happily dancing, I head into the kitchen and turn on Coco Love Alcorn's *Wonderland*. I can dance and sing while I cook!

I start water in the teapot and pull out my mason jars to make my daily herbal infusions. In one, I place an ounce of oatstraw and tops. In another, nettle forms the base, with the addition of a piece of kelp, some red raspberry leaf, and some lady's mantle. I pour boiling water over each and then these will steep through the day. I'll nourish myself with the oatstraw at lunchtime and the other one will be my dinner drink. These infusions are my daily multivitamin, giving me the vitamins and minerals I need in a way that is easy for my body to absorb and integrate.

My breakfast today will be scrambled eggs with fresh vegetables—all organic and local. The mushrooms, kale, and eggs are all from local farms, which makes my head and heart as happy as my body, which gets to benefit from all the nutrients in these yummy foods. This breakfast is nourishing on many levels. I have herbal chai in the refrigerator to warm up as my breakfast drink. I'll pour the extra into our airpot on the counter. This nourishing drink is a favorite of my whole family.

Often, I admit, I eat my breakfast standing up while helping my kids get ready for school, but today I am going to sit at the dining table looking out at the winter garden. The rhododendrons still have leaves, but most of the plants are directing their energy firmly into their roots, and tree and shrub branches are bare. There is a quiet beauty to the winter garden that I love. This view sets the tone for my lazy day of knitting and reading by the wood stove.

I'll do some yoga before I settle in, and later, I'll bundle up and go for a walk to the beach. My husband and daughter are away for the day, so I can follow my own internal rhythms and intuitions. That in itself is nourishing—a day where I need only meet my own needs, where I can follow my own bliss . . .

While some of the activities I'm describing are unique to my day of nourishment, most all of them are actually ongoing daily practices for me—the morning pages; yoga; dancing; yummy, organic, local food; nourishing infusions; herbal chai; and walking outside. I have slowly integrated these practices over the years as my children have grown. As time has freed up, I have been able to further prioritize my self-care. Now, ongoing, deep nourishment is the current that runs below everything else in my life. I've cultivated these practices because they lead to optimum health, which underlies sexual fulfillment and makes vital living possible.

SELF-NOURISHMENT AS A CORE LIFE PRACTICE

Creating your own current of self-nourishment is an act of love and care for yourself that will ripple out to the lives of all those you touch. Your health and vitality are what allow you to make the contributions you want to make in your family, your community, your profession, and the world. You will be able to support others without burning yourself out, and you will inspire others to nourish and care for themselves as well, lifting everyone up.

Wonderfully, beautifully, the creation of this current is not arduous work. It gets created slowly over time with one act of self-care after another. Each one replenishes and heals us, and we are led simply and organically to the next and the next. Let's begin together with a deep breath. Breathe in for a count of 10, letting the breath fully expand your belly and then your chest and feeling it fill your head as well. Breathe out equally slowly. Counting to 10 as the breath releases and your body relaxes. Moments like this, taking time out for a deep breath or 10 minutes of meditation or a morning at the beach, or a whole day lying in front of the fire are deeply nourishing. So much of our lives are spent rushing from one activity to another that simply stopping is a profound act of self-love.

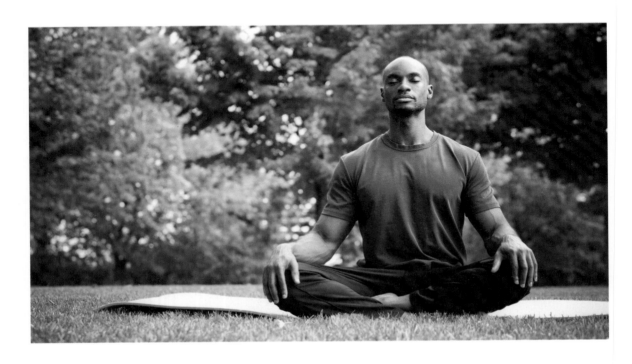

Stillness is a gardener.
She spends her days tending vegetables and flowers.
Even on the grayest days, you will find her outside,
close to the earth,
listening to the flowers grow.
She has these moments of clarity and calm
when all sense of separation dissolves
and she feels the oneness of all life.
She breathes as the ocean roils,
as the trees sway,
as beings die and are born,
as tears and laughter gather in her own breast,
as the earth spins through space.
Still she breathes,
in her bones, and her sinew,
in her tender heart,
in the marrow where she makes her blood,
Stillness feels the hum of all life and knows we are one.

—Meredith Heller, 2004
www.meredithheller.com

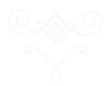

And so we've begun, in our moment of stillness, to create your current of deep nourishment. Let's consider other elements to add as you go along. Physical elements to self-nourishment are primal and immediate. Are you getting enough quality sleep? Perhaps you've already started taking a dropperful of Soothe Tincture (page 203) on days when your nerves need some calming so you can drop into sleep. Are there other steps you can take? Misting your room with the calming scent of a tulsi or lavender hydrosol as you settle in to go to sleep might be nice. Or spoiling yourself by getting some beautiful, soft sheets that you can't wait to slip between and bringing in your most comfortable pillow. Can you make a commitment to yourself to not get into work projects after dinner, but rather use that time to relax as you move toward going to bed? What else might help you?

Exercise is another element of physical self-care that is vital. My favorite form of exercise is dance. I also love hiking and swimming. When our exercise is woven in with joy, it is so much easier to prioritize! I also have a regular yoga practice and a video kettlebell workout that I do three times a week. Kind of like my daily nourishing infusion, I see these practices as my exercise multivitamin. I do them first thing in the morning; they do not take a lot of time and they provide a baseline for keeping my body flexible and strong. What is your favorite way to exercise? Can you create a rhythm around it for yourself so it is integrated into your life?

What are you eating to fuel your body for exercise and for all the activity of life? I have been curious in my own life about what food is the most nourishing for my body. There are so many options out there these days and so many studies and opinions about what and how much we should eat. Personally, I've been most inspired by eating a variety of colorful, organic foods and sourcing them locally whenever possible. I like knowing the farmers who are growing my food and have enjoyed being part of community-supported agriculture programs and farmer's markets. I shop on the edges of grocery stores, in the produce, deli, and meat sections where the food is simpler and more whole. I love creating healthy, beautiful, delicious meals for myself and my family. Gathering food, cooking, and presenting it are actually some of my favorite acts of self-nourishment. Giving myself permission to prioritize good food amid all the pressures of life can sometimes feel like a radical act of self-love.

One thing I've noticed for myself is that the physical needs of my body change over time. When I was young, my body was extremely resilient. I could have a sore muscle one day and feel fine the next. I could get hurt and heal within a relatively short period of time. With each passing decade, I'm finding that my body asks for a new level of care. When I turned 40, I noticed that aches and pains that would previously last a day or so were just not resolving. The yoga and exercise that felt optional in my 30s became a requirement, and I needed to find a maintenance exercise routine that worked my whole body. Now that I'm in my 50s, I'm finding that those restorative yoga poses that once seemed like a nice addition to my stretching routine are becoming essential as I work to restore and replenish myself after years of active mothering—giving to my family and community.

The creation of your current of nourishment will never be complete. Like everything in life, it will continually change as your needs change. Listening to your body, as we've been practicing together, will help you identify your needs. Adopting and continually returning to a commitment to deep nourishment will help you create and integrate the practices that can help you remain physically vital over the whole course of your life.

As you create your own current, I encourage you to include ways of nourishing yourself emotionally as well as physically. Emotional nourishment is equally vital. As humans we experience a rich array of emotions throughout the course of any one day. Instinctually, we may want to distance ourselves from feeling challenging emotions, ignoring them and continuing with all the things we need to do. This is how emotions get lodged in our bodies. Instead, we can ask ourselves how we can nourish ourselves. We may choose to sink

Soft Landing Tea

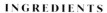

INGREDIENTS

1 heaping teaspoon
chamomile flowers

2 heaping tablespoons licorice
root, cut and sifted, or 8 slices
licorice root

1 tablespoon dried rose
petals or buds

3 cardamom pods, crushed

1 tablespoon dried oat tops

PREPARATION

1 Mix the herbs together in a quart jar or teapot.

2 Pour 3 cups of boiling water over the herbs.

3 Cover, and steep for at least 15 minutes.

4 Strain, relax, and enjoy!

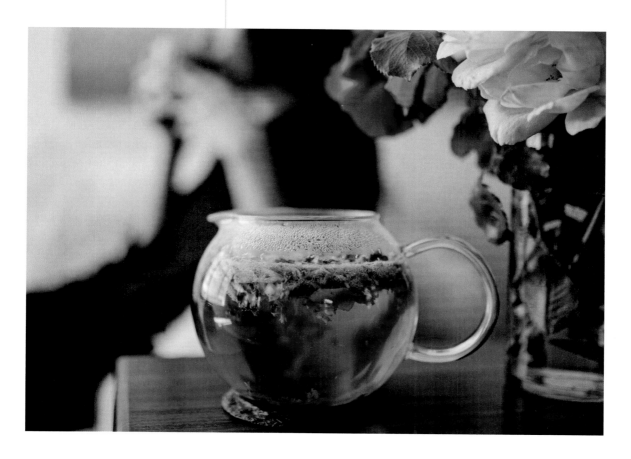

into a hot bath, wrap ourselves up in a blanket, or cozy up with a cup of Soft Landing Tea (page 229), giving ourselves tender loving care as we feel what is there to feel. Breathing deeply and focusing on body sensations rather than on our swirling thoughts can be helpful in these moments.

As we get a sense of how the emotions are affecting our bodies (maybe tightness in our belly or shoulder muscles or buzzing energy through our nervous system) we may want to choose an activity to move the energy through and out of our bodies. A cup of Grounding and Moving Tea (page 137) might help with this. Follow the tea with dancing, walking, or running outside or maybe punching a pillow. Moving and releasing the energy can be one of the most nourishing things we can do for ourselves.

Emotional nourishment may also come in the form of reaching out to a friend. Call on one of those people in your life who you know can witness your experience and provide empathy and perhaps some helpful perspective. Or someone who can just physically hold you while you cry or scream. Setting up regular appointments with a counselor or coach during intense periods in your life can be deeply nourishing emotionally. A friend asked me once if I felt I had adequate support in my life. At the time, that phrase seemed laughable—my support system was nowhere near adequate for the challenges I was facing. But that phrase stayed with me, encouraging me to add all different kinds of nourishing support to my life and to reach out and ask for help or love or care when I need it.

Spending time with friends, whether offering each other support or engaging in fun activities together, is very nourishing. Humans really do need each other and thrive when we are together.

As you continue this exploration around your sensuality and sexuality and living a more vital life, bring your friends along for the ride. Having that Aphrodisiac Circle during my year of research was so wonderful, and recently a friend and I started a sex salon, which is basically a small group of friends getting together once a month to share insights and stories about our explorations. Having straight-up conversations about sexuality feeds me. It helps normalize my choice to prioritize my sexuality, gives me new ideas and perspectives, and inspires further exploration. You could offer a pot of that Warm Nights Chai (page 171) or make a Cardamom Chocolate Mousse Torte (page 8) to help set the tone for the evening, or ask people to bring sexy treats. Sharing food with friends is always nourishing, and sharing sexy treats can help inspire conversation and connection around sexuality.

As I've deepened into sexual exploration, I've discovered practices like erotic massage and tantric breathing techniques that can highlight the spiritual nature of sexuality. Through embodiment and surrender we can reach states of being deeply connected with one another, the whole spinning earth, and universal energies. Sexual surrender is one place where we can feel our oneness with all of life.

Whether or not your sexuality becomes a spiritual practice for you, spiritual nourishment is definitely another form of nourishment you can add to your current. What does spiritual nourishment look like for you? Do you attend a church? Meditate? Pray? Walk in the woods while tuning in to the beauty and aliveness of the world around you? Dance by yourself or in community? Engage in co-created ceremonies? Whatever your form is, prioritize it! Carve out time for it in your life and bring yourself to it fully and with joy so that it can nourish you and fill you to overflowing.

Each step we take to strengthen that current of nourishment will allow us to be more the person we want to be in the world and to fulfill our commitments and dreams. We will be able to give with no strings attached because we are fully nourished and can give from the overflow without depleting ourselves. As the current gets stronger and stronger, it begins to carry us. Life gets easier, more fun, and infinitely sexier.

SEXUAL SATISFACTION AS NOURISHING PRACTICE

Sexual satisfaction itself is one of the deepest nourishing forces in my own life. I love the continued tingling in my body that can linger through a whole day after a particularly satisfying sexual experience. I love how at ease and alive I feel after an orgasm. I love how confident, happy, and beautiful I feel when I have regular opportunities to experience satisfying sex.

Since this is true for me, I have given myself permission to prioritize my sexuality. I set aside time for sex with John. We talk about what helps us be able to fully drop into the experience with each other and set up an environment that allows us both to be fully present. We also set ourselves up with elements that raise our level of arousal—elements like sensual music, candlelight, warmth, and lingerie. We seek out opportunities to learn more about sexuality, reading books, taking classes, and talking with others. This keeps us learning new techniques and bringing fresh ideas to our lovemaking. We communicate about what leads to more arousal and satisfaction and what

doesn't. And, always, always, we come back to our intention of connection rather than any particular physical result of our time together. I would say that dropping any expectation around particular physical results has been the single most helpful factor in taking all the stress out of our sex life and making it a consistently nourishing aspect of our marriage and our lives.

Removing expectations around bringing each other to orgasm is a powerful act. Both men and women can feel pressure about being "good in bed." Joe shared that he has felt a strong cultural expectation for men to make sure their female partners come to orgasmic release first. The story goes, "you're not really a man unless you can get her to release, and if you come first, you're a loser." As a woman I am aware of another cultural story that applies sexual pressure—the story that sex is primarily about satisfying the sexual urges of men. This kind of pressure is shaming and paralyzing, taking the focus away from pleasurable sensation and connection and creating unnecessary performance anxiety. Even though both partners may orgasm under such pressure, it is unlikely they will feel truly satisfied sexually.

Some relationships will feel more sexually satisfying than others, and we all go through phases where our level of sexual satisfaction varies. It is important to know this and really ride the waves of it in our lives. Fully feel the gratitude and joy of having a particularly satisfying sexual partnership in your life. Allow yourself to revel in it, get filled up, and take advantage of the creative surge that may ensue during this time.

When this is not the case, consider taking the opportunity to delve into creating a nourishing self-pleasure practice. Take time to learn about your own body and discover how fully you can please yourself. Michelle's self-pleasuring experience with rose from Chapter 4 is an example of this. She envisioned herself as the goddess and brought herself to an exquisite G-spot orgasm. Throughout the course of our aphrodisiac year together, she continually highlighted her experiences with herself as being some of her most profound experiences of sexual satisfaction.

Cultivating a sensual, erotic connection with the natural world is another avenue to keeping yourself feeling sexually alive when a partner is not present. There is a sweet, private spot right next to my garden where I can lie out and enjoy the warmth of the sunshine and the beauty of the garden plants beside me. I also find that gathering and processing plants outdoors can be an amazingly sensual and connected experience. I fall more deeply in love with the plants with each sensual experience I have with them.

If you are craving human interaction, but don't have a partner, dance can be a wonderful activity. Dancing allows us to be in sensual connection with music and other people while practicing consent and skillful, respectful relating. Tantra festivals and classes about sexuality can provide venues for learning and experiencing as well.

There are some key components to cultivating sexual satisfaction in your life whether you are in a partnership or not. One primary component is honesty with yourself about your current sexual desires. Another is knowledge about your own arousal, what brings you pleasure and what impedes your pleasure. A third is curiosity, an openness to new possibilities and the learning of new skills. Open, respectful communication and consent are absolutely essential components for healthy, satisfying sexual interactions with others. Within that, creating a shame-free environment where risk and play

can flourish will go a long way toward increasing the satisfying qualities of your sexual interactions.

If you are in a period of your life where you are not consistently feeling sexually satisfied, please allow yourself to feel the frustration and the longing, but also put energy and time into developing these key components, and watch how your life shifts. As Michelle's experience with rose and self-pleasure illuminates, the plants can be wonderful allies through these times. Let yourself fall in love with rose or tulsi or savor your Golden Oat Infusion, knowing that it is building your sexual health.

REGULAR USE OF HERBS FOR A HEALTHY REPRODUCTIVE SYSTEM AND OVERALL VITALITY

Drinking that quart of Golden Oat Infusion every day is definitely one of the most significant things you can do to keep your reproductive system healthy. Oats are deeply nourishing for our reproductive organs and are a tonic for our endocrine and hormonal systems. They help keep both vaginal juices and semen flowing abundantly and smoothly.

This practice of integrating herbs like oats into our daily routines can be powerful. Often, we wait to incorporate herbs until a health problem arises and then we want a quick fix solution to relieve our symptoms so we can get back to our daily activities. Nourishing and tonifying our body systems with herbs is a whole different way of thinking. Doing so can allow us to slowly repair and heal damaged organs or systems, strengthen weaknesses, or simply nourish our healthy systems so they stay healthy over time.

Several of the herbs highlighted in this book are classified as adaptogens—maca, ashwagandha, eleuthero, tulsi, and schisandra. Adaptogens are herbs that work in varying ways to regulate or normalize the functioning of our organs and systems. This may sound like no big deal. Stop for a moment, though, and consider the astounding healing power of our living bodies. When our organs are functioning as they were meant to, we are incredibly resilient beings. By helping our systems to function at optimal capacity, adaptogens can help us handle all kinds of environmental stressors with ease and grace.

Maca, ashwagandha, and eleuthero are all harvested primarily for their roots, and buying powdered root is an efficient way of integrating them into your life. However, I also love getting to know the plants that I am working with personally and discovered that though ashwagandha is native to India, I can grow it here in the Pacific Northwest. I stumbled upon someone selling plant starts and was able to experiment with growing it in my garden. Rosemary Gladstar let me know that eleuthero is a fairly easy shrub to cultivate as well, so I will look into the possibility of adding this native of the Taiga region of the Far East to my garden. Maca is grown high in the mountains of Peru and is being cultivated in some other mountainous areas in Bolivia and Brazil now that Western consumption of this plant is creating high demand.

On the following pages you will find two delicious recipes for integrating these herbs into your life (Dream Cream and Date Treats). The AshwaMacaMocha Shake (page 64) I introduced in Chapter 3 is another option. I recommend taking these herbs in one or more of these forms for a period of three to four weeks and then taking a break for a week, letting the tonic effects settle into your body and then choosing if you would like to start up again. If you choose to, continue for another cycle. This is how tonic herbs can be used most effectively. For myself, I have chosen to make the Date Treats as the seasons change from winter to spring and then again when they change from summer to fall. These are moments when I notice I can easily get sick as my body adapts to the seasonal change, and the Date Treats help my body adjust. I am currently drinking the AshwaMacaMocha Shake daily as I navigate the hot flashes associated with menopause. During seasonal changes or when your body is going through a period of transition or stress are great times to call on these herbs.

Each of these herbs is also restorative, helping increase our chi or life-force energy, and they are each being highlighted in a book on aphrodisiacs because they also can have a profound effect on the health of our reproductive system. In our Aphrodisiac Circle, Christina described the energy of eleuthero as sunny and growth promoting. She found it gave her more energy to fuel her healing process and helped her open more to the pleasure in her daily life. Robert found that ashwagandha gave him more staying power during sex. I've mentioned before the grounding and calming qualities that people noticed when taking maca regularly. For myself, I've noticed that in comparison with other women experiencing hot flashes, mine seem less intense with the use of maca and ashwagandha. I do not sweat during them, they move through fairly quickly, and the heat does not feel unbearable—more like a gentle reminder of the change my body is going through.

Dream Cream

This adaptogen smoothie is a great way to integrate roots like ashwagandha and eleuthero into your life.

INGREDIENTS

1 banana (or ½ banana and ½ avocado)

1 cup almond milk

½ cup plain dairy or vegan yogurt

¼ cup sunflower seed butter (or your favorite nut butter)

¼ cup coconut cream (the solid part inside a can of coconut milk)

1 tablespoon ashwagandha powder

1 tablespoon eleuthero powder

1 ½ teaspoons cinnamon

1 date (or 5 drops liquid monk fruit for less sugar)

Large pinch of salt

PREPARATION

1 Place all the ingredients into a blender (add a few ice cubes, if desired).

2 Blend until smooth.

3 Pour the smoothie into glasses. Use a spatula to get the residual liquid from the sides of the blender—there are lots of good herbs in there!

4 Drink immediately.

HERBAL TIPS

✦ This recipe contains the goodness from several powerfully nourishing roots. If you can harvest the roots yourself, it is best to do so in the fall after the leaves and flowers have died back. At this time of year, the plant has returned its energy to the roots and so they are packed with nourishment.

✦ Dried roots are storehouses of plant nourishment and medicine. Drinking and eating powdered roots are a good way to get this nourishment into our bodies.

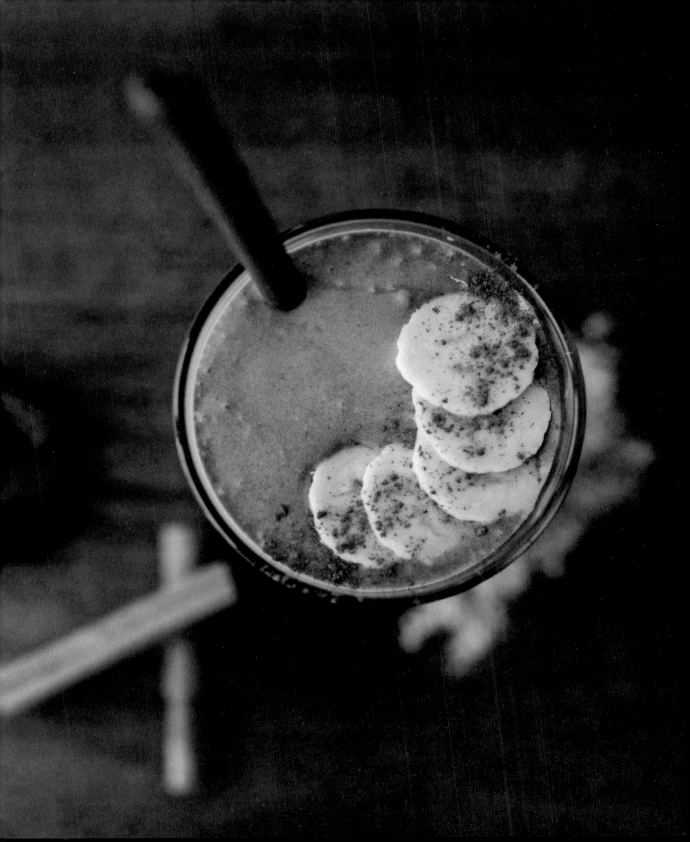

Date Treats

Rosalee de la Forêt

INGREDIENTS

1 ½ cups pitted and chopped dates

2 tablespoons cacao powder

⅓ cup eleuthero powder

⅓ cup ashwagandha powder

⅔ cup grated coconut (plus extra for rolling)

¼ cup tahini

¼ cup almond butter

2 teaspoons vanilla extract

½ teaspoon organic orange extract

1 teaspoon cinnamon

1 teaspoon ginger powder

¾ cup melted coconut oil

Pinch of salt

PREPARATION

1 Soak pitted dates in 2 cups of hot water for 30 minutes.

2 Strain dates well. (The water can be reserved for cooking sweet rice or oatmeal.)

3 Place the dates and the rest of the ingredients into a food processor. Blend until it forms a consistent paste.

4 Chill the mixture in the refrigerator for 30 minutes.

5 Roll the paste into teaspoon-sized balls and roll in coconut. Store in the refrigerator and eat within one week.

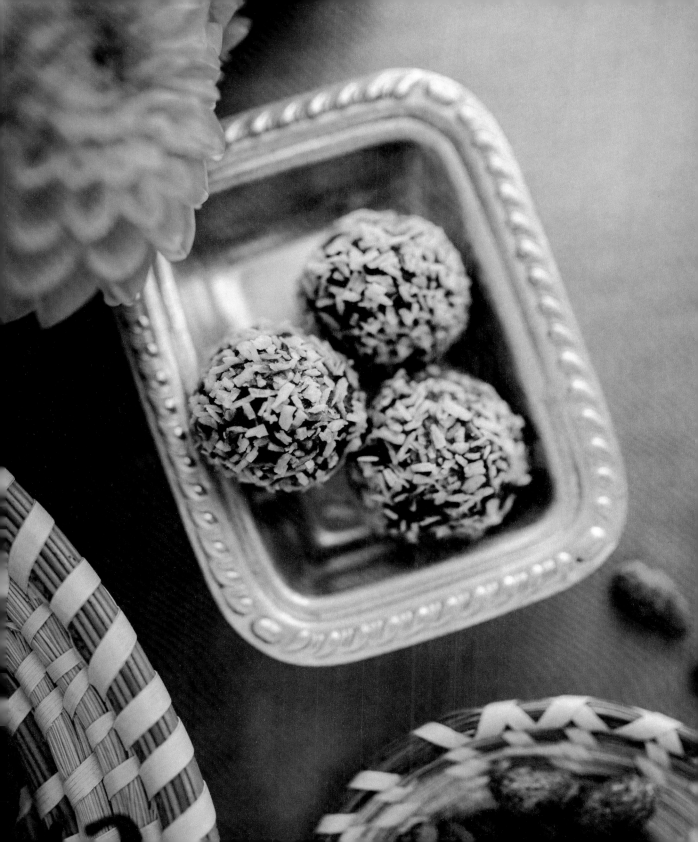

Berry Decadence Syrup

Rebecca Altman

INGREDIENTS

1 cup maple or agave syrup

¼ vanilla bean or ½ teaspoon vanilla extract

¼ cup blackberries (fresh or frozen)

¼ cup dried tulsi (or ½ cup fresh)

PREPARATION

1 Place syrup, vanilla (if using vanilla bean), and blackberries in a saucepan.

2 Cover the saucepan with a lid, and bring the syrup to a simmer for 15 minutes.

3 Add the tulsi, and replace the lid on the pot.

4 Simmer for another 15 minutes.

5 Remove the saucepan from the heat, strain, add vanilla extract (if using extract), and stir.

6 Enjoy over ice cream or another dessert, as a flavoring in soda water, in tea, or as a body drizzle.

7 Store in the refrigerator for up to 2 weeks.

Schisandra berries are adaptogens in that they tone and strengthen our organs, helping us adapt to stress and resist disease. They are a tonic for our cardiovascular, nervous, and reproductive systems. Cassie, Angela, and Christina all noted that taking schisandra regularly helped strengthen their adrenals, giving them more stamina and vitality in stressful times. They also noted libido surges over the course of the month when we were experimenting. Eating a few berries (fresh or dried) every day or taking 20 to 30 drops of schisandra tincture each day are both simple ways to try out this tonic for yourself. Brigitte Mars, in her book *The Sexual Herbal*, says that in China it is recommended to do this for 100 days in a row to experience the full tonic effects. Eating the dried berries is quite a taste sensation. Prepare yourself for all five tastes mixing together and exploding in your mouth in the same moment!

Tulsi is an adaptogen that works in a myriad of ways to help ease stress and increase our resilience. It is nourishing for our central nervous system and heart while also helping to strengthen our immune system. Tulsi promotes healthy digestion and oral health as well. Perhaps because it increases feel-good neurotransmitters in our brains, tulsi can help keep us open to the wonder of life. For ease integrating this herb into your life, tulsi can be taken in tincture form, but you

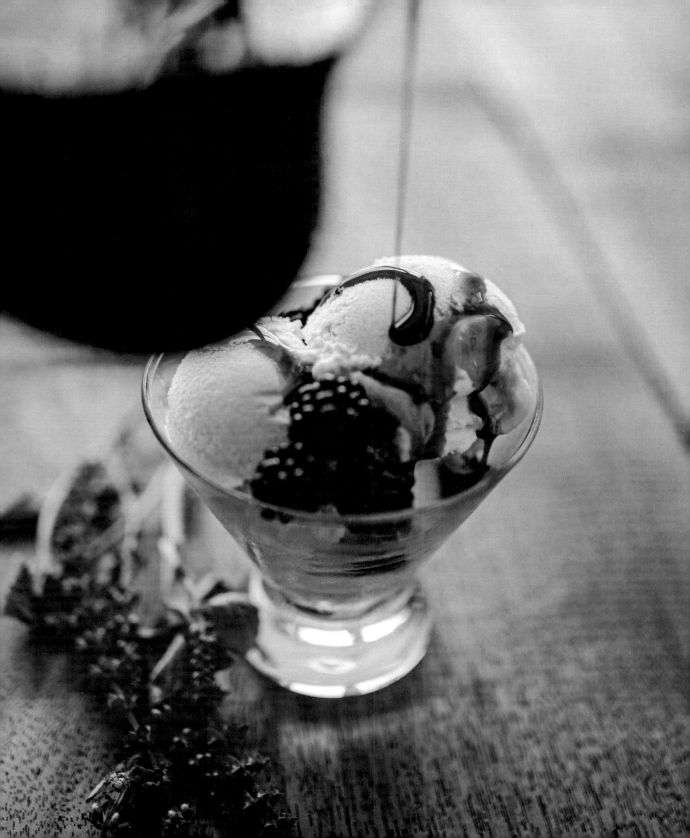

Bitter Cream Tea

INGREDIENTS

1 ounce fenugreek seeds

Honey and cream to taste

PREPARATION

1 Place fenugreek seeds and 2 cups of water in a saucepan and cover.

2 Bring the water to a boil.

3 Turn the heat down and simmer (covered) for 20 minutes.

4 Strain, reserving the liquid and composting the seeds.

5 Pour the liquid into a cup.

6 Add honey and cream to taste.

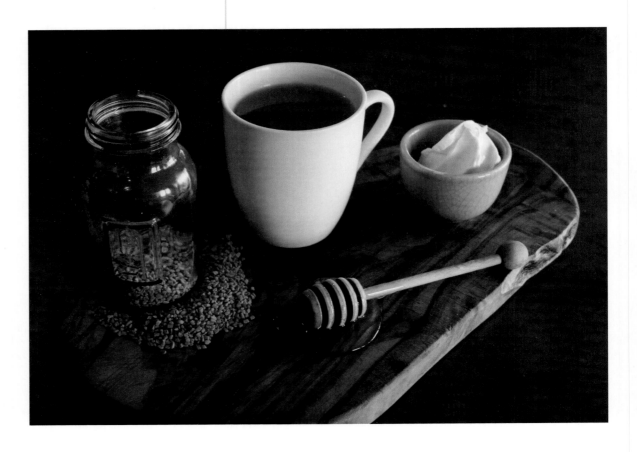

will miss out on its wonderful flavor and scent. Brewing a simple tea or including it in a syrup are two other simple, delicious ways of bringing it into your everyday life.

Hawthorn is another herb that many people in the Aphrodisiac Circle enjoyed as a tonic. Christina, Cassie, Joe, and Rebecca all found hawthorn to be a gentle, supportive herb, helping to ground and calm them through stressful times. Christina likened the support to "having fresh air to breathe." Hawthorn is particularly supportive as a heart tonic. It helps strengthen our hearts on a physical level, and on an emotional level, it can help open our hearts and heal broken hearts. If you would like to try hawthorn as a tonic, you can add flowers or berries to your Golden Oat Infusion (page 37; make it with ½ ounce oatstraw and ½ ounce hawthorn). Or take a sip of Autumn Blush Cordial each day. (You can find the recipe for that on page 39.) I also add a handful of dried hawthorn berries to my stock pot whenever I make soup stock. I love finding ways to integrate nourishing and tonic herbs into my life on a regular basis.

Fenugreek is another tonic herb that may resonate for you. It can be a supportive whole-body tonic. The seeds are high in iron, calcium, vitamins A, B1, C, and E, phosphates, fiber, and protein. They also have a high mucilage content, which makes them soothing for all our mucous membranes. Fenugreek is a digestive and nervous system tonic and it also warms and nourishes our reproductive organs and glands. It is helpful for balancing hormones, so it can be useful during menopause and can help ease menstrual pain.

Fenugreek is a uterine stimulant, so do not reach for this herb if you are pregnant. My favorite way to enjoy fenugreek is the chai blend from Chapter 6. I love the comforting maple syrup smell that the fenugreek adds. Sarah loved drinking a simple decoction of the seeds mixed with honey and cream (Bitter Cream Tea).

Ginger, another herb in that chai blend, can be a powerful tonic, especially in the colder months or if your body runs cold. Ginger is so warming. It increases our circulation by energizing our heart and dilating our blood vessels. Several Aphrodisiac Circle participants noted the warming effects of ginger during the winter and feelings of more vibrancy than usual for the time of year. Christina found that it kept her internal heat up, making her more comfortable and open in her body. She wrote that she "felt more connected to herself as a sexual being" and that her "erotic energy was like a warm, steady hearth fire."

I have highlighted many plants in this section. Each may offer you unique benefits at different points in your life. There is no need to try to integrate all of them right now. Pick one to experiment with, feel how it works in your unique body at this moment in your life. With regular use over time, your relationship with it will grow and you will know when to call on it again in the future. I truly love how the plants are a continual source of deep nourishment for us. When we remember to integrate them into our current of nourishment, they contribute so much to our vitality and health.

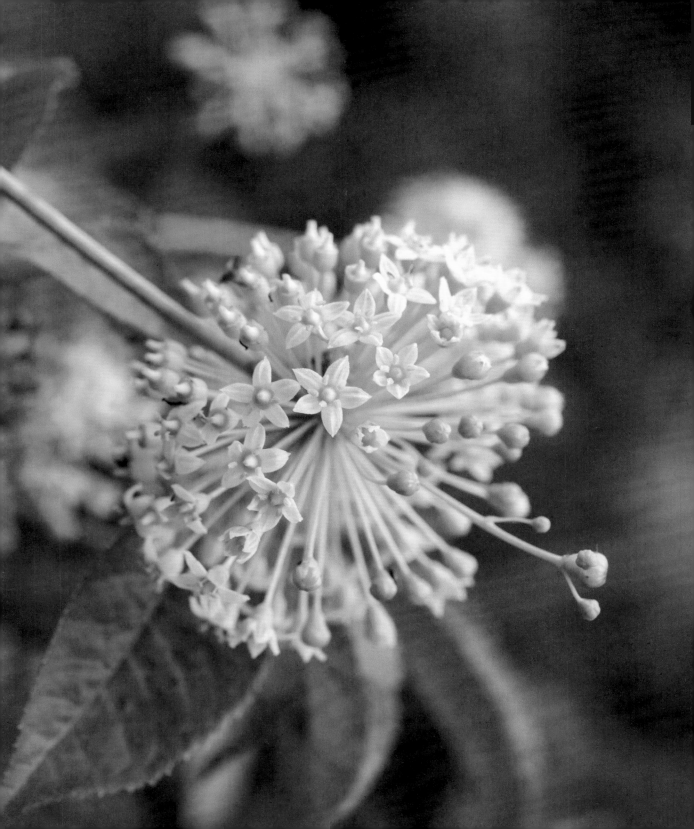

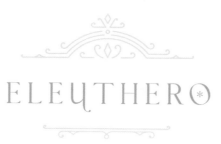

ELEUTHERO*

Eleutherococcus senticosus

Eleuthero increases the amount of chi in our bodies, increasing both our energy and stamina. This herb is deeply restorative when we are recovering from physical illness or struggling on an emotional level. It also provides a steady stream of energy to keep our internal fire burning bright through challenge and change.

How Does Eleuthero Work in Our Bodies?

Eleuthero is an excellent adaptogen. Adaptogens are herbs that assist with overall healthy organ and system functioning. This leads to greater physical resilience. Ginseng family plants are particularly potent is this regard because they contain a high number of active constituents that are all working together. Eleuthero has seven eleutherosides that help reduce stress and stress-related anxiety and depression.[1]

Eleuthero works in several ways to increase our energy and stamina. Syringin, a constituent in eleuthero, triggers the release of acetylcholine, which supports our energy level and helps us maintain a healthy metabolism.[2] When used as a regular nutritive tonic over time, eleuthero strengthens our immune system, protects and nourishes our nervous system, relieves fatigue, and supports our adrenal glands.[3] In particular, eleuthero relieves fatigue (sometimes called adrenal exhaustion) from any sort of chronic stress or ailment.[4]

Ruth Trickey recommends it as a general tonic for women who are overworked or "burning the candle at both ends."[5] Although eleuthero is an energy booster, it is also a nervine that, when used over time, can help with insomnia, improve the quality of our sleep, and prevent us from waking in the night.[6]

Eleuthero is also great for our hearts, relaxing our arteries, lowering high blood pressure, reducing heart enlargement, and decreasing heart disease.[7] Syringin, one of the main eleutherosides, protects our heart cells from pressure and regulates healthy regeneration of cardiovascular cells, helping to both protect and heal our hearts.[8]

A Bit about Eleuthero Plants

Eleuthero, a ginseng family plant, is a large, relatively fast-growing shrub that is easily cultivated and can be sustainably harvested. Though not in the *Panax* genus like Panax and American ginseng, eleuthero has similar (though milder) properties and effects to these other overharvested ginsengs.

Herbal Shorthand

APHRODISIAC ACTIONS: *adaptogen, endocrine system tonic, energy building, ergogenic, nervine, neuroprotective, restorative*

ENERGETICS: *warming, dry* **TASTES:** *acrid, bitter, slightly sweet*

NOTABLE APHRODISIAC CONSTITUENTS: *Seven primary eleutherosides, including syringin, vitamins, and minerals (including calcium, iron, zinc, and vitamin C)*

DOSAGE SUGGESTIONS: *Eleuthero is a tonic herb and should be taken in a medium dosage on a regular basis for a specific period of time. A basic tonic dose would be one to nine grams of powdered root per day or a dropperful of tincture three times per day.*

SPECIAL CONSIDERATIONS: *High doses can cause overstimulation in sensitive people (insomnia, jitters, rapid heartbeat, or headache). Lower the dose or discontinue use if you experience these symptoms.*

Don't mix with digoxin. (Though studies suggest that the incompatibility with this drug may be due to adulteration of eleuthero with P. sepium, *it is best to err on the side of caution. Also, know your source and be sure you are getting pure eleuthero.)*

How to Use Eleuthero

PARTS USED: *root, root bark, and sometimes leaves*

Eleuthero is wonderful when used as a tonic during times of stress or change. Here are some ways to integrate eleuthero into your diet as a tonic:

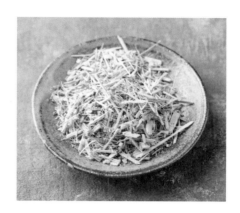

*Make and keep a batch of **Date Treats (page 236)** in the refrigerator and eat a couple a day.*

Mix eleuthero powder with honey and fruit concentrate and spread on toast.

Add eleuthero root to a tonic soup or tea blend.

*Add eleuthero powder to a smoothie—**Dream Cream (page 234)***

Take a daily dose of tincture.

Participant Experiences

During this month I gave participants a choice to experiment with ginseng or eleuthero. We experimented as winter was turning to spring, and in general did feel like these plants gave us an energy boost and helped us stay healthier through this time. For me, the energy boost from eleuthero in my body felt aligned with the bursting spring energy. I also call on eleuthero as summer turns to fall or if I am going through a particularly stressful time or feel like I need an energy boost.

Two participants were already taking eleuthero as part of a regular tonic blend, one to help regulate her hormones during menopause and one as adrenal support.

Christina reported the most profound effects with this herb, saying, "The energy of eleuthero feels sunny and growth promoting, like the energy of springtime that makes the plants emerge from their winter stillness. It seemed to give me more energy to fuel the healing processes I am engaged in. I felt more energy after only a few days on the eleuthero capsules. I started wanting a more sensual experience of the herb itself, so I started emptying the capsules and mixing the herb into nut butter as a simple variation on the energy balls recipe. I think I got even more energy from eating the herb this way—still a feeling of inner vitality to counteract past feelings of fragility that required armoring to protect myself. This definitely helped me feel more open to pleasure in my daily life and to connecting with others."

SIMPLING

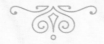

The concept of herbal simpling comes into play as we begin to explore deep nourishment and healing. *Simpling* is about using just one herb at a time as you work to nourish or heal yourself. Often herbs are blended together into tea blends, combination extracts, or other herbal recipes. Sometimes this is a good idea as herbs can help enhance each other's effectiveness, but more often than not, these blends represent a sort of scattershot approach to herbalism. People combine a bunch of herbs that are good for coughs in the hopes that one of those included will be the one you need and make a difference for you. One downside to this scatter-shot approach is that you never really know what is making the difference for you.

In the Aphrodisiac Circle, we studied one herb each month, really incorporating it into our diet and into our lives in a variety of ways so we could get a sense of the effect of that particular herb in our bodies. Trying out herbs in this way can be a great way to really get to know them. As you go deeper into nourishment and seek out herbs for healing, find simple recipes or try just one herb at a time for one particular issue so you can track the results. This is the concept of simpling, and I have found it very helpful as I have deepened my connection with the plants over the past 15 years.

This book gives you lots of ideas and recipes. I encourage you to take it slow. Find one or two that interest you, and give them a try. Try them a few times; notice the effects. Find another one. Try it for a while. Simple and slow. Remember, there is exquisite eroticism in slow, deep exploration!

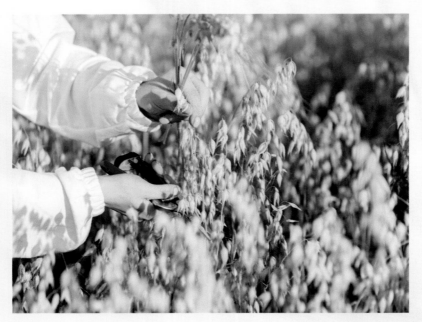

Building Your Personal Current of Nourishment

1   Settle yourself into a comfortable place and take 10 deep breaths.

2   Practice a sensory meditation to bring yourself into a present and embodied state.

3   Consider all of the different forms of nourishment we explored in this chapter. Ask yourself if there is an idea (or two) that will be deeply nourishing for you to add to your personal current right now. Note what arises.

4   Look over any notes you took as you read through this chapter on deep nourishment, noting any ideas you had along the way that would help build your current.

5   Close your eyes and visualize yourself going through your life with these nourishing practices in place. Notice how you feel in your body, notice how you interact with others and the environment, and notice how your daily rhythm adjusts and changes.

6   Capture this vision in your own creative way—writing, singing, dancing, etc.

7   Now, choose one new practice that you are excited to bring into your life—a new form of exercise, a regular herbal addition, or a way of nourishing yourself emotionally or spiritually.

8   Follow through on adding it to your routine.

9   Notice how you feel after a week or month with this addition, and choose whether to keep it or let it go.

10   From a centered, embodied place, choose another practice to try out and follow the steps again.

11   Repeat these steps over and over again throughout your life, and over time you will feel your current strengthen and begin to lift and carry you. As you continue to adjust it over time, it will continue to serve your health and vitality even as you navigate life changes.

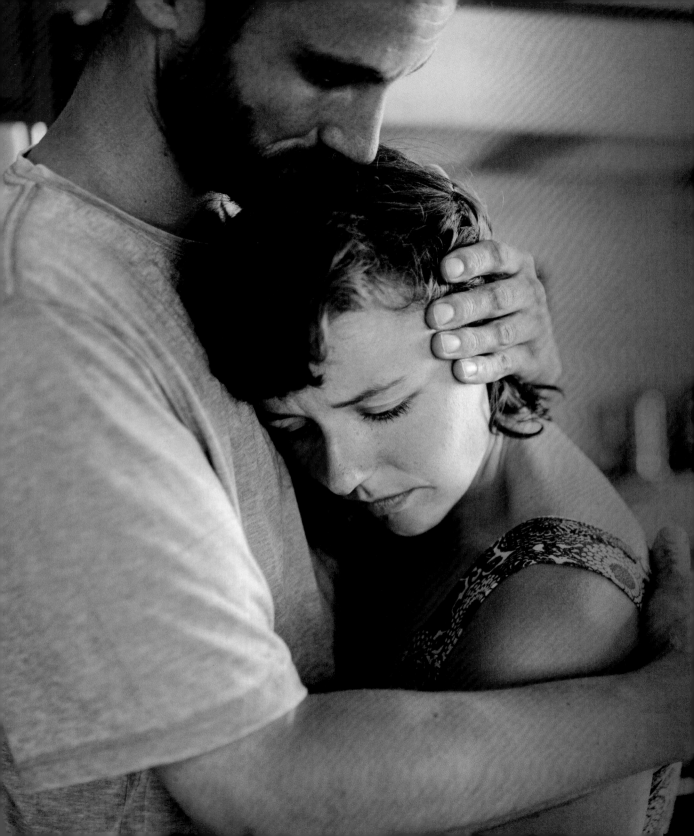

~

TEN

NAVIGATING
TIMES
OF
CHALLENGE
AND STRESS

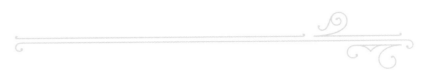

Experiencing times of challenge, stress, discomfort, and unhappiness is a normal part of life. One thing I've noticed is that when I'm experiencing challenging emotions or difficult life circumstances, I often tell myself I must have done something wrong, or that something is wrong in my life and it needs to change. One of the challenges of having freedom and choice in our lives is that if we haven't created the perfect life for ourselves where we are always happy, we can feel like we have done or are doing something wrong. This kind of thinking can lead us into reactive mode. We might choose to engage in negative self-talk, blame someone else (probably someone we love) for our problems, or rush into making changes that may only make things worse. Instead, let's explore some ways we can support ourselves as we move through the challenges.

The current of self-nourishment we began to develop in the last chapter can be a saving grace in such times. Times of challenge and stress are times when that current is particularly helpful. We can pause and recognize that we are in a moment of challenge and ask ourselves, "How can I nourish myself right now?" We can avoid spiraling into reactivity and self-protection. As we nourish and care for ourselves, we naturally slow down and create a safe place for ourselves to fully feel the emotions that are surfacing. We may be moved to reach out for support from those we love. As we move through the challenging emotions, we are able to gain perspective and see things with greater clarity. We may choose to make changes in our lives, but these changes will not be coming from desperation, but rather from a place of grounded clarity. Damiana bitters (page 252) can be just the right thing in such times, soothing us as we sink into the "bitters" and feel all that we need to feel.

Sensuality and sexuality are keys to self-nourishment, and yet they may be the furthest thing from your mind when you are stressed. For me, at least, self-nourishment often looks like gifting myself with a delicious, sensual experience: sinking into a hot Seda Blanca Bath (page 61), going for a brisk cold-water swim, taking a walk outside, wrapping myself in a soft blanket, or seeking solace in the arms of my lover. These are the kinds of activities that can help me endure the difficult emotions I need to feel, move through my pain, and reclaim my sense of equilibrium.

Times of challenge come, and they last for as long as they last. Times of comfort and joy also come and last for as long as they last. Change is the only constant in life. It is our task as humans to fully feel and enjoy the times of comfort and joy and to nourish ourselves through the times of challenge—allowing, embracing, and fully feeling both. This is a key to vibrant living.

I have learned a new definition of the word joy. I had thought joy to be rather synonymous with happiness, but it seems now to be far less vulnerable than happiness. Joy seems to be part of an unconditional wish to live, not holding back because life may not meet our preferences and expectations. Joy seems to be a function of the willingness to accept the whole, and to show up to meet with whatever is there. It has a kind of invincibility that attachment to any particular outcome would deny us. Rather than the warrior who fights toward a specific outcome and therefore is haunted by the specter of failure and disappointment, it is the lover drunk with the opportunity to love despite the possibility of loss, the player for whom playing has become more important than winning or losing.

The willingness to win or lose moves us out of an adversarial relationship to life and into a powerful kind of openness. From such a position, we can make a greater commitment to life. Not only pleasant life, or comfortable life, or our idea of life, but all life. Joy seems more closely related to aliveness than to happiness.

— Rachel Naomi Remen,
Kitchen Table Wisdom

Damiana Bitters

INGREDIENTS

2 tablespoons dried damiana leaves

4 teaspoons fresh rosemary leaves

5 dried figs

Vodka or brandy to fill a pint jar
(about 2 cups)

HERBAL TIPS

✦ Be sure the alcohol completely
covers the herbs and figs in
order to prevent mold.

PREPARATION

1 Place the figs and herbs in a pint jar.

2 Fill the jar with vodka or brandy.

3 Stir well and cover with a lid.

4 Allow the herbs to infuse into the alcohol in a jar on your
counter for 2 to 4 weeks, stirring daily for the first week.

5 Strain when the flavors have infused to your liking, reserving
the liquid and composting the herbs.

6 Add the bitters to fizzy water or a mixed drink recipe or
simply sip it straight.

7 Store the bitters in a dark bottle or dark location, and use
within a year.

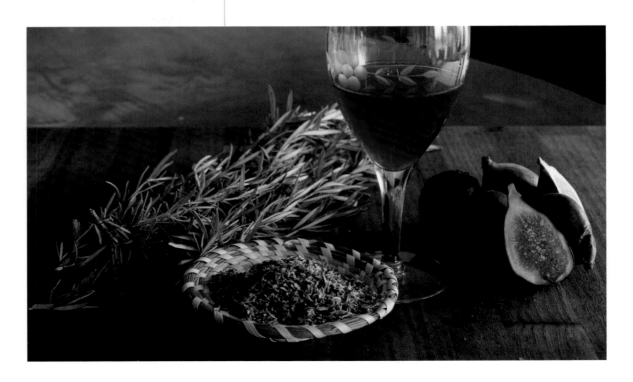

NOURISHING THROUGH CHALLENGES

Over the course of our year together, several participants faced significant life challenges, and we really noticed how the herbs were a wonderful source of nourishment and support. Angela, in particular, comes to mind. She started out the year feeling vulnerable about joining the circle. Having only recently taken the step to marry her long-time partner, she was interested in exploring some of her blocks about initiating sexuality. She felt shy in her body as a result of childhood sexual trauma and was seeking to loosen up, be more embodied, and raise her libido so she could be more available for sensual and sexual connection.

Angela had been raised within a biker gang with misogynistic attitudes, and both she and her sister suffered sexual violation as children by a neighbor living down the street. She was highly active sexually as a teenager, but there was no emotional connection involved in the interactions. They were more a way of masking her pain. With her husband, this was changing. Sex and emotion were now intertwined, and this year of focusing on herbs and eroticism took her into a place of inner turmoil as she began to face the pain of what had happened to her.

Though she is an inherently sensual being, Angela had grown up with the story that a woman who prioritized her sexuality was a bimbo or whore. She was wanting to repattern her beliefs around the erotic, and yet erotic energy felt dangerous to her. She admired others who were sexually empowered and yet had the feeling that this was not for her.

Angela was mothering two young children (ages 6 and 13). That limited her time and energy for sensual and sexual expression. In the second month of the study, it became clear that she was going to have to find a different living situation for her family. She became wrapped up in the stress of moving to a tiny home as they worked to build a yurtlike structure on their land. She mothered her family through the emotional stress of the moves while also engaging in the hard physical labor of building their new home. At the same time, she and her husband were questioning the work they were doing. She had been working at a restaurant for many years, and he was working in construction. Shifting homes and jobs are two of the most stressful things a person can face.

In her shares about the project, Angela regularly expressed gratitude for her involvement and for the support of the herbs through these challenges. Oats helped her to stay levelheaded and grounded as she grappled with the fact that her family was going to have to move. Roses helped soothe her frayed edges and remind her of the beauty of life, even in the turmoil. A friend offered a jar of hawthorn honey as they moved into the tiny home—a gift of heartsease during the transition. Kava proved an excellent remedy, working to calm her nerves, as she navigated the extreme pain from a back injury. Schisandra offered her vitality and strength and had a pronounced positive effect on her libido.

As the herbal path, coupled with the deeply connected sex with her husband, led to the surfacing of her pain from her childhood trauma, Angela began to find ways to heal. Singing offered a way to express and release some of the pain, and she engaged in grief and gratitude rituals in her local community that were powerfully healing. Though the experience was intense, she is glad to have gone into the shadowy places because the healing she has found has led her to feel increasingly embodied and empowered sexually.

During the month we experimented with damiana, Angela was going through another rough time. As she engaged with this herb, she found herself feeling more embodied, and it helped bring her and her husband together for a deeply connected lovemaking session, which felt nourishing amid the stress. During this month she had a breakthrough realization about a career shift that would require a big leap of faith but would also allow her and her husband to do the work they felt most called to do. At the end of the study, Angela said, "My life has changed on so many levels, our whole center is shifting. The herbs have supported me in so many ways through one of the hardest phases of my life. I feel systemically, the way that our lives are shifting will ultimately lead to a life with more space and health to actually cultivate sensuality and eroticism!"

Another Aphrodisiac Circle participant, Rachel, started the project just after a painful end to a long-term partnership. Her engagement exploring personal sensual pleasure during a time of acute grieving felt affirming of her body and life. And often, she found the rawness of her own experience, in contrast to the other participants' experiences of relaxing and reveling in their expanding sensuality, deeply stimulated her sense of loss and aloneness.

Staying with the project, Rachel noticed and came to appreciate the ways that the herbs supported her process of being with and moving through these emotions. For instance, she found the daily practice of drinking oatstraw and milky oats to be particularly grounding and nourishing, softening the hard edges of self-protection. Though roses were wrapped up with past memories, she found that having rose oil lovingly rubbed on her back helped her to open into the vulnerability of her situation and spurred a deeper receptivity to the wild roses in her yard. Through her experiences with roses, she came to appreciate how her involvement in the project helped her stay connected to her sensuality and be kind to herself in the midst of her grief. Schisandra was another herb that stood out for her, helping to fortify her. Finally, she found that a mix of hawthorn, milky oats, and damiana nourished her heart and nervous system while encouraging her to stay in her body and senses during this time when she might normally have shut this part of her away for quite a long time.

For me, in December of our year-long project, my mother was diagnosed with ovarian cancer. For the next six months, my siblings and I were traveling back and forth to Phoenix to be with her as she underwent surgeries, spent nearly a month in an ICU, moved to long-term care, a rehab center, home, and then back into an ICU before being placed on hospice and finally dying in June. These were an intense series of months, worrying about her, watching her struggle, trying to be supportive from many states away, flying back and forth, and ultimately letting her go and being with my family in our collective grief.

I stuck with my nourishing routines and with the project through this time. My daily nourishing herbal infusions, my exercise routines, my ocean swims, dance, my sensual and sexual connection with myself, my husband, and the natural world—these are the things that carried me through. I began to drink tulsi rose tea (Aphrodi-Tea page 21) during that time. Tulsi is an adaptogen that is adept at supporting our bodies through stress, having a calming effect on our nervous system and strengthening our confidence in ourselves to move through the challenges we are facing. Tulsi combined with the gentle love of rose was deeply soothing for me, and I will forever associate the taste and smell of this tea with my mother and the depth of my love for her.

Rebecca also went through a crisis with a parent's health during the study. As her father underwent open-heart surgery, we were working with oats, and she found that they helped her maintain her energy and balance her stress. Her dad came through the surgery well, and she found new motivation to include Golden Oat Infusions (page 37) in her daily routine once more.

In all of these situations, we were using the herbs because we were involved in this Aphrodisiac Circle. During times of stress and challenge, it can be difficult to reach for nourishing herbs or to take time for our nourishing routines. We become lost in our pain or grief. Each participant mentioned how grateful they were that they were involved in this project so that the herbs were present in their lives during the stressful times in their year. Which leads me to ask, what external structures can we set up for ourselves to remind us to reach for nourishment when we are stressed? Perhaps a little note on your bathroom mirror with the question, "How can I nourish myself today?" or an agreement with a friend to remind each other.

My current of nourishment has become very strong in my life. This is because I have chosen nourishing activities that I love doing, like dancing and ocean swimming, and because I love the way I feel in my body and in my life when I stick with them. They have become core practices, and I don't let much get in the way of me doing them. Cultivating these kinds of routines when we are feeling good can go a long way toward our being able to sink into them when we are stressed and need them most.

I remember that when my mom was finally home from rehab, she was trying to find something nourishing to eat that also tasted good to her. I suggested chicken broth with miso in it.

Set yourself up so that deep nourishment comes with ease when you need it most.

That is the most nourishing thing I can think of and so easy on our digestive systems. Well, that did not sound good to her at all. In that moment, I felt so glad that I taught my body to love chicken broth with miso and nourishing infusions. Those are my favorite things when I am sick or stressed. They taste like healing nourishment, and because I rely on them regularly in less intense times, they have become my "comfort food."

So, take a moment to consider how you can set yourself up so that deep nourishment comes with ease when you need it most. What foods or drinks would best serve as your comfort foods? Choose one or two to integrate into your diet now. Have you started to build your own current of nourishment, integrating some routines that you love? Perhaps you want to return to the exercise for building your current of nourishment from Chapter 9 and add another practice to your current. Make it something you love. Find a time to begin, and follow through.

HORMONAL CHANGES

Our current of nourishment will also be helpful when our bodies are going through hormonal changes. Puberty and menopause affect our physical bodies in ways that impact all aspects of our lives. Moving through pregnancy, childbirth, and transitioning to parenting, we experience profound changes. Each of these periods of hormonal fluctuation marks a transition from one phase of life to another—child to teen, young adult to parent, adult to elder. Both men and women experience physical and emotional challenges during these transitions.

When faced with change, and when our bodies start to behave in ways that are unfamiliar, we may find ourselves resisting, wanting to hang on to childhood or to not transition to becoming an elder. Menstruation, wet dreams, hot flashes, irregular bleeding, moodiness, cramping—all the various symptoms associated with hormonal changes will likely feel inconvenient at best and sometimes incapacitating. During these times, be

kind to yourself, ask over and over again, "How can I nourish myself right now?"

One of the phrases that stuck with me from my herbal training was, "What your body does is right." It may, at times, feel infuriating, uncomfortable, or even extremely painful, but our bodies are always doing what they need to do to maintain optimum health. They are constantly responding to external and internal factors and working to keep us alive. Our illnesses or symptoms are a result of their rebalancing efforts. Working with our bodies and nourishing ourselves through transitions, rather than resisting and just trying to suppress symptoms, can help us ride the wave of change in a healthy, vital way.

Call on the adaptogen herbs during these periods of transition. They are here to support us through times of change. They can work with our bodies in broad ways, including helping to regulate our hormone levels, boost our immune systems, and calm our nerves. Those Date Treats (page 236), a glass of Dream Cream (page 234), or your AshwaMacaMocha Shake (page 64) could be

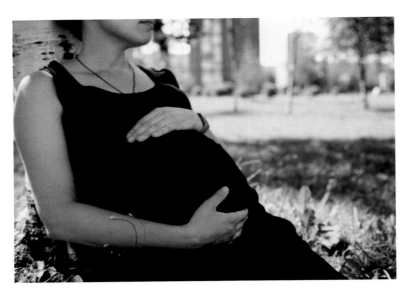

the perfect choice to help you sail through the transition with minimal symptoms and maximum ease (If you are pregnant, please skip the ashwagandha in these recipes and always check to be sure the herbs you are using are safe for you and your growing baby.) If you can increase the amount of time you spend in nourishing routines, that can be very helpful too. Giving yourself time to tune in to your body and its changing needs is important, as is time to rest and integrate the changes that are happening. Add some restorative yoga poses to your daily routine, go get a massage a couple of times a month (using your Sensations Massage Oil, page 224), or take some long walks through your neighborhood, in the forest, or on the beach. Taking quiet time in nature can be wonderfully nourishing.

SELF-COMPASSION

Self-compassion is definitely a primary tool for vital living. Sometimes stress and challenge happen due to physical changes in our bodies, but other times they happen because of a choice we've made. Perhaps we choose to change jobs, end a relationship, or move our family to a new area. Though we've made the choice out of a desire to make things better in some way, our choices can require transition periods that are often more stressful than we anticipate. When that happens, our voice of self-criticism can get very loud. You know that voice? It's usually not very kind. Mine tells me that I am stupid, not good enough, and too much. This is the voice of shame.

The truth is, that if you are vitally alive and interacting with others, you are bound to make some mistakes. Living life requires making choices, and we will not always choose perfectly. Even our best choices may have some negative consequences. Relating authentically with others requires vulnerability and risk—the vulnerability to speak the truth and risk that the truth may lead to painful feelings for ourselves or someone we love.

Our self-critical voice is desperate to keep us safe. It encourages us not to take risks so we don't have to experience unpleasant emotions. That voice will keep us small and separated from life if we let it. No one is ever successful at anything without making some mistakes along the way and experiencing some uncomfortable and unpleasant emotions. Remember Courtney Walsh's poem from Chapter 5 about being human and experiencing "messy love, sweaty love, lived through the grace of stumbling. Demonstrated through the beauty of messing up. Often." That's a good poem to read to help inspire self-compassion. Remind yourself that making imperfect choices is a part of being human.

Transforming self-criticism into self-compassion is a skill you can cultivate. Giving yourself permission to be imperfect and human is the first step. Next, ask yourself, "How can I nourish myself right now?" Giving yourself the gift of nourishment is a very compassionate act. Take a dropperful of De-stress Elixir (page 259) and settle yourself into a Seda Blanca Bath (page 61). The herbs are here, ready to support you. As you settle into the bath, you will likely begin to get some new perspective. Maybe you will remember or get some new clarity about why you made the choice you did. Perhaps this will help you settle into it despite the challenges it has created. As you settle into self-compassion, forgiveness may be able to emerge, and you may also see some action you can take to bring healing or ease to the situation.

Living life requires making choices, and we will not always choose perfectly.

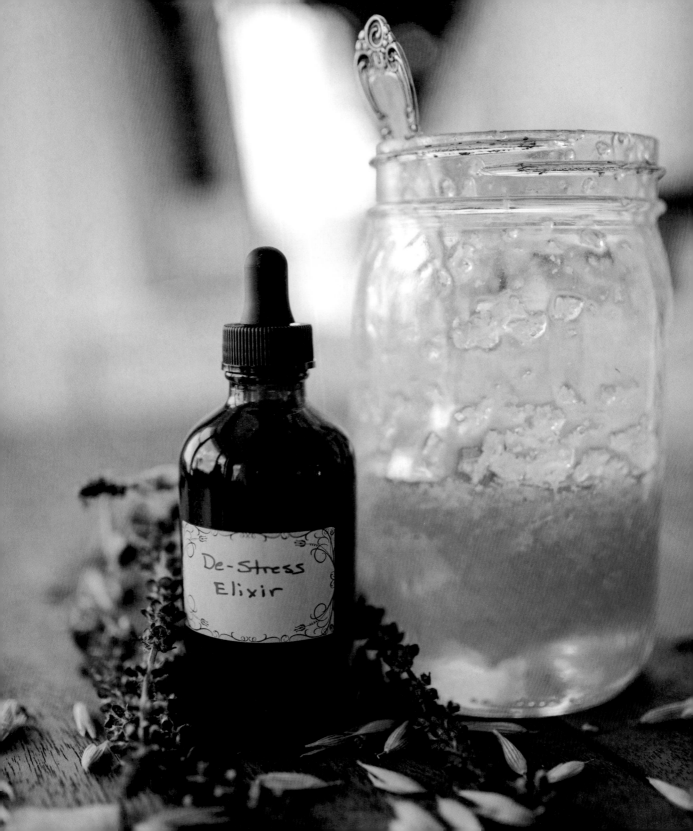

De-stress Elixir

INGREDIENTS

½ pint fresh (or ¼ pint dried) tulsi leaves

½ pint fresh milky oat tops

1 pint 100-proof vodka

Honey, to taste

HERBAL TIPS

✦ While dried plant material is often preferable when making herbal oils, fresh plant material is almost always preferable for tincture making. The water content in fresh plants will not cause a tincture to spoil (as is the danger with oils) and alcohol is very effective at extracting constituents from fresh plants. This is particularly important with milky oat tincture. You will get a much less desirable result (not milky at all) if using dried oat tops.

✦ You can also make this elixir by buying pre-made milky oat and tulsi tinctures and mixing them together with the honey.

PREPARATION

1 Prepare two separate tinctures with the tulsi and the oat tops as directed in the Soothe Tincture Recipe (page 203).

2 Mix the tinctures together in equal parts.

3 Add honey to taste (try 2 teaspoons per ounce of tincture).

4 Take by the dropperful as needed for stress.

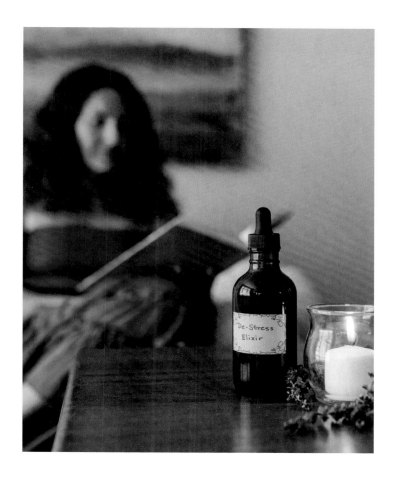

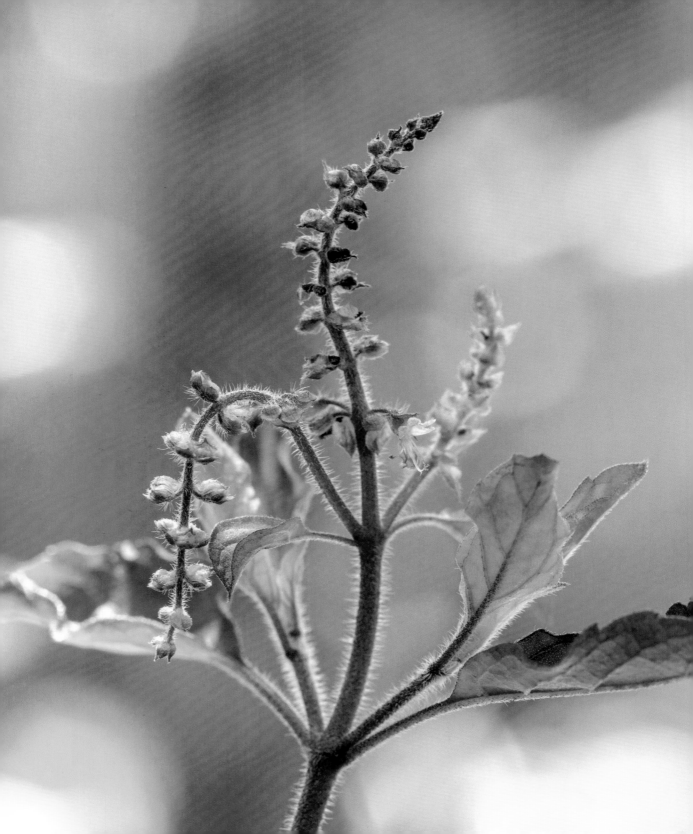

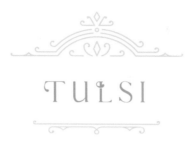

TULSI

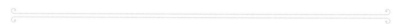

Ocimum sanctum, O. gratissimum

Mmmmm. I have fallen in love with the scent and flavor of tulsi. For me, it is soul soothing and sensually stimulating. Being enveloped in this scent when bathing with the Divinity Soak bath salt blend (page 102) is a truly divine experience, and the taste of tulsi in creations like Berry Decadence Syrup (page 238) is truly mouthwatering.

How Does Tulsi Work in Our Bodies?

Tulsi can help bring you into the present moment and expand your perspective. As a central nervous system stimulant, tulsi can help sharpen your awareness and promote clear thinking.[1] In her e-mail newsletter, Rebecca Altman of Kings Road Apothecary said it "opens us up: opens our senses to experience more deeply, opens our eyes to see things more clearly, opens our minds to understand more, and opens our hearts to help us connect more deeply to the world around us."

In *Adaptogens*, David Winston and Steven Maimes say tulsi "nourishes a person's growth to perfect health and promotes long life".[2] As an adaptogen, tulsi has a positive effect on the hypothalamic-pituitary-adrenal (HPA) axis, which helps us handle life stress with less anxiety and depression.[3] To receive these benefits, tulsi needs to be taken as a regular daily tonic for two months or more. Over time, tulsi helps us build resilience, and it is safe to take as a daily tonic for extended periods, and so can be a good ally to see us through stressful life events.

Tulsi also helps strengthen our immune systems and has been shown to be a COX-2 inhibitor, which makes it useful for inflammatory conditions. It can help prevent and address upper respiratory viruses like colds and influenza.[4] Tulsi has also been used effectively to help treat sores from herpes virus outbreaks.[5] Its high eugenol content makes it pain relieving as well.[6] It specifically helps with neuropathic pain by its antioxidant and neuroprotective actions.[7]

Tulsi is wonderful for our heart health. It slightly thins our blood, helping our circulation, and helps regulate both our blood sugar and cholesterol levels.[8] It prevents the negative effects of stress on the cardiovascular system.[9] In addition, the ursolic acid found in tulsi protects both our liver and heart cells.[10]

Tulsi has also been found to support our oral and digestive health. Tulsi tea's warming, pungent qualities can improve digestion, helping to relieve bloating, gas, and nausea.[11] Regular use of tulsi prevents stress-induced gastric ulcers and improves the mucous membranes and natural protective secretions of the gut.[12] When consistently used as a mouthwash, the extract can help reduce bacteria and plaque, and prevent bleeding gums.[13]

Within our brains, tulsi increases feel-good neurotransmitters,[14] and the rosmarinic acid within tulsi protects our neurons while also helping to relieve depression.[15] K. P. Khalsa said that tulsi "opens the heart and mind, encourages devotion and supports the energy of attachment."[16]

Herbal Shorthand

APHRODISIAC ACTIONS: *adaptogen, antidepressant, aromatic, cardiotonic, nervine, neuroprotective*

OTHER ACTIONS: *analgesic, antibacterial, antioxidant, antiviral, digestive, expectorant, antioxidant, immunomodulator*

ENERGETICS: *warming, drying*   TASTES: *pungent, sweet*

NOTABLE APHRODISIAC CONSTITUENTS: *essential oils like rosmarinic and eugenol, ursolic acid, flavonoids*

DOSAGE SUGGESTIONS: *Tulsi is a tonic herb so should be taken in medium-level dosages on a regular basis over a period of time. (A medium dose could look like several dropperfuls of tincture or a cup or two of tea throughout the day.)*

SPECIAL CONSIDERATIONS: *Tulsi has antifertility effects that make it inadvisable for couples trying to conceive and for pregnant women.*

Tulsi can help control blood sugar levels, so insulin intake may need to be adjusted for those with diabetes.

A Bit about Tulsi Plants

Tulsi or holy basil is a mint family plant in the same genus as culinary basil. The two plants are of different species, however, and are not used in the same ways. Some of the other names for this plant include "Elixir of Life," "Queen of Herbs," and "Mother Nature's Medicine." In Sanskrit, the word *tulsi* means "beyond compare." It is one of the most sacred and powerful herbs in the Ayurvedic tradition of India.[17]

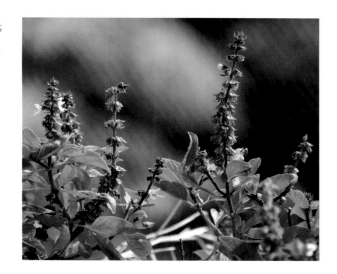

How to Use Tulsi

PARTS USED: *leaves, flowers*

TULSI TEA: *Steep 1 teaspoon of fresh (or ½ teaspoon of dry) tulsi leaves in 2 cups of boiled water for 5 to 10 minutes. It is also a wonderful addition to tea blends as in **Aphrodi-Tea (page 5)**.*

Tulsi's flavor makes it a wonderful addition to syrups and drinks like juleps or mojitos.

Tulsi's scent and relaxing qualities also make it a wonderful air freshener and bath salt.

Tulsi tincture is a simple way to get the tonic benefits of this herb, but taking it this way, you miss out on the divine smell and taste.

Participant Experiences

Those of us who experimented with tulsi found it to be a gentle, calming herb with an intoxicating scent. Michelle drank a cup of tulsi rose tea each morning (delivered in the hands of her lover) and she describes the feeling it gave her as "powerful well-being." Artemis drank it as a tea, added it to her Golden Oat Infusion, and took it in tincture form. She noticed it connecting her to her feminine/yin essence, and helping her heart feel restful and light. Tulsi helped carry me through the illness and death of my mother. Besides drinking tulsi rose tea, I have found bath blends and air fresheners with tulsi to be profoundly relaxing.

THE HEALING POWER OF SENSUALITY AND TOUCH

That Seda Blanca Bath (page 61), massage, or walk in nature are all healing, sensual experiences. Often when we are caught in a situation of stress or challenge, we are stuck in our heads amid swirling thoughts. Immersing ourselves in sensual experience can bring us out of our heads and down into our bodies. Becoming aware of the physical sensations accompanying the swirling thoughts or difficult emotions can be the beginning of moving through them in a healthy way. As you are immersed in that slippery soft bath, listening to soothing music, or walking among the trees, drinking in the smells, sights, and sounds of the forest, you can breathe into the knots in your stomach or those tight shoulder muscles. Visualize them loosening. Rub your belly, or roll your shoulders. Allowing our bodies to move in ways that release the tension can help move the energy and transform the situation. Jump up and down, splash the bath water against the wall, dance wildly, tense your muscles and then release them, and sink into deeper relaxation.

Allowing yourself to be touched, massaged, held, or even sexually stimulated can also be healing. Touch connects us not only with our own sensual body but with another. When we are feeling stressed, challenged, or ashamed, we often want to hide away by ourselves, but reaching out to a loved one can be a much more healing choice. As social beings, humans take comfort in the presence of others. It can be powerful to be witnessed in our upset and to still feel loved. Just the presence of another human body next to ours is relaxing and healing. If you have a willing partner or friend, ask for the kind of touch you want—a gentle caress,

being held tight, or a deep, muscle-relaxing massage—maybe even a hard spank or deep penetrating intercourse. Communicating clearly will help you get the touch you most need in the moment.

Touch can also bring up the need for physical emotional release. As our muscles are loosened with massage or our bodies are held in tight embrace, we may begin to cry or shake or even need to get up and stomp or wave our arms around. Being present for each other in moments like this, witnessing and holding space, is intensely vulnerable and deeply connecting. If we can trust that the sounds or movements we make are part of helping us to heal, we give one another a deeply healing gift. If you are the one providing witnessing, it is important not to take the release personally, as if you did something wrong to cause it. Check in with your partner, ask if there is anything you can do to help support their release. If you both stay with it, this kind of release can happen fairly quickly and bring deeper connection between the two of you.

Sometimes these needs for emotional release can happen unexpectedly. When Lisa and her husband were experimenting with cacao, they made a chocolate body drizzle and were enjoying licking it from each other's bodies. As their lovemaking progressed, perhaps because of the heart-opening power of cacao, Lisa found herself crying in the midst of their union. Her husband checked to be sure he hadn't done anything to hurt her, and once reassured, was able to be present and hold her until the tears passed. She could not bring words to what the tears were about, but the two trusted that the energy release would be freeing, and their connection that day felt deeply loving.

MAKING A PLEASURE PLAN

If you find yourself in a time of challenge or stress, consider making yourself a *pleasure plan*. When we feel challenged, we can go into survival mode. Every action we take feels like it needs to be about merely getting by, feeding ourselves and our families, and making sure we have a roof over our heads. We each have a different threshold for when we get triggered into this kind of state, and once we are in it, it may feel impossible to get out.

Making a pleasure plan can be a way of claiming your power to shift out of survival mode and into vital living. Many things might be part of a pleasure plan, and one key is to start very simply. Creating an elaborate plan that you don't follow through on is not helpful. Perhaps your pleasure plan is simply to begin each day with one minute of pleasurable self-touch—a foot massage or belly caress, something that feels nourishing and awakens your sensual body. Follow through on that one action for a week or a month, and notice what changes.

A pleasure plan should be highly personalized to fit your life. Perhaps you want to create a pleasure nest for yourself. Carve out a corner of space in your home or yard that is just for pleasure. Bring soft cushions and blankets and items to delight your senses, perhaps some incense to delight your sense of smell or a soft body brush to run over your skin. Gift yourself with time in your nest, even 10 minutes a week. Let

it be time out of the daily grind, time dedicated to pleasure. Time spent creating your nest and anticipating your time there may begin to shift your attention out of survival and into vital living.

Perhaps you would like to make a weekly date with yourself that is time dedicated to your pleasure. Set aside an afternoon to do something that nourishes and delights you. Maybe you will spend time in nature or go dancing or spend time with friends or have sex. Your date can be different each week, but the focus is on your pleasure. This is time for you to delight in being you, in having a sensual body, in whatever way feels good. Set aside the time and then let yourself dream into what you will do with it. When you have an idea, let yourself enjoy the anticipation of fulfilling on it. Like setting up physical space, setting aside time for pleasure shifts our attention and calls us out of stress and into gratification and vitality.

Simple rituals can also be part of your pleasure plan. Perhaps it's pausing at certain points during your day and noticing something beautiful in the world around you—really taking it in. This

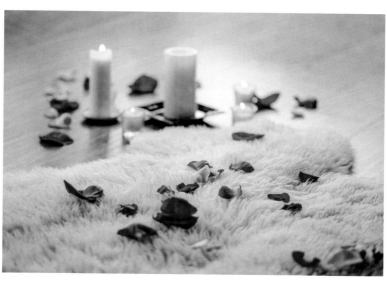

morning the full moon was framed in my kitchen window. When I caught sight of it in the midst of my morning rush, it stopped me in my tracks. I paused to take in the beauty, letting it fill me with delight. Pausing in simple moments of beauty and taking a couple of deep breaths to bring the experience into our bodies can be a beautiful simple ritual. Taking a sip of hawthorn or kava cordial after a stressful experience could be a pleasurable simple ritual as well, especially if it is done with intention and attention. Sit in a comfortable place, pour the cordial into a special glass, enjoy the smell of it, the feel of it on your tongue, the taste, the warmth that spreads through your body.

A pleasure plan is simply a way of prioritizing pleasure, setting aside time and space for sensual delight. You don't need a lot of time or a lot of space, just an intention to allow yourself to experience pleasure even in the midst of challenge. With each pleasurable experience, our bodies relax, our senses open, and new possibilities emerge. As this happens, you will likely feel inspired to create another experience for yourself, and as you dream and imagine your next pleasurable experience, your anticipation builds. As more of your attention gets drawn toward pleasure, the pleasurable part of your life will expand.

NAVIGATING TIMES WHEN SEX FEELS CHALLENGING

Sexual connection might be part of your pleasure plan. Sex can be a source of both nourishment and support, but at times sex itself can feel challenging. This can happen for all sorts of reasons. We may have a health issue connected to our genitals (like a yeast infection) that makes sex uncomfortable. We may be in a period in our lives when our libido is low. Perhaps we are in an argument with our partner and not at all interested in intimate connection, or our heart has been broken after ending a relationship. Maybe we are so busy that having time and energy for sex feels downright impossible. Whatever challenge you are facing, know that you can find your way to a place where sex is again nourishing and supportive.

The first step to getting through a challenge is turning toward it, rather than running from it or stuffing it under the rug. When we turn toward the challenge, we are able to identify it and get curious about it. This will likely require some courage, so bring along some Five Springs Tea (page 73). Once the issue is identified, we can begin to grapple with it and move through it. If it is a physical challenge we are facing, we can set ourselves on a path toward healing. If our libido is low, we can begin to explore why that might be the cause for us. Perhaps there are underlying physical or emotional factors that we can address once we identify them. Giving yourself some time and space to name and explore the issue will often help reveal a path through it. Make this time pleasurable—slip into a Divinity Soak (page 102) or sit in a cozy spot with a cup of Soft Landing Tea (page 229)and your journal.

Sometimes the path will require multiple steps before you reengage with sexual exploration. Allowing time for these steps without self-judgment is a sweet gift you can give yourself. Let your current of nourishment carry you through these times, and make a pleasure plan so you are still experiencing pleasure in all kinds of ways until healthy, nourishing sex becomes possible again.

Sometimes, it may also be a good idea to just go ahead and engage with your partner even if it is feeling challenging. Taking time to set up a space for intimacy and simply slipping between the sheets and connecting physically may ease the mental challenges that were keeping you from engaging. Or perhaps you need to make some agreements first, like setting aside your differences of opinion while you are making love or agreeing to only give each other positive feedback, setting judgments aside. Take time to pause and breathe when you need to, ask for what you need and want. Be curious about your partner's needs and wants as well. Breathe together or just hug without a sexual agenda as ways to gently attune yourselves to each other's bodies. Perhaps you will be inspired into a further dance of connection, or perhaps you will get clear that you need some time apart. There is no right or wrong outcome. The art is in being with the dance of challenge and breakthrough, breakthrough and challenge.

OPPORTUNITY FOR CULTIVATING EROTIC ENERGY FLOW

Turning toward the Challenge

1 Find a comfortable spot and take a few deep breaths.

2 Take a few sips of Five Springs Tea (page 73).

3 Practice the sensory meditation or another way of bringing yourself into a sensual, embodied place.

4 Ask yourself, "What challenge am I facing?" and allow an answer to arise.

5 Write the answer in your journal, draw, or dance it.

6 Get curious about this challenge. How long have you been experiencing it? Have you experienced it before? Is there something underlying it?

7 Write, draw, or dance it.

8 Get curious about your path forward. What would help you move through this challenge? Do you feel drawn to making a pleasure plan? Would getting back to your plan help? Maybe you just need to take some time in a warm bath to fully feel your emotions.

9 What is a first step you can take?

10 Take it.

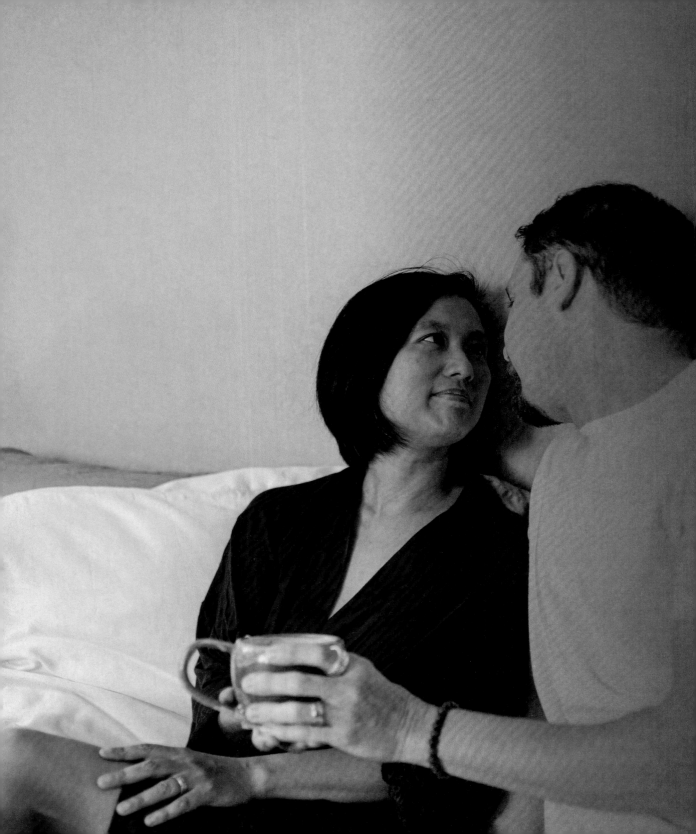

ELEVEN

HEALING

Sexual fulfillment and physical health are deeply intertwined. When we are physically healthy, we have more energy, feel more attractive, and have greater interest in and capacity for sexual interaction. Just as it is normal to go through times of stress and challenge, it is normal to go through times when our physical health is less than optimal. Fortunately, our human bodies are incredibly resilient and have a profound capacity for healing. One of the ways that herbs can act as aphrodisiacs is by helping us to heal. Whether we are dealing with a physical challenge that directly impacts our genitals, reproductive systems, or some other aspect of our body, we will feel increasingly excited to engage sexually as we heal.

As we fall in love with our bodies, honor them, and learn to listen to them, we are taking steps toward becoming empowered self-healers.

In our Western culture, we tend to respond to illness by engaging in a fight with it. We feel personally attacked by uncomfortable symptoms and might even wonder what we did wrong to deserve to feel this discomfort. We want to fight off the illness and win, making the symptoms go away as quickly as possible so we can continue with our likely overly busy lives. This can lead us to pursue remedies targeted at symptoms rather than root causes and possibly remedies that do little more than suppress symptoms, often derailing our body's natural healing responses.

As we slow down, listen to our bodies, and honor the messages they are giving us, we will likely find ourselves responding very differently to signs of illness. We will be moved to slow down even more when we feel ill. Give our bodies time to rest. Lying down with a lavender pillow over your eyes may be just the thing for that headache. Maybe you will come back to that question, "How can I nourish myself right now?" When we love our bodies and are committed to honoring them, feeling into different answers to that question is the most natural thing in the world. Sometimes simple nourishment and rest are all we need for full restoration.

We may continue to experience symptoms even after we have given ourselves the gift of rest. Recognizing that this is so, we have an opportunity to stay slowed down and get curious about what is going on. Rather than jumping reactively into choosing remedies that repress symptoms, potentially prolonging or even worsening the illness, we can start to ask ourselves questions that can help us get to the root of what is going on, and allow us to choose remedies that can truly support healing. Honoring and caring for our bodies also takes us out of shaming and blaming

ourselves or others for the fact that we are feeling this way. Honoring and nourishing energy is the antithesis of shame and blame.

HEALING SHAME

Often the first step to healing issues that have to do with our sexuality is overcoming the shame associated with the condition. Any health issue can have a layer of shame associated with it, but when the issue has to do with our genitals, there often is an extra layer of shame. We live in a time when the majority of prevailing religions see sexual desires as sinful. Denying ourselves bodily pleasures is seen as an essential component of some religions. This has led to a tremendous amount of repression and shame. Our genitals are our "private parts," and should be kept hidden and not talked about. So if our vaginas or penises are feeling itchy or dry or we are experiencing discomfort or pain during intercourse, our first response may be to just bear it, don't think too much about it, and hope it goes away on its own.

It is not my desire to argue with anyone's spiritual or religious beliefs, but I am passionate about healing and moving beyond the shame and repression associated with our sexuality and our genitals. Our desire for sexual fulfillment is a natural part of being human. I think that anyone who has experienced having a healthy flow of erotic energy in their life or a period of time when their sexual needs were fully met would agree that these periods of time were the healthiest and happiest of their lives. We are wired for sex as a means of reproduction and also as a source of pleasure, comfort, connection, confidence, and creativity.

So how do we heal shame? Well, one of the first steps is to recognize it for what it is, and question it: "My genitals are feeling itchy and uncomfortable." That's a fact. How long have you let that be true without taking action to alleviate the itch? Is it because you are experiencing some level of shame? Do you feel like you must have done something wrong to bring this condition on yourself? Or are you feeling embarrassed to talk about it? These are two (of many) ways that shame can show up. Once you've recognized that some level of shame is present, I recommend pulling out my favorite question: "How can I nourish myself right now?" Healing and moving beyond the shame is going to require courage, so taking some time to nourish yourself is a good first step. (Be sure you are choosing a nourishing activity rather than spending time numbing or avoiding the issue. Those choices are just more shame playing out.) Nourishing yourself will help you build up the life-force energy you will need for the next steps.

What are these steps? Well, first is to talk about it. Find someone you trust (a health care practitioner or a good friend) and let them know what is going on with your body and that you are concerned and want to find a way to address the issue. Choose someone who you know will listen and be willing to help you. Our shame is telling us to hide, be silent, just bear it. Talking about it will feel like the very last thing you want to do, until you find that trusted person and go for it. You will experience an instant feeling of relief, just having spoken it. Now you can begin to gather information. Listen to their ideas about what you might do next. If they don't know how to help directly, they may be able to offer information

about someone who can and will likely be able to support you as you get the help you need.

ASKING QUESTIONS TO GET TO THE ROOT OF A HEALTH ISSUE

Once we've moved past the shame and have acknowledged that we have physical issues that need attention, we will want to take steps toward healing. Before considering a remedy, it is important to engage our curiosity so that we fully understand what is happening. Then we can choose the most appropriate remedy for our unique situation.

So we've already asked, "How can I nourish myself?" Asking that question and taking action is a great place to start. When you return home from your walk, get out of the bath, or wake up from your nap, sit down with a paper and pen and consider some more questions:

1 What is the issue? Give it a name or describe it in words.

2 When did you start experiencing this issue?

3 What was going on when it started? Did any stressful events take place around the time of the onset? What was happening in the months leading up to this situation beginning for you?

4 Does there seem to be any connection with your menstrual cycle (if you have one) or any other cycles like the time of year?

5 Is there is pain associated with the issue? Rate it on a scale of 1 to 10.

6 Is there anything that eases the discomfort or that makes it worse?

7 Are there other symptoms associated with this issue? Describe any symptoms you are noticing.

8 Has this ever happened to you before? How did you handle it?

9 Consider the perspective that what your body does is right. What is right about this issue? Is it your body's response to something bigger? Is there a gift in it for you?

These questions will help you to get to the root of what is going on for you so you can choose the right remedy and course of action for your situation. If you write your answers down, you can revisit them after a period of experimenting with remedies so that you can check for healing progress. The period of time you set for a check-in will vary depending on the intensity of the issue. If it is an acute situation, you may want to check in after an hour has passed or the very next day. For less intense issues, you may check in after a week or a month. It is important to give remedies some time to work before giving up on them or switching tracks.

There are a wide variety of issues that we might want to address that are related to our sexuality, and herbs can be incredibly effective healers. While it would be wonderful to be able to simply give you a list of herbal remedies that are appropriate for a variety of ailments, it would be irresponsible of me to do so. Any time we are experiencing physical challenge, there are many factors at work, and choosing the right herbal remedy for you requires an understanding of your particular story and the underlying factors that are at play in your specific situation. What I can

do here is walk you through a couple of examples of how you can approach your health issues herbally, so that you feel empowered to utilize available resources to achieve the healing you are seeking.

First, let's look at the issue of low libido. (Step 1: Name the issue.) This is an issue that both Rebecca and Angela from the Aphrodisiac Circle identified for themselves. Steps 2 and 3 are about when the issue began and what was happening at the time. Rebecca associates her issue with the onset of perimenopause, whereas for Angela, it seems to be related to a "shyness" in her body. With this issue, it feels important to consider what a "low" libido means to you. We consider our libidos to be low because we are comparing them to some other state. For Rebecca, that would be her level of libido before perimenopause began. For Angela, it may be a comparison to what she perceives as the level of other people's libido or an imagined ideal libido. If we consider that what our bodies are doing is right, we can see that during this time of transition for Rebecca, her lower libido may be signaling her that her body is busy dealing with hormonal changes, encouraging her to deeply nourish herself and look inward toward her own needs. As Angela considers the onset of her lower libido, she may find the traumatic event in her childhood to be the root of her shyness.

When considering step 4, whether the issue is related to any cycles, Rebecca may find there are times in her perimenopausal cycle when her libido is higher than at other times. Angela may find a seasonal connection to increased lower libido that coincides with the time she experienced the sexual abuse. This information can help the women when making healing choices.

They may choose to nourish themselves more in the times when their libidos are particularly low, and prioritize pleasure in their schedules when it increases.

Moving on to step 5, the women notice that there is no physical pain associated with the low libido, but there is a level of emotional pain present. Both would like their libidos to be higher than they are and are feeling frustrated. They could rate the intensity of the emotional pain on the 1 to 10 scale to give themselves an idea of how much they want to prioritize finding a solution. Step 6 asks them to consider if there are elements that ease their discomfort or make it worse. This could be a generative exploration for each woman as she considers elements in her life that lead to sexual stimulation and elements that turn her off. An exploration of other symptoms, when consid-

Addressing a Health Issue

1 Set yourself up in a cozy spot with paper and pen, or better yet, dedicate a notebook to your health and well-being.

2 Do a sensory meditation or use another practice to bring yourself into a state of sensual embodiment.

3 From this place, consider if there is a health issue relating to your sexuality that you would like to address or consider a recently resolved issue just for the exercise.

4 Take yourself through the questions from earlier, writing your answers to each one in turn. Put a date and time at the top of the page so you can track your progress over time.

5 After answering the questions, do you have any new insights about this issue? Can you see the next step you want to take toward healing? Do you need to move through shame or gather more information, or is there a remedy you want to try?

6 Set a timeline for yourself about when you will take this next step and/or how you see yourself proceeding with a healing plan.

7 Make a commitment to yourself to revisit this page within a specific time frame (not more than a few days) to check in with your progress on your healing journey. Keep adding to your notes and making new healing commitments as you take healing steps.

ering question 7, could lead Rebecca to get really present with her perimenopausal symptoms. Angela might list the overall stress she is feeling in her life with all the changes that are going on for her—moving, new job, recent marriage. She might also list her ongoing minor colds and her back injury. Considering question 8, if this has ever happened before, Angela may be aware that this has been an issue for her as long as she can remember. Rebecca may remember other times in her life when her libido was low. Seeing that it changed with time may help her be patient with her body during this cycle.

I could imagine that this questioning process might lead both women to a new level of patience with their situation. The issue of low libido has been a gift because it was a signal from their bodies of deeper issues going on, and now they each can take the time to really address those root causes. Rebecca may choose to let her libido be low for a while as her body goes through its hormonal changes. She could focus on deep nourishment from oats or maca, take some long walks, and get in touch with herself and her needs and desires. Similarly, Angela might decide to let her libido continue to be low as she navigates all the change in her life. She noticed during our study that she really benefited from the adrenal support offered by schisandra berries, so she could make a plan to include those in her daily diet. She might also want to integrate eleuthero. As a chi builder and adaptogen, this herb could really help her be resilient through the changes and help support her energy level as she tackles all the hard work before her.

Both women may be able to recognize some elements that lead to sexual stimulation and some that turn them off. They could begin to con-sciously increase the frequency with which they experience the turn-ons and minimize the turn-offs. They can also add to their lists over time. With intention and attention, they can continue to build on the elements that support the level of libido they are seeking. These solutions are not quite as simple as making a libido boosting brew and drinking it down, but I hope you can see how following this process can lead you to effective solutions that really get to the root of the issues and help you make empowering changes in your life.

For men, low libido might be an underlying cause of erectile dysfunction, but going through this series of questions may bring other possi-bilities to light as well. By tracking when he is experiencing difficulty getting or maintaining an erection and when he started experiencing this as an issue, he can gain some valuable insights. If the difficulty is occurring during times when he is feeling particularly stressed or nervous about his sexual performance, he may get curious about how he can relieve that stress. If, on the other hand, the issue has slowly built over time, and happens regardless of external circumstances or his level of relaxation, he may want to consider what physical issues may be contributing to lack of adequate blood flow to his penis. Erectile dysfunction can indicate a buildup of plaque on the artery walls, and as such can be an early sign of heart disease. Other health issues like diabetes and endocrine disorders may also be underlying causes.[1] Seeing a trusted professional to gather information may be his next appropriate step toward healing.

Gathering information is an important step in the healing process. Answering these ques-tions for yourself is a critical part of information gathering. They will help you get very clear about your symptoms. Making a visit to your doctor, talking with friends, reading articles on the internet from reliable sources, and pulling out your favorite herbal books can all be sources of information as well. It can be very empowering to go to the doctor with this mindset. Rather than looking to your doctor for a cure, you can use the visit to further your understanding of your health situation. In the case of erectile dysfunction, tests might be able to tell you if fats and cholesterol are building up in your arteries and if your risk of heart disease is increasing. If so, the erectile dysfunction gave you the gift of alerting you to this larger issue.

Now, you can choose your own course of action, perhaps following the doctor's advice or perhaps doing your own research and choosing something different for yourself. A change in diet or exercise routine might be in order, and you might look to herbs like ginger for support. Ginger can help break down plague deposits in the arteries and increase circulation. However, if you are a person who runs hot, ginger might not be the best option for you. Considering what remedies work well in your particular body is an important part of this process. In her book *The Sexual Herbal*, Brigitte Mars recommends ashwagandha, damiana, eleuthero, fenugreek, maca, and milky oat seeds to increase sexual energy and improve circulation. In *Down There*, Susun Weed adds schisandra, oatstraw, and hawthorn to the list of useful herbs for erectile dysfunction. Perhaps, with research, one of these might be a better choice.

Once you have gathered the information, it becomes much easier to home in on a course of action. Ginger might be your perfect choice if the underlying cause is plaque buildup in the arteries, but if the underlying cause seems to be stress or anxiety, you might want to nourish with a Golden Oat Infusion (page 37) or Dream Cream (page 234) with herbs like ashwagandha and eleuthero that can help increase sexual energy while also helping your body deal with stress more easily. Adding exercise or other self-care routines might also be useful, and communicating with your partner about your struggle can be very empowering. Simply opening the conversation and exploring pleasure options like focusing on connection rather than penetration and orgasm can relieve stress and anxiety. As with shame, getting the issue out in the open and talking about it goes a long way toward relief and healing. Remember that once you have chosen a course of action, it is important to give it adequate time to work before changing course.

Healing often does not happen overnight. Being patient with ourselves and our bodies through the process can be challenging, but the deep healing that comes from following through on healing options that actually address root causes is its own reward. Remember to take time to rest and nourish yourself, to gather information, and to choose a healing path that is appropriate for your body. Give your chosen remedy time to work, to heal the root causes of your symptoms. Note and celebrate improvements and also notice if, over time, it becomes clear that a different course of action is in order. You may need to adjust dosages or choose a different set of herbs entirely. Working with a qualified clinical herbalist can be helpful and likely essential when dealing with chronic or particularly difficult health challenges. This path to healing is effective and empowering and can be followed for any issue affecting your full sexual fulfillment. It puts your health squarely in your own hands with encouragement to seek all the support you need. In the end, no one knows your body better than you, and only you have the power to make healing choices and follow through on them.

SEXUALLY TRANSMITTED INFECTIONS

When we engage intimately with one another, there is risk of passing sickness and infections between us. Taking responsibility for your own health and vitality includes acknowledging this truth, educating yourself, and taking action to protect yourself and your partner(s). Sex is a beautiful expression of love, attraction, and joy. The fact that diseases and infections can be passed between us as a result of this kind of expression can feel frustrating, sad, and downright frightening, so much so that we may want to avoid thinking about STIs altogether.

If we are to truly engage in healthy sexuality, these kinds of infections need to be openly acknowledged, freely spoken about, and understood. A little bit of knowledge goes a long way toward prevention and empowerment. The kinds of infections we can pass range in severity between something like crabs (or pubic lice), which can be irritating and cause intense itching but are fairly easy to treat, to HIV, which is life-threatening. Before engaging with a new partner, it is important to have open, honest communication about any infections they know they are carrying and for you to share honestly about any you are carrying. We should never knowingly put a lover at risk by withholding information. If

you are exploring sexually with multiple partners, you should get tested regularly for STIs, to be sure you are infection free. This is part of loving and taking care of each other.

Crabs can be spread by skin-to-skin contact, but most sexually transmitted diseases are passed through fluid exchange—saliva, sexual fluids, or blood. Condoms (both the male and female varieties) provide a great deal of protection, helping to prevent the passing of these infections during intercourse. There are also many pleasurable ways to engage in intimate exchanges that do not involve fluid exchange, including hugging, eye gazing, and massage.

One level of prevention is keeping yourself healthy and your immune system strong. Keeping your current of deep nourishment strong in your life helps keep you at maximum health so that infections are less likely to take hold in your body. This is important but does not take the place of having open communication, engaging in safe forms of intimate contact, or using condoms until you can be sure you and your partner are STI free.

If you do contract an STI, you will likely go through a series of emotions as you come to terms with this new reality. Disbelief, shame, anger, and sadness all are likely to be part of your experience. As you adjust to the news, practice the steps for healing shame (from earlier in this chapter), and educate yourself about the disease. Learn what you can do to heal it and how to protect your intimate partners. Contracting an STI does not mean the end of your sex life, but it will likely require you to make some decisions and adjustments. Your knowledge and open, immediate, and direct communication with your intimate partner(s) is essential to making certain that the disease does not spread past you.

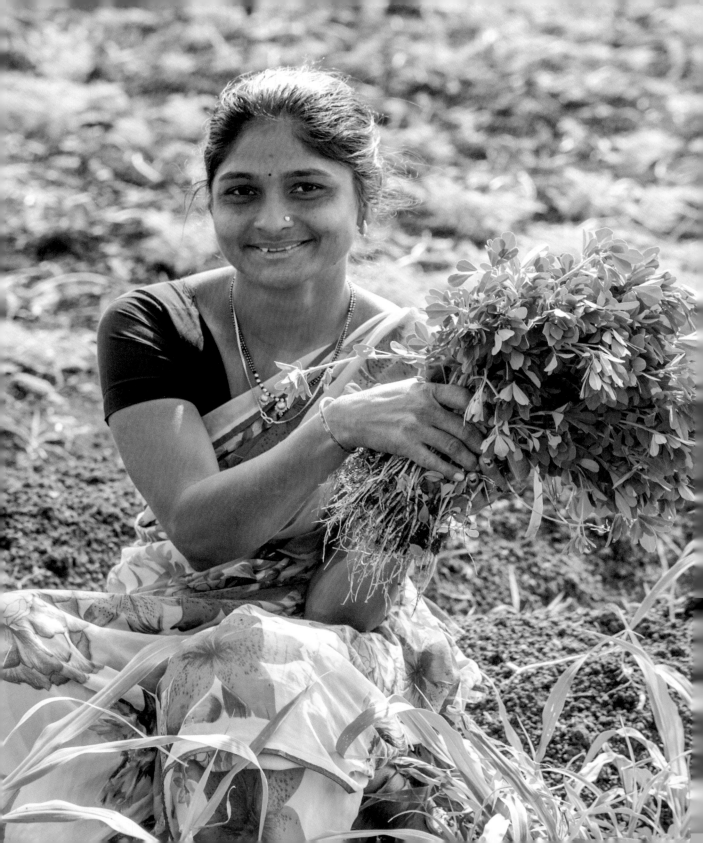

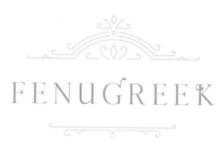

FENUGREEK

Trigonella foenum-graecum

I fell in love with fenugreek when I added the dried seeds to my herbal chai blend (Warm Nights Chai, page 187). Fenugreek added a heavenly maple syrup smell and a new depth of richness to the tea. Drinking it, I felt I was wrapped in cozy comfort. This is an herb that gently awakens our senses and encourages deep connection and snuggling.

How Do Fenugreek Seeds Work in Our Bodies?

When taken regularly over time, fenugreek is a nourishing and rejuvenating whole-body tonic.[2] Fenugreek warms and nourishes our digestive tract, lungs, kidneys, reproductive organs, glands, and immune system.[3] The seeds are high in iron, vitamins A, B1, and C, phosphates, fiber, and protein. They can help regulate our blood sugar levels and improve insulin sensitivity if we can consume as much as 15 grams per day.[4]

In addition, fenugreek seeds are calming and restorative for our nervous systems and nourishing for our hearts. Their effects on our nervous system are due to their ability to regulate sugar and lipid levels in our blood, their antioxidant qualities, and their modulating effects on our immune system. These effects can help prevent neurodegenerative diseases and depression.[5] Isovitexin, a flavonoid polyphenol compound in the seeds, both protects and strengthens our hearts.[6]

Some of the aphrodisiac actions attributed to fenugreek include sweetening the breath, increasing the libido, and improving sexual functioning. For women, fenugreek can help to normalize the menstrual cycle, stabilize our emotions, soothe our nerves, and restore energy.[7] In addition, they can increase breast size and enhance female fertility.[8] Fenugreek is also great for hormonal balancing during menopause, especially helping to inhibit the excess activity of testosterone and treat vasomotor symptoms and hot flashes.[9] They are effective for improving sexual functioning for postmenopausal women. Their high mucilage content makes them soothing for all our mucous membranes,[10] and can also help with vaginal dryness.[11]

Fenugreek seed is a uterine stimulant, so it should be avoided during pregnancy until you are ready to give birth, and then it can help bring on contractions.[12] The seeds also are rich in minerals, and drinking fenugreek tea before nursing can help with plentiful milk production.[13] So this is an herb to turn to before and after, but not during, pregnancy.

For men, fenugreek seed is a general male reproductive system tonic.[14] When taken in medicinal doses, it can improve sperm count and sperm motility, improve mental alertness and mood, and help with erectile dysfunction, premature ejaculation, impotence, and overall performance.[15]

A Bit about Fenugreek Plants

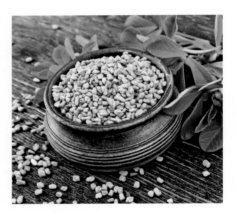

Fenugreek is native to the Mediterranean coast and is a commonly used seasoning in Egypt, India, and the Middle East. It is related to red clover and looks somewhat like it. It grows to about two feet tall and has the small, round, green leaves of a plant in the pea family. Fenugreek seeds are light brown and deeply furrowed into two unequal pieces.

Herbal Shorthand

APHRODISIAC ACTIONS: *aromatic, cardioprotective, demulcent, energizing, ease menstrual pain, hormone balancing, nutritive, reproductive system tonic, restorative*

OTHER ACTIONS: *antioxidant, anti-inflammatory, digestive tonic, expectorant, galactagogue (stimulates lactation), immunomodulatory, uterine stimulant*

ENERGETICS: *warming, moistening*   TASTES: *bitter*

CONSTITUENTS: *flavonoid polyphenol compounds such as rhaponticin and isovitexin, iron, phosphates, fiber, and protein*

DOSAGE SUGGESTIONS: *Fenugreek is a tonic herb and should be taken regularly in medium dosages for a specific period of time. A tonic dose could look like 1 to 2 capsules or a dropperful of tincture 3 times daily or a daily cup of tea (1 tablespoon of seeds in 1 pint of water steeped for 10 minutes).*

SPECIAL CONSIDERATIONS: *Avoid taking fenugreek during pregnancy as it is a uterine stimulant. It can affect blood sugar levels.*

How to Use Fenugreek

PARTS USED: *seed and fresh leaves*

To access the tonic effects of this herb, it is important to integrate it into your life on a regular basis over an extended period of time (try one month)

Fenugreek Tea: 1 tablespoon seeds in 1 cup of hot water steeped for 10 minutes. You can strain the seeds or eat them as you drink. Add cream and honey to taste.

Add seeds to soups, stews, or stir-fries.

Add fresh leaves to dishes as a garnish near the end of the cooking time.

*Add ground seeds as an ingredient in baked treats like **Golden Sunrise Cake (page 296)** and **Bitter Maple Oat Squares (page 306)**.*

Many who have consumed fenugreek know about the sweet maple smell that comes from this plant. One study notes the major compound responsible for this is 2,5-dimethylpyrazine.[16] The smell and sometimes bitter taste can be modified by adding mint leaves to any fenugreek preparation.[17]

Participant Experiences

Participants who connected with this herb found that they felt an increased desire for snuggling. Several of the women reported increased breast and overall body sensitivity. For one, this led to vulnerable, sensual lovemaking. Sarah was drinking it as a strong tea with cream and honey and wrote, "I like the tingling taste and it relaxes my mind similar to damiana. I feel all warm and sensitive in my breasts and skin."

Herbs can offer healing and support for STIs. Continuing with herbal infusions and other nourishing practices will be important. Dream Cream adaptogen smoothies (page 234) or Date Treats (page 236) would be a good addition to your diet as you navigate this period of stress and change. Maybe you will want to make yourself an herbal spa and pamper yourself so you remember that you can still experience all sorts of sensual pleasure. For remedies specific to your situation, consult a local clinical herbalist or your doctor or naturopath to gather information. Choose a course of action that feels right to you, and give it time to work. Give yourself time to adjust to your new reality, staying present to any gifts (insights or changes in behavior, etc.) that may emerge along the way.

THE HEALING POWER OF PLEASURE AND SEXUALITY

When faced with any kind of physical or emotional challenge, pleasure can be a healing balm. Pleasure is available to anyone anywhere. We need only turn our attention toward it. It can be as simple as pausing and running our finger slowly over our lips, tuning in to the exquisite feel of slow, gentle touch on this sensitive part of our body. Or we can go outside and lie in the sun, feeling the warmth sink through our skin, warming our very core. Pleasure is free and available every minute of every day, and feeling it stimulates the pineal gland to release chemicals like dopamine that help make us feel good. As we reach for and find pleasure in these simple acts, our pain may become more bearable and anxiety and depression can give way to gratitude and increased vitality. As we turn again and again toward pleasure, we increase the flow of erotic energy in our lives, energy that can be channeled into healing.

Sex itself can be a healing force. Feeling erotic energy moving in us is, like oxygen or food, an element we need to feel vital and alive. Erotic energy is powerful energy. Selah Martha, a therapist and former co-director of the Body Electric School, explains that this energy is powerful because it has charge, momentum, and force; it is energy in motion. I interviewed Selah for this section and am excited to be able to share some of her wisdom here. This idea that sex has the power to heal and transform has been one of the discoveries that has fascinated me most on my own exploration of sexuality.

Selah describes sexual energy as "strong water that can open doors and move things around" inside of us. Trauma or unprocessed emotions can get stuck in our muscles and energetic body systems. During sex, anything that has become stuck can get released as the wave of sexual energy moves through us. If we are willing to work with the energies that are released, being curious and giving ourselves time and space to fully feel and experience what comes up, we open to the real possibility of transformation and deep, core-level healing. Breath is a primary tool to facilitate this kind of healing. Pausing and breathing deeply together can be stabilizing as stuck energy begins to move. Quicker breathing, coupled with physical movement like kicking or pushing against something with your feet, can help to move the energy out of your body.

This kind of healing happens on a nonverbal level, in the arena beyond intellect and words.

Selah explains that this kind of healing can reach levels that are hard to get to with the tools our culture more commonly turns to—tools of the mind like thinking, discernment, and categorizing, or even tools of the heart that work on an emotional level. This kind of healing is working at a primal level, deep down in the roots of our humanity, in our lower energy centers or chakras. Healing at this core level can impact our lives in profound ways, helping to clear up physical ailments or allowing us to see new possibilities within our relationships and our lives. This kind of healing may be able to happen within our intimate relationships, but there is also support available from professionals like sexological body workers.

Angela's story illuminates how this kind of healing can happen. As she engaged sexually with her husband, pain from her past sexual trauma began to rise up to be healed. As he remained present and patient with her through the year, she engaged with nourishing and healing herbs and with song and grief rituals. Slowly, over time, this helped her become increasingly embodied and sexually empowered. Golden Oat Infusions (page 37) and adaptogens like ashwagandha and tulsi can be helpful allies through these kinds of healing processes as they help calm our nervous systems and support us through change. They can be useful for our partners as well while they build the resilience and agility to remain present with us through our healing.

Selah quotes one of her colleagues, Alex Jade, as saying that healing sexual experiences are "the application of love on the body." This application of love slowly, over time, can be a significant healing force, moving us toward the kind of sexual fulfillment and vital living we crave.

CULTURAL HEALING FOR HEALTHY SEXUALITY

One of my core questions as I began this book project was, "How would healthy sexuality look and feel?" Our culture is plagued by such sexual repression and shame that the answer to this question is not obvious. To truly find out what it will look and feel like, we need to do some deep healing. One aspect of this is healing our shame around our sexuality, which we touched on earlier in this chapter.

There are many ways that this shame may show up for us. One woman I spoke with connected shame to these kinds of questions about rape: "Did I ask for it? Was I leading him on?" This kind of shame can lead women to overeat, dress in clothes that don't show off their bodies, or put their sexual nature on a shelf and not engage with it at all. Consent violations can lead people of all genders to become afraid and shameful about their sexuality—about wanting sex or looking sexy. This can lead us to being hesitant to initiate even simple connections with each other (such as asking someone to dance) and can keep us from getting our needs for intimacy and sexual fulfillment met. This can spiral into desperation and people getting their needs met in unhealthy ways (such as violating the consent of another).

We may also feel shame about our sexual orientation or desires. Shame about something we did or did not do in our interactions with another. Shame about how our bodies look. The list goes on . . . and on . . . and on. Do you know how it feels in your body? Take a deep breath and consider that question. How does shame show up physically in your unique body? What actions do you impulsively want to take when you feel it?

I know these feelings well. I dance with shame often. For me it can feel like heat rising through me, like a swirling mind, an inability to focus, knots in my stomach, and energy running through my nervous system. It can lead me to want to hide or to seek validation or to try to do something to quickly fix or change the situation. One thing I've found is that when I act from shame, my actions never make things better but rather only add to the chaos. So, taking that time to nourish myself and to talk to someone I trust have proved essential to truly healing and moving beyond the shame.

The steps I discussed earlier in this chapter about shame are, in my experience, invaluable. As we talk about the situation, the shame, the consent violations—new ways of being with one another emerge. We begin to feel proud of our sexual orientation, how we look, and who we are. We develop skills to take responsibility for our actions and hold others accountable. We build vocabulary and habits that reflect our expectation of respect and consent in our interactions with others. We learn that we can speak up and help each other learn these new ways.

As we heal and move beyond shame, whole new possibilities emerge.

Imagine a consent-based culture where we feel safe and confident—one where we could fully enjoy looking sexy and having a wide range of sexual desires. Imagine being able to be sexually fulfilled while also being deeply spiritual. Imagine the possibility of being able to easily get the skilled, effective help we need to heal any physical, emotional, or psychological issues that are in the way of sex being a completely ecstatic experience.

HEALING FROM POWER-OVER DYNAMICS

This is another area where significant healing needs to happen if we are to experience truly healthy sexuality. The genuine, mutual consent that underlies healthy sexuality is not possible when power-over dynamics are at play. We are blessed to be living in a time when people are questioning the health of any one group of people having power over others. For thousands of years we have been living in a patriarchal culture where men have been in power over women. This dynamic has been damaging for both genders. It has stifled women and put undue pressure and responsibility on men. Culturally, we have identified with different racial, religious, or political groups and fought for power over one another. We have seen ourselves, humans, as the dominant species on earth with power over other species and the earth itself.

Power-over dynamics have impacted all of life on earth in terrifying ways, wiping out whole species, laying waste to whole ecosystems, and instilling deep trauma wounds in people. Actions like the witch burnings and the lynching of Black men are horrific examples of what we have done to one another in the name of power. There are a million appalling actions, large and small, that have instilled trauma that keeps us from relating in healthy ways. If we want to experience truly healthy sexuality, we must provide each other with the holding, compassion, and empathy that allow us to heal from the impacts these kinds of actions have wrought.

As we pursue this healing and let go of power-over dynamics, all sorts of new opportunities emerge. As individual people stand in their own personal power, not defined by gender or race, and begin to cooperate, there is the possibility for a great weaving of ideas and actions. We can move from a time focused on independence and domination to a time of interdependence and reciprocity. Strong masculine principles like logic, intellect, assertiveness, and doing can weave in with strong feminine principles like intuition, nurturing, allowing, and being. We can benefit from the skills, creativity, and gifts of people from diverse cultures and backgrounds and even from other species with whom we share the earth.

As always, the herbs are here to support us through the changes.

Sexual intercourse is a physical merging of different people with different energies. When both are in their personal power and it is a fully consensual merging, it becomes a living example of the beauty of what can happen when we engage in *power-with* dynamics. People reach heightened states of pleasure and ecstasy and deep, core-level healing occurs.

When cultures, genders, races, and species work together, respecting each other's power and gifts (even when we don't fully understand them), that is when we experience our true potential for vital living. We can see this happening right now in many areas of our culture. Perhaps the best living examples are in Native cultures and on per-

maculture farms across the earth where diverse people are working with nature in reciprocal and creative ways. They are contributing to the health and vitality of the land, other species, and themselves in turn. People are also exploring power-with dynamics in intentional communities, in relationships, in artistic performances, and even in some corporate cultures. Brené Brown's book *Dare to Lead* gives a template for integrating these dynamics into successful workplace cultures. This is the kind of culture I am developing at LearningHerbs, the company I co-own with my husband, John.

All of these examples are indicative of the positive shift that is happening toward health and vitality. The healing of power-over dynamics begins as we embrace our interdependence and work cooperatively to restore, replenish, and creatively build a new kind of future together. It happens slowly over time as we engage in mutually consensual sexual relations and build healthy relationships. As always, the herbs are here to support us through the changes. Dream Cream adaptogen smoothies (page 234) and nourishing infusions will help provide the solid foundation of nourishment, strength, and resilience needed for this transition. Kava, oats, and tulsi can help us deal with our stress as we navigate the changes. Schisandra can give us courage and help us stand in our power. Hawthorn and rose will protect our hearts while helping us to keep them open. Ultimately, the transition is the healing.

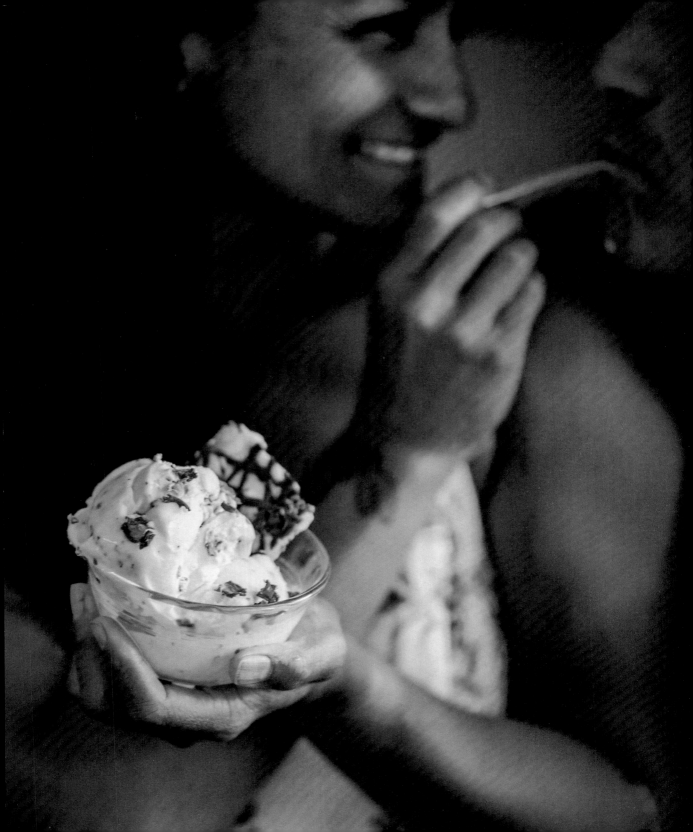

TWELVE

SHARING

DELICIOUS

DELICACIES

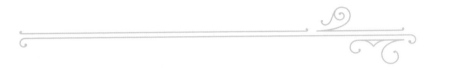

Over the course of this aphrodisiac journey together, we have explored many ways that herbs can help support our sexual healing, empowerment, and enjoyment. We've explored the power of loving ourselves, being tuned in to our bodies, and being in healthy relationship with each other. Now, let's just drop into pure pleasure. Preparing, serving, and enjoying delicious herbal delicacies can allow us to spoil ourselves and our lovers while delighting all of our senses.

Imagine getting a call from your sweetheart, inviting you to an evening of sensual decadence. Their rose wine is ready, and they would like to share it with you on their cozy couch in front of the fire. Or perhaps it is summer, and they entice you with homemade coconut rose ice cream drizzled in Berry Decadence Syrup (page 238). What about an evening of feeding each other chocolate-covered strawberries?

Holy moly, just reading these words makes my mouth water with anticipation. Imagining the night that could follow makes my pussy juices flow. Add to that all that we have learned about how these herbs act in our bodies and about healthy sexual interactions, and the true potential of aphrodisiac treats begins to become clear. The treats on the pages that follow are more than the love potion libido boosters you may have imagined aphrodisiacs to be when you picked up this book. They are herbal support for decadent pleasure and deep sexual fulfillment.

You can engage with the recipes on the pages that follow to create aphrodisiac treats for yourself or to share with a lover. Either way, you will be increasing the flow of erotic energy in your life, especially if you engage as we did in Chapter 1, making the preparation an aphrodisiac experience. Remember to center yourself with an erotic intention that you add as an ingredient, stirring it in with the herbs. Bring your full attention to the process of making the treat, engaging your senses so that you enjoy maximum sensual stimulation from working with the different ingredients. If it is possible to gather the herbs yourself, enjoy the stimulation of being out in nature—the warmth of the sun on your skin; the smell of the earth, flowers, and leaves around you; the sound of birdsong. Move slowly, drinking in the sensation. Each ingredient is worthy of your attention. Smell, taste, feel, listen, and fully enjoy the visual beauty of each one, the mix of them together, and the finished delicacy you create.

Perhaps there is an added thrill to be working with an herb or ingredient that you don't know well, one that feels exotic. In general, I am an herbalist who allies mostly with the plants that grow around me, but when it comes to sexuality and pleasure, I do think there is also turn-on and allure in trying something exotic. I encourage you to be playful and experiment. Let yourself get to know and enjoy an herb or ingredient from a faraway land. Savor the use of them as the gifts they are, giving thanks for the faraway hands that tended the plants and the resources involved in bringing them to your doorstep.

Seductive serving of your treats can add to their aphrodisiac quality as well. Use your skills developed in Chapters 2 and 4 to create an erotic environment. Bring in elements that you know will add pleasure to the experience. Candlelight? Flowers? Consider what you want to wear. What can you put on that arouses you and/or your partner? What scents do you want to add on your body or in the room? It is equally wonderful to treat your partner and/or yourself. Either way, set aside time so you can go slow and be fully present. If you are inviting your lover, consider what stages you want to share with them. Do you want them to come for just the dipping of the strawberries or for the mixing of the chocolate sauce? Perhaps you will gather the hawthorn flowers for the soda together and share in the anticipation during the fermentation process. Anticipation, delighting in sensual experiences, and seductive flirtation throughout the process all build erotic energy, keeping the flow strong in your life. Remember this flow can be source energy for confidence and creativity. My wish for you is that creating and enjoying these treats tap you in and bring you fully *alive*.

Hawthorn Flower Soda

INGREDIENTS

3 cups hawthorn flowers (Use fresh flowers if possible. You can include some leaves as well)

1 cup granulated sugar

⅛ teaspoon champagne yeast

PREPARATION

1 Bring 5 cups of water to a boil in a saucepan, then remove it from the heat.

2 Dissolve the sugar in the hot water.

3 Add hawthorn flowers to the water. Stir, then cover and let it steep for 4 hours.

4 Strain the liquid into a half-gallon jar, and add enough water to fill the jar. Compost the flowers.

5 When the mixture is at room temperature, add ⅛ teaspoon champagne yeast, and stir well.

6 Cover the jar with cheesecloth or a dish towel.

7 Leave the jar on the counter for 2 days, stirring daily.

8 Pour the liquid into clean plastic soda bottles with screw-on lids or clean glass swing-top bottles.

9 Store bottles at room temperature for 1 to 3 days. (Warning: if the pressure builds too much, glass bottles can explode—I like to put mine in a cooler so they are out of direct sunlight and are also in a contained space. Plastic bottles will become firm as pressure builds and can act as tester bottles in this way. You can also release the top from a swing-top bottle daily to check for fizz.)

10 When the soda is fizzy, transfer the bottle(s) to the refrigerator.

11 Drink the soda within 2 weeks. (Fermentation will continue, though slower, when the sodas are chilled. To prevent exploding bottles, do not forget your soda in the back of the fridge!)

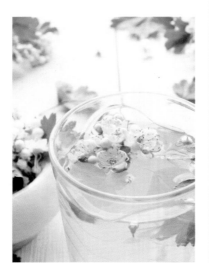

Rose Petal Wine

Emily Han

INGREDIENTS

2 cups fresh rose petals
(or 1 cup dried)

¼ cup Cognac or Cognac-
style brandy

1 bottle (3 ¼ cups) dry white wine

¼ cup mild honey

PREPARATION

1 If using fresh rose petals, pat them with a clean, dry towel to remove any moisture.

2 Put petals in a quart jar, and pour the Cognac and wine over top of them.

3 Cover the jar tightly, and give it a good shake to combine.

4 Refrigerate the jar for 1 week.

5 Strain the mixture through a fine mesh strainer, and discard the solids.

6 Put the strained wine and honey in a clean jar. Cover the jar tightly, and give it a good shake.

7 Age the strained wine for at least one more week before serving. Serve chilled.

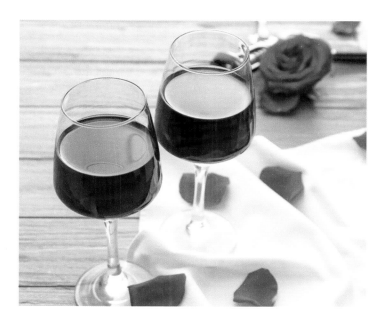

Sweetheart Shrub

INGREDIENTS

1 cup fresh rose petals
(or ½ cup dried)

1 cup fresh hawthorn flowers
(or ½ cup dried)

1 cup fresh or frozen strawberries

½ cup honey

About 1½ cups white wine vinegar

PREPARATION

1 Put flowers into a pint jar.

2 Add ½ cup honey to the jar.

3 Pour vinegar over the flowers to fill the jar and stir.

4 Cap with a plastic lid (vinegar will corrode a metal canning jar lid and destroy the drink).

5 Let this infuse on the counter for a week, stirring daily.

6 Strain, reserving the liquid and composting the flowers.

7 Add 1 cup of chopped strawberries to the infused vinegar and allow the mixture to infuse on the counter for another week, stirring daily.

8 Strain, reserving the liquid and composting the strawberries.

9 To serve, add 1 to 2 tablespoons of shrub to 8 ounces of water or sparkling water.

10 Store the shrub in the refrigerator for up to 6 months.

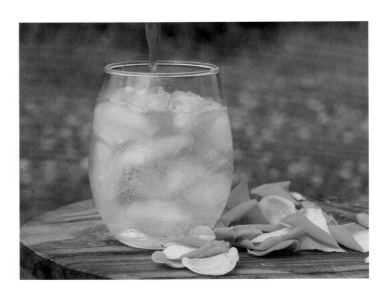

Love Drunk
Drinking Chocolate

This is a super thick drinking chocolate. You can adjust the thickness according to your taste by adding more or less water or adding half-and-half instead of cream.

INGREDIENTS

2 tablespoons coconut oil

3 ounces dark chocolate (your favorite chocolate bar, 70% or higher)

½ cup heavy whipping cream, coconut cream, or nondairy creamer

Pinch of salt

Pinch of cinnamon or cayenne (optional)

PREPARATION

1 In a heavy-bottomed saucepan, melt the coconut oil and chocolate on low heat, whisking periodically until it is well combined and smooth.

2 Add ¼ cup of water, ½ cup of creamer, and a pinch of salt.

3 Stir the mixture until combined and even. If at any point the chocolate is sticking to the bottom of the pan, remove the pan from the heat immediately and keep whisking.

4 For some added flavor or spice, try adding a pinch of cinnamon or cayenne.

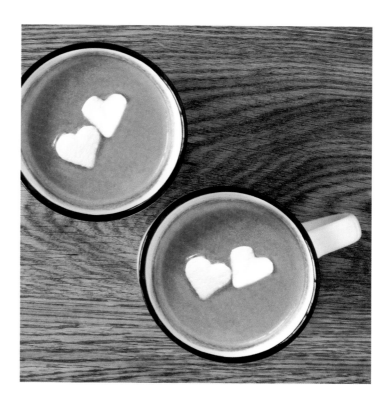

Coconut Rose Bark

Hanna Nicole

INGREDIENTS

Coconut oil to grease the pan

1 cup melted cacao butter (roughly 1½ cups unmelted)

½ cup maple syrup

1 cup cashew butter (roughly 2 cups raw cashews, blended till smooth)

1 teaspoon ground cardamom

¼ teaspoon salt

2 tablespoons cacao nibs

3 tablespoons dried rose petals, lightly crushed

3 tablespoons coconut flakes

PREPARATION

1 Grease an 8 x 8-inch or 8 x 9-inch baking dish with a little coconut oil, then press a piece of parchment paper down onto the oil to hold it in place.

2 Melt cacao butter using a double boiler or low heat on the stovetop. Remove the double boiler from the heat.

3 Add maple syrup, cashew butter, cardamom, and salt to the cacao butter and whisk together.

4 Add cacao nibs, rose petals, and coconut flakes. Stir to evenly distribute them through the mix.

5 Pour the mixture into the parchment-lined baking dish, and spread it evenly across the bottom. You can vary the thickness of your bark by pouring in just the amount you would like, using a larger pan or multiple pans for a thinner bark.

6 Transfer the dish into the freezer for 40 minutes, until hardened.

7 Cut the bark with a knife or break into pieces for serving.

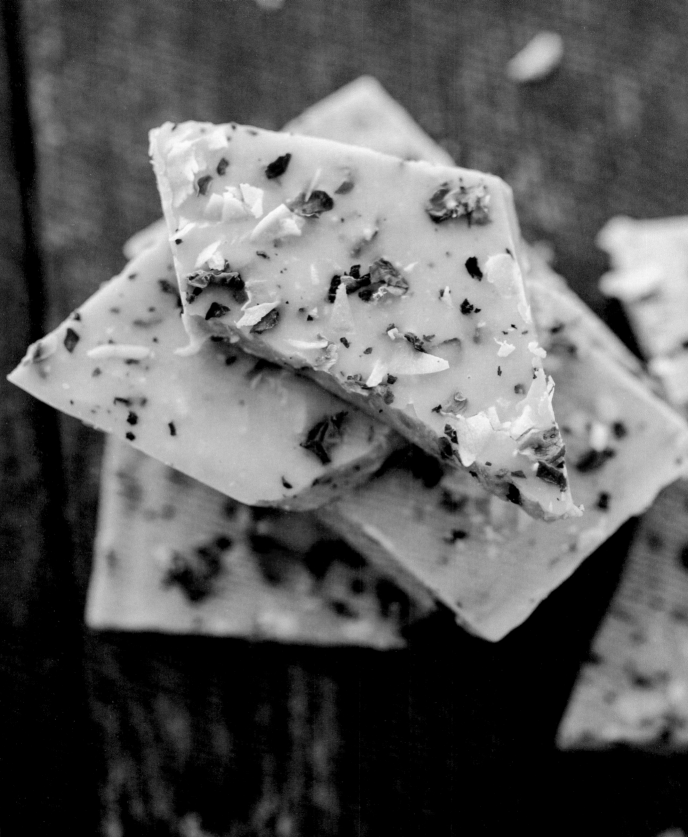

Golden Sunrise Cake

Hanna Nicole

INGREDIENTS

3 tablespoons fenugreek seeds (grind 1 tablespoon into powder in a coffee grinder)

1 to 2 tablespoons of tahini (enough to grease the inside of the cake pan well)

1 cup coconut sugar

Juice from half a lemon (straining seeds out) (2 tablespoons)

Zest of one lemon

¼ teaspoon almond extract

¼ teaspoon vanilla extract

3 cups almond flour

1 tablespoon turmeric powder

1 ½ teaspoons baking powder

¼ teaspoon salt (or a touch more)

½ cup coconut oil (melted)

½ cup butter (melted)

¼ cup pistachios, chopped

PREPARATION

1 Boil ¾ cup of water, and then place 2 tablespoons of the fenugreek seeds in a bowl and pour the boiling water over top. Let the seeds soak for 10 minutes.

2 While the seeds are soaking, grease a 9-inch cake pan, or a parchment-lined springform pan with tahini.

3 Once the fenugreek has finished soaking, strain the water into a bowl, and compost seeds.

4 Preheat the oven to 350 degrees F.

5 Add coconut sugar, lemon juice and zest, almond extract, and vanilla extract to the boiled fenugreek water, then whisk until completely dissolved, and set aside.

6 If you haven't already, place the final tablespoon of fenugreek seeds in a coffee grinder and blend until powdery.

7 Mix almond flour, turmeric, baking powder, fenugreek powder, and salt in a bowl until well blended. Use a fork to press out any clumps.

8 Create a hole in the center of the dry ingredients and pour in your melted butter and oil. Mix well.

9 Once oil and dry ingredients are completely combined, slowly add the water mixture, ¼ cup at a time, and whisk until the consistency resembles yogurt (loose but not runny).

10 Pour the batter into your tahini-greased cake pan, and sprinkle with pistachios.

11 Bake for 30 to 35 minutes until the top is browned and a toothpick poked into the center comes out clean. (Pulling out the cake as soon as it's done and then letting it cool will give you a moist texture that is ideal for this recipe.)

12 Allow the cake to cool almost entirely, and serve with chilled whipped cream or drizzle with honey for added sweetness.

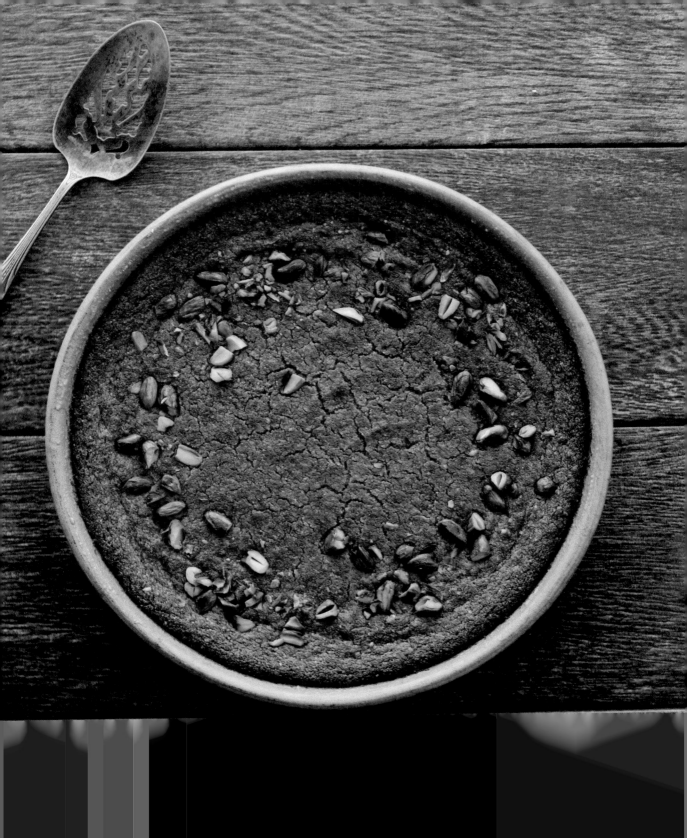

Dusty Rose Petal Truffles

Rosalee de la Forêt

INGREDIENTS

8 ounces dark chocolate

2 teaspoons vanilla extract

1 teaspoon cinnamon

½ teaspoon nutmeg

⅔ cup full-fat coconut milk

powdered cacao and powdered roses for rolling

PREPARATION

1 Begin by chopping or pounding the chocolate into pea-sized pieces.

2 Place pieces into a medium-sized bowl along with the vanilla, powdered cinnamon, and nutmeg.

3 Warm the coconut milk slowly until it just starts to simmer.

4 Pour this immediately into the bowl with the chocolate.

5 Let this mixture stand for one minute, and stir with a whisk until the chocolate is melted and has a smooth consistency. (Note: Most of the time this process works great. If the chocolate does not melt fully, place the mixture in a double boiler and heat slowly until melted.)

6 Cool the truffle sauce to a semi-hard consistency in the fridge or freezer and check it frequently. It needs to be soft enough to form into balls, yet hard enough to roll without falling apart.

7 Scoop the mixture into bite-sized pieces and roll it into balls.

8 Roll the balls in powdered cacao or rose petals.

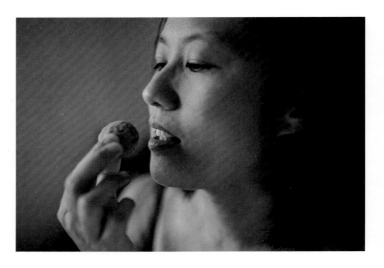

Chocolate-Covered Strawberries

INGREDIENTS

24 strawberries (approximately)

1 cup cacao butter

5 drops liquid monk fruit or ¼ cup honey

½ teaspoon vanilla extract

½ cup cacao powder

2 teaspoons coconut oil

Cacao nibs and/or coarse sea salt for sprinkling (optional)

PREPARATION

1 Place the strawberries in the freezer while you complete the next couple of steps.

2 Melt the cacao butter slowly in a double boiler.

3 When melted completely, add the monk fruit or honey and vanilla, and whisk until evenly combined.

4 Pour 2-3 tablespoons of this mixture out into a small pot, and set aside for later.

5 Add the cacao powder and coconut oil to the double boiler, remove it from the heat, and stir until melted and combined.

6 Let the mixture cool in the double boiler, off the heat for 5 to 10 minutes so the cacao can thicken.

7 Pull the strawberries from the freezer and dip them one at a time into the melted chocolate.

8 Place the dipped strawberries neatly on a flat surface (plate or board) and return them to the freezer. If you like a thin layer of chocolate on your berries, then one dip should be fine. If you like the chocolate layer to be nice and thick, repeat this process a couple of times, making sure to freeze your berries for about 10 minutes between dipping so the previous chocolate layer is nice and hard before adding the next.

8 When you have finished layering with dark chocolate and you have returned the berries to the freezer for their final 10 minutes, warm the melted cacao butter that you saved from earlier on the stove, until it is just melted again.

9 When the cacao butter is melted, scoop some of the butter up using a spoon and drizzle your dark chocolate–covered strawberries with diagonal lines.

10 Sprinkle with cacao nibs and/or salt, or enjoy as they are.

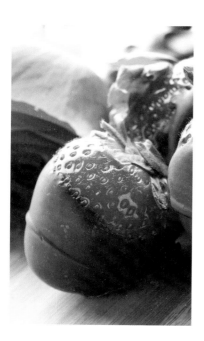

Eros Cream

Hanna Nicole

INGREDIENTS

2 cans full-fat coconut milk

½ cup honey (or ½ cup rose honey)

¼ cup rose water

Pinch of salt

10 drops liquid (or ¼ teaspoon powdered) monk fruit (optional)

1 teaspoon vanilla extract

2 teaspoons orange extract

1 small handful of fresh or dried rose petals

¼ cup chocolate sauce (see recipe for Chocolate Body Drizzle, page 173)

PREPARATION

1 First, if you are using an ice cream machine, make sure you have frozen the inner basket for at least 24 hours (ideally 2 days) beforehand.

2 In a medium-sized bowl, empty both cans of coconut milk and stir gently until evenly combined.

3 Combine honey and rose water in a saucepan over low heat. As soon as the honey is loose and the rose water is well combined, remove from heat.

4 Add salt, monk fruit, vanilla extract, and orange extract to the honey mixture. Whisk until combined and set aside to cool slightly.

5 When the honey is cool but not stiff, add it to the coconut milk, stirring it in slowly.

6 Place the mixture of coconut milk and honey into the fridge for 2 hours or freezer for 40 minutes.

7 Get your ice cream machine ready to go. Turn it on and get it spinning before you pour your honey and coconut mixture in. When you do, pour slowly and use a spatula to get everything out of the bowl.

8 Let the mixture churn for 30 to 40 minutes or until your ice cream has set. Once the ice cream begins to harden, slowly drop your rose petals into the mixture (and if you would rather have your chocolate ribboned throughout the ice cream instead of on top, now is the time to add it. The chocolate should be loose but not hot. And poured in slowly).

9 When the ice cream is very thick and your machine is working hard to keep turning, turn it off and serve.

10 Store any leftover ice cream in a glass container with a secure lid and keep it in the freezer.

11 If you didn't opt for ribboning your chocolate drizzle throughout the ice cream, serving it warm and on top is a great addition.

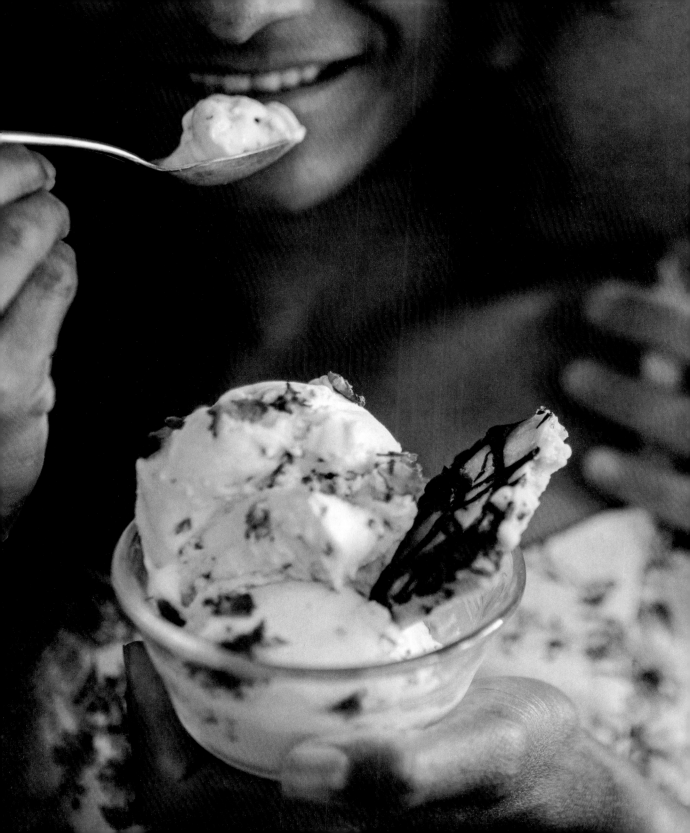

Schisandra Mocha Truffles

Hanna Nicole

INGREDIENTS

¼ cup dried schisandra berries

8 ounces plain dark chocolate (60 to 70%)

1 single-serving packet of instant coffee (caffeinated or decaf)

⅔ cup full-fat coconut milk (13.5 ounces)

½ teaspoon cinnamon

Pinch of salt

½ cup cacao powder

8 ounces plain dark chocolate (80 to 90%)

2 tablespoons coconut oil

Cinnamon, coarse salt, or shaved chocolate for sprinkling (optional)

PREPARATION

1 Soak the dried schisandra berries for 6 hours or overnight.

2 Strain well and smash the fruit with the back of a spoon to remove as many of the seeds as you have the patience to. (This is an optional step that creates a smoother center.) Place mashed berries in a strainer and press to remove as much moisture as possible. Set aside.

3 Chop the 8 ounces of dark (60 to 70%) chocolate into pea-sized pieces and place it in a bowl with the instant coffee.

4 In a heavy-bottomed pot, heat the coconut milk until it just begins to boil.

5 Pour coconut milk over the coffee and chocolate. Let the hot milk melt the chocolate, and when the chocolate is silky enough, whisk it all with a fork until smooth.

6 Mix in mashed schisandra berries, cinnamon, and salt with a fork until well combined.

7 Place this mixture in the fridge for 1 to 2 hours until creamy and solid.

8 Put the cacao powder into a bowl.

9 Pull your creamy chocolate mixture out of the fridge and, using a mini ice cream scoop or spoon, create a small bite-sized ball by rolling it briefly between your palms.

10 Roll each ball in the cacao powder until lightly dusted. Transfer these onto a parchment-covered tray or plate and put it in the freezer.

11 While the truffle centers are firming in the freezer, melt 8 ounces of the darker chocolate with the coconut oil in a small pot. Whisk until well combined.

12 When this chocolate is silky and loose, remove it from the heat, before it sticks to the bottom. Set this chocolate to the side, and let it cool on the counter for 5 to 10 minutes, stirring occasionally, until thick but runny.

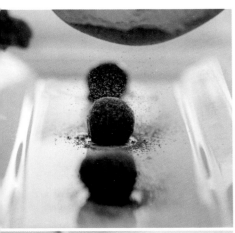

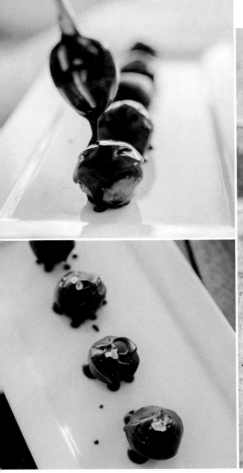

13 Pull your truffle centers from the freezer. Dip the truffle centers into the warm chocolate using 2 small spoons for a thick coating and set them back down on the parchment tray.

14 Sprinkle the top with a little cinnamon, coarse salt, or shaved chocolate for aesthetics, and transfer into the refrigerator to set.

15 These truffles will take up to 10 minutes in the refrigerator to firmly set. You can test them by lightly touching their outer shell for solidity.

16 Store the truffles in the refrigerator to prevent melting.

17 Enjoy!

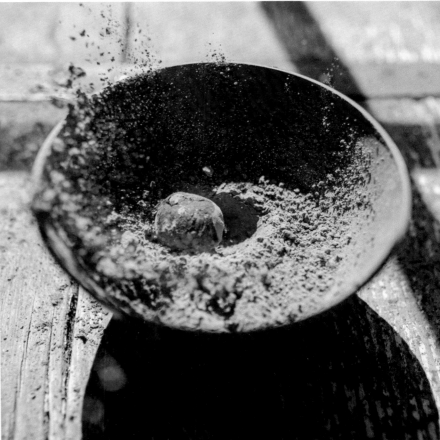

Maca Butter Barz

Hanna Nicole

INGREDIENTS

½ cup almond flour

½ cup powdered maca root

1 cup coarsely
chopped almonds

2 tablespoons chia seeds

1 heaping
tablespoon cinnamon

¾ teaspoon salt

3 tablespoons coconut oil

1 cup almond butter

1 teaspoon vanilla extract

¼ cup maple syrup

PREPARATION

1 Combine all the dry ingredients in a medium-sized bowl.

2 Melt coconut oil over low heat and pour into another small bowl with the almond butter, vanilla extract, and maple syrup.

3 Combine the wet and dry ingredients, and stir until well combined, with the chopped almonds and chia seeds evenly distributed in the batter.

4 Pour this into a parchment-lined 9 x 9-inch baking dish, and using a spatula, smooth out the edges until it is even.

5 Place the mixture into the fridge for 1 to 2 hours until set.

6 Use a clean, sharp knife to cut the bars into whatever size suits you.

7 Store the bars in the fridge for up to 10 days.

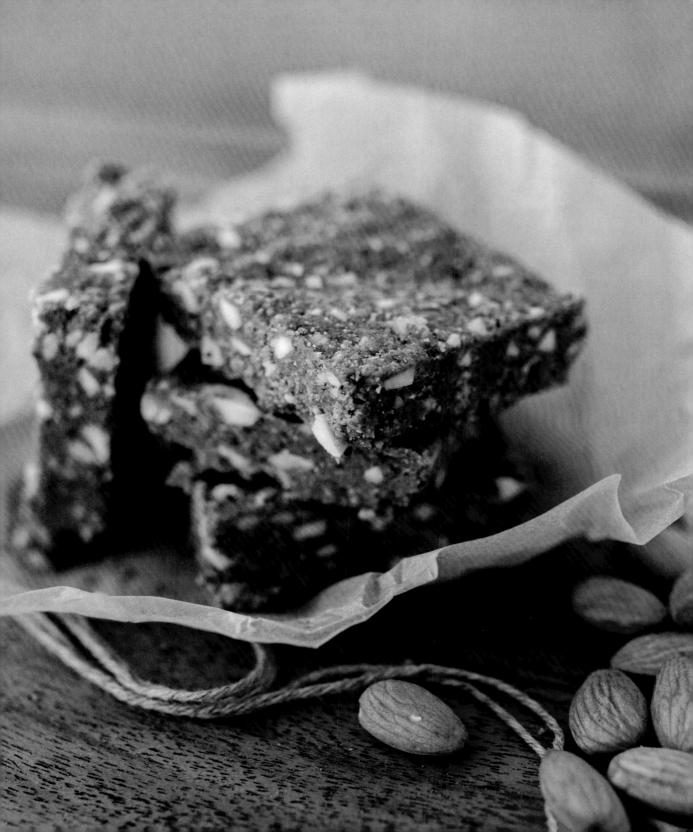

Maple Oat Squares

Hanna Nicole

INGREDIENTS

2 cups rolled oats

1 cup shredded coconut flakes

1 cup sesame seeds

2 cups chocolate chips (optional)

¾ teaspoon ground cardamom

1 ¼ teaspoons cinnamon

½ teaspoon salt

⅓ cup melted coconut oil

½ cup maple syrup

1 cup tahini (room temperature)

¼ cup chia seeds (blended with ½ cup water into a slurry)

½ cup canned coconut fat (just the fat)

1 teaspoon vanilla extract

1 banana

PREPARATION

1 Preheat the oven to 350 degrees F.

2 In a medium-sized bowl, combine all of the dry ingredients.

3 Melt coconut oil over low heat, and pour it into a bowl with the other wet ingredients.

4 Whisk wet ingredients together until smooth, smashing the ripe banana into the mix.

5 Pour the wet ingredients into the dry ingredients, and mix until all the oats are well coated.

6 Lightly grease a 9 x 13-inch baking dish, then press a piece of parchment down until it sticks to the bottom and sides of the dish evenly.

7 Pour the oat bar mixture into the baking dish, and press down evenly.

8 Bake the mixture for 20 to 25 minutes, until lightly browned on top.

9 Pull the dish out of the oven, and allow it to cool for 10 minutes.

10 Slice the mixture into bars and store them in the fridge for up to 10 days.

Variation: These bars can be made into Bitter Maple Squares by substituting ¼ cup of ground fenugreek seeds and ⅛ teaspoon of powdered monk fruit (or 5 drops liquid) for the chocolate chips. This is a lovely way to incorporate fenugreek into your diet.

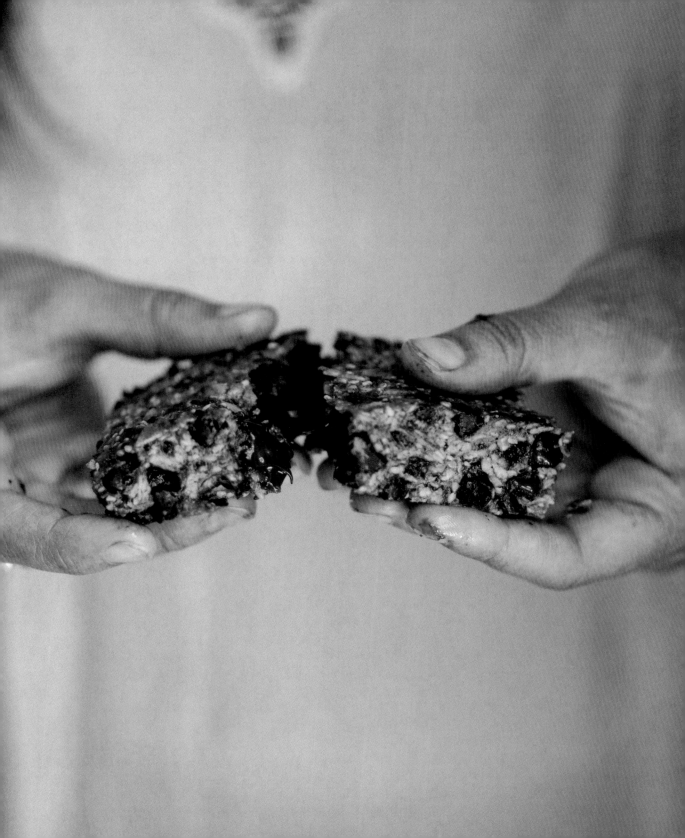

Schisandra Jelly

INGREDIENTS

½ cup dried schisandra berries

1 small red apple, chopped

½ cup granulated sugar

PREPARATION

1 Place schisandra berries, chopped apple, and 1½ cups of water in a small saucepan.

2 Bring the water to a boil. Turn the heat down to low, and simmer for 20 minutes.

3 Strain the mixture through a cheesecloth or jelly bag, reserving the liquid and composting the fruit.

4 Add the sugar to the liquid and return it to the saucepan.

5 Heat the liquid until the sugar is fully dissolved, then bring it to a rolling boil. Boil for 5 minutes.

6 Check for set point by putting a small amount of the liquid on a spoon and putting it in the freezer for a few minutes to see if it gels. If it does not, boil the liquid for a few more minutes, and check again.

7 When the liquid reaches set point, place it in a jar and refrigerate until it sets.

8 Store the jelly in the refrigerator and serve it on Maple Oat Squares, muffins, or toast.

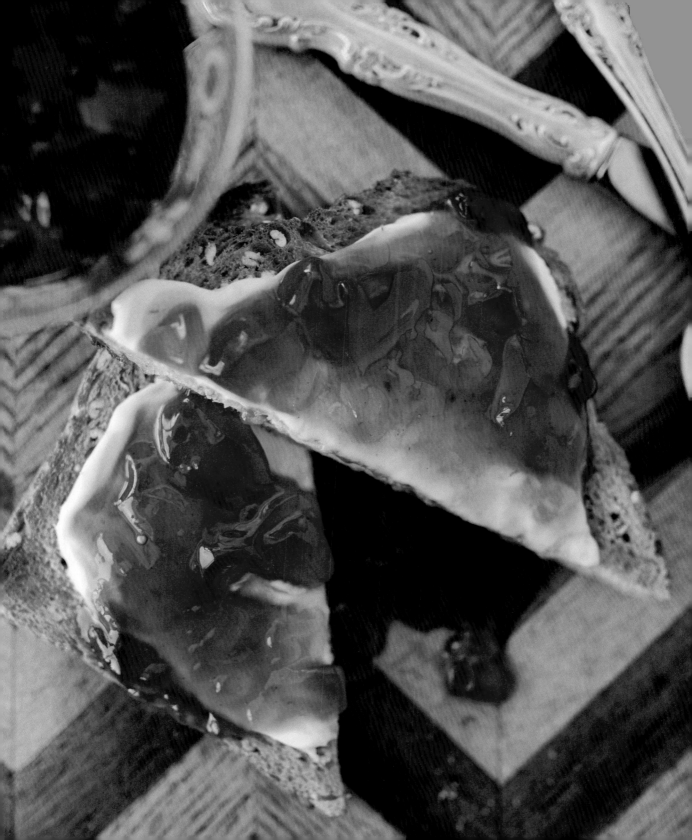

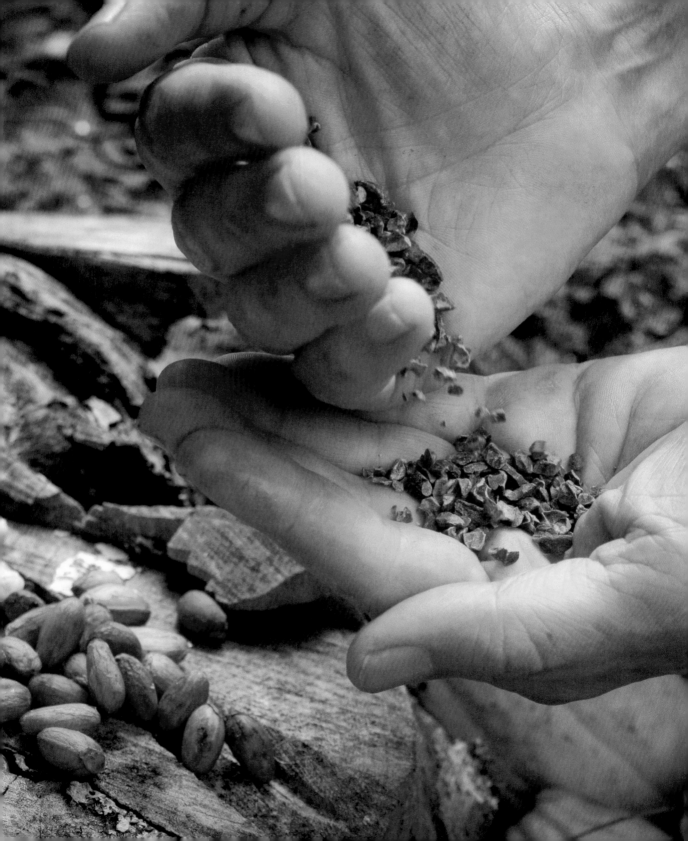

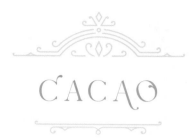

CACAO

Theobroma cacao

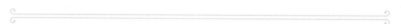

"Food of the Gods." This is the translation for cacao's genus name, *Theobroma*. As thick, rich, creamy chocolate, cacao becomes an absolute delight for our senses. If you are a chocolate lover like me, just the smell of chocolate can be intoxicating. The dark, creamy smoothness of melted chocolate or seeing it baked into or drizzled on treats is a feast for our eyes. And the taste, so utterly, irresistibly delicious . . .

How Does Cacao Work in Our Bodies?

When we eat chocolate, we feel energized and uplifted. This is partly due to the caffeine in cacao, especially in combination with theobromine,[1] but it also nourishes our bodies with minerals like potassium, magnesium, phosphorus, and calcium.[2] The synergistic effects of these and other constituents like anandamides and phenylethylamine likely contribute to its mood-elevating effects as well.[3] The phenylethylamine compound is also natural in the brain, and research shows that trace amounts of it are released when we are in love and during orgasm.[4]

These compounds also act to protect the cardiovascular system, which may contribute to the heart-opening sensations some experience in the consumption of chocolate. Cacao is both heart opening and an excellent ally for physical heart health. It has been shown to protect the cardiovascular system and reduce the risk of heart disease by favorably influencing vasodilation, reducing inflammation, decreasing platelet aggregation, reducing lipid oxidation, and reducing insulin resistance.[5] It also can lower high blood pressure, and the theobromine in cacao dilates the coronary arteries and improves blood flow to the brain.[6]

It is both cardio- and neuroprotective, meaning it helps tone and protect our hearts and nervous systems while also providing endocrine, immunological, respiratory, reproductive, and dermatological health benefits.[7] Cacao is a stimulating nervine, and both the caffeine and theobromine within it have neuroprotective properties, nourishing and strengthening our nerve cells.[8]

Herbal Shorthand

APHRODISIAC ACTIONS: *cardioprotective, energizing, nervine, neuroprotective, nutritive*

OTHER ACTIONS: *antioxidant, inflammatory modulator*

ENERGETICS: *warming, moistening*

TASTES: *bitter*

CONSTITUENTS: *anandamides, calcium, caffeine, flavonoids, phenylethylamine, phosphorus, potassium, magnesium, theobromine*

DOSAGE SUGGESTIONS: *Cacao is a tonic-level herb and should be consumed in medium dosages (2.5 grams of high-flavonoid cocoa powder or 10 grams of high-flavonoid dark chocolate per day). I recommend developing a taste for dark chocolate to minimize your sugar intake.*

SPECIAL CONSIDERATIONS: *Cacao may lead to insomnia, nervousness, or anxiousness in some people due to its stimulating effects.*

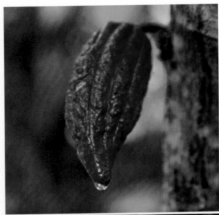
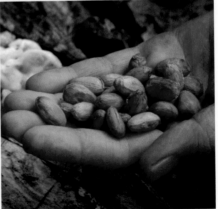

A Bit about Cacao Plants

Cacao plants are native to the deep tropical regions of Central and South America, and yet chocolate is consumed in countries across the globe. When we unwrap our favorite chocolate treats, we do not often think about the cacao plant, trees that grow 20 to 30 feet tall, have glossy, bright green leaves that droop from the branches, and small pink flowers that blossom throughout the year. The trees produce fruits called cacao pods that can be up to a foot long and three inches in diameter. They can be green, red, yellow, or yellow-brown when they are ripe, depending on the variety. Inside the pods are the cacao beans (seeds) surrounded by a mucilaginous, white pulp that has a flavor that is both sweet and sour.

In order to make chocolate, the cacao pods are harvested and split open. The beans are removed from the pods and fermented. During the fermentation process, the white pulp turns into liquid and drains off, and the unique chocolate flavor develops in the beans. The beans are then dried and sorted. The nibs are removed from the seed shells and roasted. As they roast, they darken in color and their flavor deepens. The roasted nibs are ground in stone mills where friction and heat turn them to a thick liquid, which is the basis for chocolate and cocoa products. This liquid mass is pressed to extract cocoa butter and then either powdered or used to make various chocolate products.

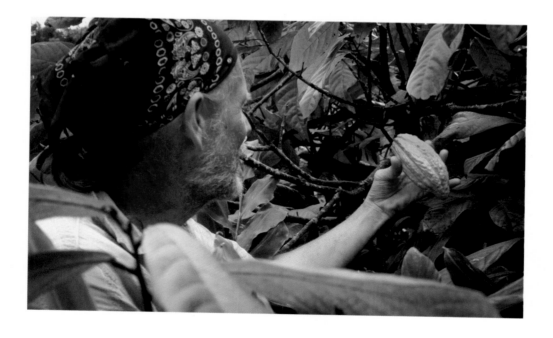

How to Use Cacao

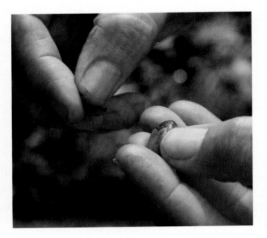

PARTS USED: *fermented seeds*

Cacao can be enjoyed in a myriad of ways. Generally chocolate treats are made with added ingredients, especially sweeteners, since it is quite bitter in 100 percent cacao form.

CACAO VS. COCOA: *The main difference between the two is that cacao butter and powder are made in processes using lower heating methods so they are more nutrient rich than cocoa butter and powder, but either type will be effective for recipes in this book:*

As an ingredient in sweet treats like candy bars, truffles, cakes, and cookies

In liquid form as a drink ingredient or as a syrup to be poured over other treats or as a body drizzle

As an ingredient in body-care products like lip balms or body butters

Participant Experiences

Cacao was the first herb we played with in the Aphrodisiac Circle, and it brought a sense of inspiration, joy, and pleasure right away. For a few participants, it was overly stimulating, and several people remarked about what a powerful herb they found it to be. Chocolate is a regular part of many of our lives, and our circle agreed that they would engage with cacao in a more conscious, respectful way going forward. Participants particularly noted feeling increased body and sensual awareness and arousal. We also felt more open hearted and comfortable in our vulnerability with greater intake of cacao.

There was a quality of indulgence and delight in our cacao experiments. We tried various cacao drinks, truffles, mousse tortes, chocolate pancakes, and body drizzles. Angela added cacao nibs to a bath salt blend. Gabrielle made a simple, private, daily ritual for herself of eating and savoring bites of a 100 percent cacao bar. Artemis made a ritual of a nightly cacao drink with cinnamon, cayenne, almond milk, and maple syrup, smelling, stirring, and slowly sipping by candlelight. We noticed a grounding quality in the earthy, exotic flavor and enjoyed the increased eroticism flowing in our lives throughout the month.

Delicious Delicacy Date Night

1   Plan a date night for you and your lover or all for yourself.

2   Choose some recipes from this chapter to prepare for the date.

3   Check the length of time needed for preparation (include time for gathering the ingredients as well as preparing the treats).

4   Choose a date and invite your lover, enticing them with the names and/or descriptions of the delicacies you will prepare.

5   Put the date on your calendar so you can enjoy anticipating it.

6   Enjoy the process of gathering your ingredients, especially if you get to harvest some yourself.

7   Make the preparation of the delicacies an aphrodisiac experience, delighting your senses and heightening the anticipation.

8   Fully revel in the sensual delight on the night of your date!

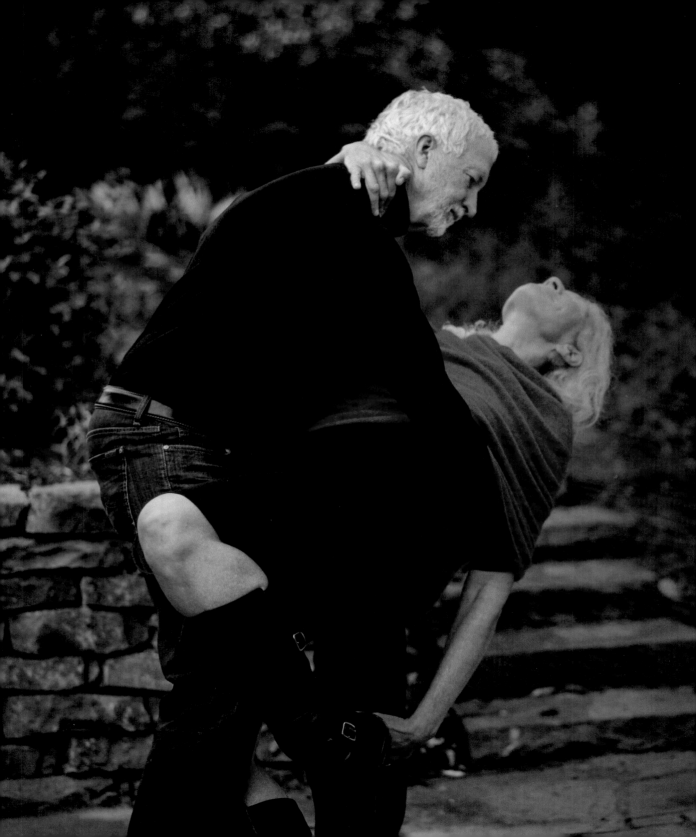

THIRTEEN

WELCOME

TO

VITAL

LIVING!

emember that first invitation, way back at the beginning of the book, to run your finger lightly and slowly over your lips? Take just a moment now to do that again. Feel the delicate curve of them. Notice how sensitive they are, how much sensation arises in your body from the lightest touch. Can you feel how this brings you fully into the present moment? Into delicate, beautiful sensation?

We have explored so much together through the pages that followed, from creating environments where love and eros can flourish to building healthy, erotic relationships, to navigating times of challenge. I wonder what exercises touched you most deeply, which recipes you tried and loved, which plants you've fallen in love with. I wonder how your life has changed.

Through it all, the simplest key to vital living can be found in that very first activity. Running your finger lightly and slowly over your lips. Letting it bring you present, into the moment, into sensation. Our ability to feel pleasurable sensation is one of the greatest gifts of being alive in a human body on this beautiful earth. Reveling in it brings joy and vitality.

The plants with their beautiful flowers, alluring scents, and essential nourishing and healing qualities can support that reveling in so many simple and profound ways. As we prioritize sensual and sexual experiences, recognizing them as the gifts they are, and call on the plants to help nourish these aspects of our lives, we begin to heal from the shame and repression that has kept us from healthy expression. With each healing step, reveling becomes more and more a part of our everyday lives and we find ourselves within a healthy flow of vital, erotic energy that brings out our confidence and creativity.

HEALTHY SEXUALITY

Sexual experiences are a natural part of that erotic flow. Let's look at some key elements of healthy sexuality.

One key aspect is personal self-care—cultivating a current of deep nourishment in our lives and integrating ways of taking exceptional care of our physical and emotional health. We need to make sure our bodies are getting the nutrients they need, and that we are getting enough rest and exercise. Herbal infusions can become a daily part of this self-care. Dream Cream adaptogen smoothies (page 234) can be integrated in times of stress. Beyond basic care, simple,

pleasurable rituals like taking time to drink a cup of Day Bright Tea (page 189) in the morning or massaging Love Your Body Lotion (page 86) into your skin before you go to bed can nourish your sensual, sexual self. Self-care also involves being continually engaged in our own personal growth and emotional healing. When we care for ourselves in this way, our self-acceptance and self-love grows, and we become less reliant on our partner and their response to our desires for our feelings of self-worth. This leads to cleaner and more nourishing connections.

Another key aspect is increasing our knowledge about ourselves as sexual beings. Learning all we can about our bodies, about the workings of our sexual organs and body systems and about how our bodies like to be pleasured, helps set the stage for healthy sexual connection. We can also learn about how our bodies communicate with us about what they like and don't like. We can listen for and voice our bodies' yes's and no's, holding strong boundaries for ourselves, and engaging with enthusiasm when we feel a full yes. We can begin to claim our erotic energy as source energy and grow our skills at communicating with our partner about what brings us deeper into arousal. We can help our partner communicate with us by being curious and asking questions. The more knowledge, consciousness, and openness we can bring to our sexual interactions, the healthier they will be.

Knowing our own bodies well also allows us to take responsibility for our own pleasure. This takes a lot of pressure out of sexual interactions. When we know what we like and are able to ask for it or give it to ourselves, then we are more likely to experience the pleasure we are seeking in our interactions. Sometimes, when we are deeply connected, the energy or experience that emerges is something different from what we expected or thought we wanted. Knowing that we can pleasure ourselves can allow us to relax into what is emerging without fear of ending up sexually frustrated.

Building our self-pleasuring skills also allows us to ask for what we want without making demands of our partner. Those participants exploring consensual nonmonogamy also found that having multiple sexual relationships took pressure off any one partner to meet their sexual desires. This form of relationship requires strong and effective communication skills and deep trust. When handled well it can open up the possibility of a wide variety of sexual experiences. When we know we can get our own needs and desires met through self-pleasure or with another partner, we can more easily make requests without attachment to our partner's response. This can help us to more graciously accept and honor our partner's authentic no. Consent is truly at the heart of healthy, sexual interactions, and underlying consent is deep respect. Going slow, attuning to ourselves and one another, and being willing to stop or adjust what's happening as needed allows true, healthy connection to emerge. Whenever we step beyond the bounds of consent, we are outside the realm of healthy sexuality. Within the realm of consent, there are endless opportunities for healthy forms of sexual expression.

As we learn more and more to connect within this realm of deep respect, attunement, and consent, trust and safety emerge. Greater safety allows us to be vulnerable with each other and take risks with our expression that can lead to heightened arousal and more profound levels of connection, sensation, healing, and sexual experience. As trust and safety grow between us and we become increasingly willing to be vulnerable and adventurous, shame dissolves and we come more and more into the fullness of our personal sexual expression. How this looks can vary day to day and even moment to moment. Sometimes sex can be slow and tantric, sometimes animalistic, sometimes playful or kinky. As we relax into the present moment and sink into our connection with each other, all different forms of sexual expression emerge, and our experience of sexual fulfillment expands, helping us drop our goals of orgasm or any particular outcome.

All of this leads to great sexual satisfaction more often. Healthy and satisfying sexual experiences leave us feeling both relaxed and vital, which can lead to even more healthy and satisfying sexual experiences. This is another naturally expanding feedback loop!

Where do the herbs fit into all this? Well, in all the ways we've learned throughout the book. They are an integral part of self-care; they can help us relax and drop into our bodies and help us to set up and revel within sensually and sexually pleasurable experiences. They can support our self-pleasuring practices and help us relax into our partner's occasional no's. They can also support us when we mess up and don't do all of this perfectly. Remember, we are coming from a culture of repression, shame, and exploitation around sexuality, so we cannot expect ourselves or our partners to do any of this perfectly. Giving ourselves and our partners space to experiment and sometimes fail is another aspect of healthy sexuality during this time of transition. Reach for oats and tulsi to calm your nerves, adaptogens to help with resilience through the learning process, and herbs like maca to help center and ground you in the truth of who you are.

HOW TO CHOOSE THE RIGHT HERB FOR YOU

As we have seen through our exploration together, herbs can do so many things to help support healthy sexual fulfillment. I hope you have experimented with some along the way and have a sense of how they work in your body. As you continue on your personal journey, it is likely that you will find yourself craving herbal support. The first step in choosing an herb is to identify what kind of support you are looking for. This will help you set an intention for working with them. Here are some questions you can ask yourself to help solidify your intention:

1　Do I have a flow of erotic energy in my life that helps me feel confident, vibrant, and creative?

2　As I think about my unique journey of sexual empowerment, can I see a next step for myself?

3　What do I love about my sensual/sexual life right now?

4　What do I wish were different?

5　Am I needing any kind of healing right now? (If you need healing, that will likely be the first step in moving toward fulfillment.)

6　What would help me most to be more available for intimacy? (Relaxation? Better communication with my partner? A beautiful space for intimate connection? Or something else?)

7　What do I imagine would help to increase my pleasure during sensual or sexual interaction?

8　Is there a particular desire I have been reluctant to pursue that I would like to explore?

9　Would I like to do something special for my partner?

You may want to ask more questions or different questions entirely. Throughout the book, we have practiced bringing ourselves present and allowing answers to arise. Whatever questions you choose to ask, you can use this technique to find answers. The important part is to discover and articulate your intention for yourself. Remember some of the intentions from the Aphrodisiac Circle participants? Michelle was looking to "continue to open [her] heart, and experience the strength/creativity [she gains] through vulnerability with a loving, strong, powerful male partner." Joe was looking to increase his connection with his wife of 15 years and "rekindle their fire." Rachel had just ended an eight-year partnership and was looking to intentionally find pleasure again. The more care you take with this step, identifying how you would like to call on the herbs for support, the more successful you will be at choosing the right herbs and preparations for you. I believe that working with herbs with a strong intention will help make them more effective as well.

Once you have clarified your intention, begin considering the herbs. I have highlighted 13 different herbs in this book and there are many, many more that also have substantial gifts to offer in the realm of sexual healing and empowerment. Often, the first place I start when considering which herbs I want to turn to is my own experience. Have I used an herb before that helped me in the way I am currently looking to be supported? If so, I will likely turn to that herb again. There is no better source of knowledge than body wisdom.

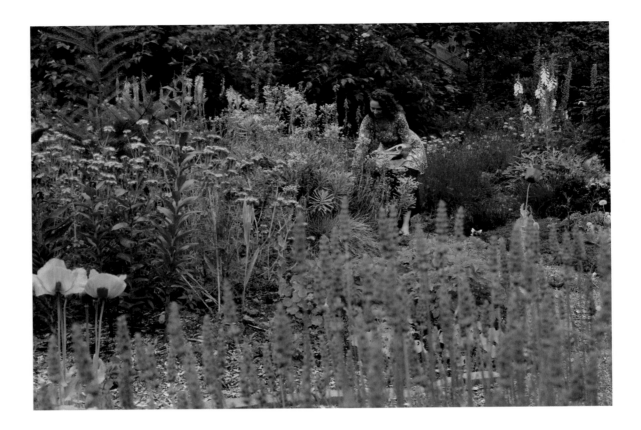

If you are looking for a new sort of support and don't have body knowledge to base your choice on, asking an herbalist for suggestions can be a wonderful next step. Herbalists will have had their own body experiences with herbs and also have knowledge of the effects the herbs have had on their clients. They can draw on this wide base of knowledge to also help inform your choice.

Seeking out information like that included in the herbal monographs in this book can help you make an informed choice. You can find similar monographs and information in herb books and on herbal websites. Looking for information about the actions associated with the herbs you are considering and about the plant constituents will help you understand how the herbs are likely to affect your body. You also know to look for information about an herb's energetics (whether it is warming or cooling, drying or moistening), and information about dosages, preparations, and using the herbs safely.

As you make choices about herbs that you want to engage with, remember that you don't have to get it exactly right. Experimentation is good, and it is fun! You may just have an attraction to a particular plant or an intuitive hit to try something out. Go with that, always. Check about dosage so you get a sense if this is a nutritive herb like oatstraw that you can take in large quantities or more of a medicinal herb like damiana that you want to take in smaller doses. Find a preparation that appeals to you or is convenient for your current life circumstances and try it out. With each experience you gain your own body wisdom about how an herb works for you. Over time, you will find yourself instinctively reaching for particular herbs to help support you in your unique circumstance. You will find your favorites that you call on again and again and will likely reach outside of these from time to time as you encounter new situations.

As you are making your choices, please remember to consider issues of sustainability and overharvesting. For regular use, choose herbs that grow near you in abundant supply. If you do choose to engage with an exotic herb, do so consciously, and preferably for a limited time. Educate yourself about a plant's availability. You may find outstanding results with ginseng, but when you learn that it has been overharvested, you may choose to look to eleuthero instead.

If you find yourself calling on certain herbs over and over again, look for ways that you can help support their health and well-being. Plant and tend them in your garden, get involved in helping protect wild areas where you harvest them, or help other people learn about the importance of keeping them healthy. We are in relationship with these plants, and just like with our partners, we must never take them for granted. All healthy relationships require continual gratitude and respect.

We are in relationship with these plants, and just like with our partners, we must never take them for granted.

HOW TO ENGAGE WITH THE HERBS

Once you have chosen an herb to work with, you will want to consider how you want to prepare it. Throughout the course of this book, I have included recipes for you to try and herbal tips so that you have been learning herbalism experientially. That is my favorite way to teach—one experience at a time. These various preparations are your toolkit. You can use them as a base to experiment with more herbs.

Let's take a look at some of the different preparations we have explored. We started with a simple tea, Aphrodi-Tea (page 5), made with tulsi and rose petals. Teas are a basic herbal preparation that most of you were probably already familiar with before you started reading. With teas you can vary the combination and amount of herbs you use and the steeping time to dial in the taste you find most pleasing and the strength of the herbal actions. Sometimes herbs are best used with a relatively short steeping time—5 to 20 minutes. Generally, longer steeping times will allow more of the herbal constituents to be drawn into the water. This is ideal when you want to draw out the vitamins and minerals from nourishing herbs like oatstraw.

These strong teas are referred to as infusions, and a general rule of preparation is an ounce of herb to a quart of water, steeped for at least four hours. Infusions are sometimes used for a more medicinal dose of tonic or medicinal herbs as well.

Generally, teas and infusions are made from dried leaves and flowers of plants. If you want to draw out constituents from the harder plant material like roots, bark, or berries, you might make a decoction. The Warm Nights Chai recipe (page 171) in this book is an example of a decoction. We placed the plant material in a pot, poured water over it, and brought it to a boil, then turned down the heat and simmered it for an extended period of time, at least 20 minutes. Again you can adjust herb combinations, amounts, and simmering time to adjust the taste and strength of the decoction. Decoctions can also be used for leaves and flowers if you want to get a dose of their qualities more quickly than an infusion allows. Teas and decoctions can be consumed straight or used as a base for making syrups like the Berry Decadence Syrup we made in Chapter 9.

Teas, infusions, and decoctions are all ways of extracting plant constituents into water. We can also extract constituents into other menstruums including oil, alcohol, vinegar, and honey. Each menstruum pulls out slightly different constituents and is used in different ways.

Oils, like our rose petal massage oil, are probably the trickiest to make because the water content in the plant material can easily make the oil go rancid. Gentle heating using the slow cooker or stovetop is a fairly reliable way to get a good result. Making sure every piece of equipment you are working with, from your double boiler pan to your stirring stick, are bone dry is essential to preventing rancidity. Heat can also cause your oil to go off, so low heat is key here. You can also use the heat of the sun, putting your oil outside for a few days. Just be sure to bring it in at night so dew does not get into the oil. This is my favorite way to infuse summer flower goodness into oil. I do it with fresh rose petals, calendula, and St.-John's-wort flowers. You can vary the plant

material, the kind of oil you use, and the amount of time you infuse it for varying results. Some oils, like almond or jojoba, soak into our skin more easily than others, like olive oil. Some oils have stronger scents than others as well. It is fun to experiment and create infused oils that you love. These oils can be used straight for massages but can also form the base for many herbal body preparations like lip balms, body butters, lotions, and lubricants.

Alcohol and vinegar extractions are very simple to make, basically filling a jar with finely chopped plant material and pouring alcohol or your vinegar of choice over top to fill the jar, stirring and allowing it to sit for six weeks. Alcohol extractions can be used as tinctures, like we did with our milky oat tops. For these you want to use strong alcohol like 100-proof vodka. Other alcohols like brandy make wonderful cordials, bitters, or elixirs. Herbal vinegars can be used as salad dressing ingredients or also in herbal shrubs like the Sweetheart Shrub (page 292). The trick to remember when infusing herbs in vinegar is to make sure the vinegar does not come in contact with metal while you are infusing or storing it. (Use a plastic lid on your mason jar or put a layer of plastic wrap between the metal lid and the jar.) Vinegar corrodes metal, and this will ruin your preparation.

Of course, we cannot forget honey extractions. These are, in my opinion, one of the most divine ways to enjoy herbs. Honeys are best made with aromatic herbs or berries and can be used in all kinds of imaginative ways. You can simply spread them on crackers or toast, add them to teas, use them in skin-nourishing masks, enjoy them by the fingerful, or lick them off the body of your lover. Use them in ways that appeal to you in the moment to bring that flow of erotic energy into your life!

Besides honeys we also learned to make all kinds of delicious herbal treats, some sweet, some more savory. Some herbal treats involve using our infusions or vinegars or honeys. Others involve mixing herbal powders into the treats like the Dream Cream smoothie (page 234) or Date Treats (page 236). Powders can also be rolled onto the outside of treats like the rose petal powder on the outside of Dusty Rose Petal Truffles (page 298). As you make these treats, remember to slow down and engage your senses so you turn your treat making into an aphrodisiac experience. Preparing them with other delighted friends can also heighten the flow of erotic energy. I tested the recipes for the book with two wonderful girlfriends, and we created so much beauty, laughter, and love together in my kitchen!

Speaking of creating beauty, we also learned about using herbs to help create sensual space. You might try putting rose petals on the bed or a beautiful bouquet on the headboard. A bottle of massage oil, a plate of chocolate truffles, or some chocolate body drizzle next to the bed can help increase anticipation and arousal. Herbs can also be used to create an intoxicating scent. You can now make hydrosols and incense and have a beginning sense of herbal perfume making.

Herbal baths and steams are also delightful preparations for sensual and sexual interactions. Remember the Divinity Soak from Chapter 4? Different herbs have different effects—from deeply relaxing to warming and invigorating. You can vary the herbs used for the effects you want to achieve: skin toning, moisturizing, or nourishing. Steams can be used on our faces, genitals, or in a sauna to nourish the skin on our whole bodies.

The recipes in this book are more than just instructions about how to make specific herbal preparations. They contain the information you need to work with all kinds of herbs in a confident and empowered way. The herbs are, and have always been, the people's medicine. Each time you try out a recipe, you are deepening your relationship with the plants and building your skills and confidence in being able to choose and make herbal preparations that are just right for you and those you love.

OTHER TOOLS FOR SEXUAL EMPOWERMENT

Beyond working with the plants, in our journey together, we have looked at many other tools that can lead to increased sexual empowerment. This began with the simple idea of slowing down and acting with intention and attention. I offered ideas like creating simple rituals for yourself that bring you into your senses and help increase the flow of erotic energy in your life. We explored the idea of making a pleasure map of your body and of reading books or taking classes to learn more about your body and its capacity for pleasure. Pleasure maps can be continually updated as your understanding grows. We also explored setting up environments where love and eros can flourish and learning about what increases and decreases arousal for yourself and your partner so you can pamper and pleasure one another. Within the realm of relationship, we explored tools for increasing our skills at healthy relating like the Relating Meditation and the Wheel of Consent.

On a personal level, we explored the importance of creating a current of self-love and nourishment to help build and maintain vibrant health, and the idea of making a pleasure plan to carry you through times of stress. We looked at questions you can ask when you feel your health faltering to help you choose the right remedies for healing. We explored how creating a self-pleasure practice can be a tool for self-nourishment and pleasure. It can also help you to meet your partner in sensual/sexual activity with less expectation and pressure and instead with openness and curiosity. Creating a network of friends who support one another in getting empathy and support helps with this as well and is a profound act of self-love.

SEXY DEVELOPMENTS FOR APHRODISIAC CIRCLE PARTICIPANTS

The Aphrodisiac Circle was a support network of its own, encouraging exploration and development around sexuality and vital living. As we reflected at the end of our year together, we all noticed a greater sense of empowerment in the realm of sexuality in our lives and in engaging with the herbs. Sarah spoke of a deeper connection to herself that allowed her to move away from following the lead of a man in her sexual explorations. She found a new freedom and vitality in her body and a deeper connection to her own desires in the moment. Christina, who had been healing from past sexual trauma, described feeling more open and willing to connect. She also celebrated the deepening of her connection with the herbs. Michelle also celebrated that deepening. She described herself as an herbal novice at the beginning of the project and noticed

the shift to feeling empowered to try out different herbs and feel into the effects on her body. Before this project, she would look to experts to tell her what herbs or supplements to take. Through the project, she deepened her relationship with the plants and her confidence in being able to choose herbs that are right for her.

For several participants, the project led to big lifestyle changes. Rebecca and Simon realized changes would have to happen if they were to have the time and space for intimate connection that they were both craving. Checking back with them a year later, they had downsized their business and were making choices that greatly reduced the amount of stress in their lives. They were separating work from their home lives more and more, giving themselves the freedom and ease they had been craving. Angela shifted her career and settled into her new home and is now finding the time to do the deep healing work around her childhood sexual trauma that will help her open to the level of intimacy she desires with her husband. James ended up getting a divorce in order to honor his truth about being polyamorous. He and his ex-wife are co-parenting their newborn son, but they have ended their intimate relationship. Sarah successfully opened her marriage, and both she and her husband are exploring intimate connections beyond their marriage while keeping that primary relationship strong.

Each of us found particular herbs that are strong allies for us. Joe and Cassie both had profound experiences with oatstraw, Joe finding it took the pain from his intense ejaculations and Cassie enjoying the lubrication it brought to her vagina. Oats will definitely be a continual ally for both of them. Several of us fell in love with roses. Christina described rose as a friend and ally in her self-care journey. Michelle and Gabrielle both developed profound self-pleasuring practices with rose as an inspirational ally. Sarah reflected on the beauty of connecting with her own sexuality as she rubbed powdered rose petals and oats on her body in the shower. Simon noticed a surprising connection to ginger after brewing his coffee with ginger in the winter and finding the ritual of sitting and drinking it opened space for relaxation and connection. Christina came to see ginger as a "feminine power ally." Cacao became a favorite for Joe, Cassie, Christina, and Simon. Artemis formed strong, ongoing relationships with oats, ashwagandha, tulsi, and hawthorn. They have become regular parts of her self-care routines. Damiana, she will call on for wild nights with a trusted lover where she can fully surrender into her body's desires.

In relation to his intention of finding deeper connection with Cassie and rekindling their fire, Joe wrote,

The herbs truly have made an impact on our relationship, and what's great is that it happened in a way that was unexpected. Previously, when I thought of the idea of using an aphrodisiac, the image I held was more like popping a pill, and voila!, my libido would be kickin'. But what I learned over the course of this year is that the vast majority of herbal aphrodisiacs don't work this way at all. Instead, at least for me, it's the little things stacked together that led to a gradual deepening sense of connection with Cassie.

First, I believe our intention and dedication for over a year to explore and give ourselves time, patience, and grace to grow together was key. We allowed ourselves to connect when it felt authentic, and we didn't push each other to do anything

when one of us felt that it didn't feel right. We created safety for each other.

Additionally, just the act of playing together with the herbs helped rekindle our fire—each herb gave us something new and different to look forward to. For example, as we prepared our damiana tincture, we'd ask ourselves, "How would this herbal ally change our experience? Will it affect us differently than the others?" As a result, it brought variety and a sense of newness and fun exploration.

And last, I believe the aphrodisiac qualities of the herbs themselves supported our desire to deepen our connection. They made us feel more relaxed and safe being vulnerable, as if we were being held by something greater than just ourselves.

The herbs helped us break free from the mundane routine from which we had gotten stuck. And in this way, the herbs helped us come more fully alive and present with each other. Our fire is now shining bright again. For that, I am deeply grateful!

I am delighted by these kinds of results. The plants have become beloved and effective allies for me in my own life, and I love witnessing others as they form their own unique relationships with herbs. The Aphrodisiac Circle opened up new possibilities and perspectives for us all. With the plants as allies, we deepened our relationships to ourselves and our sexuality, and we were able to witness and support one another along the way.

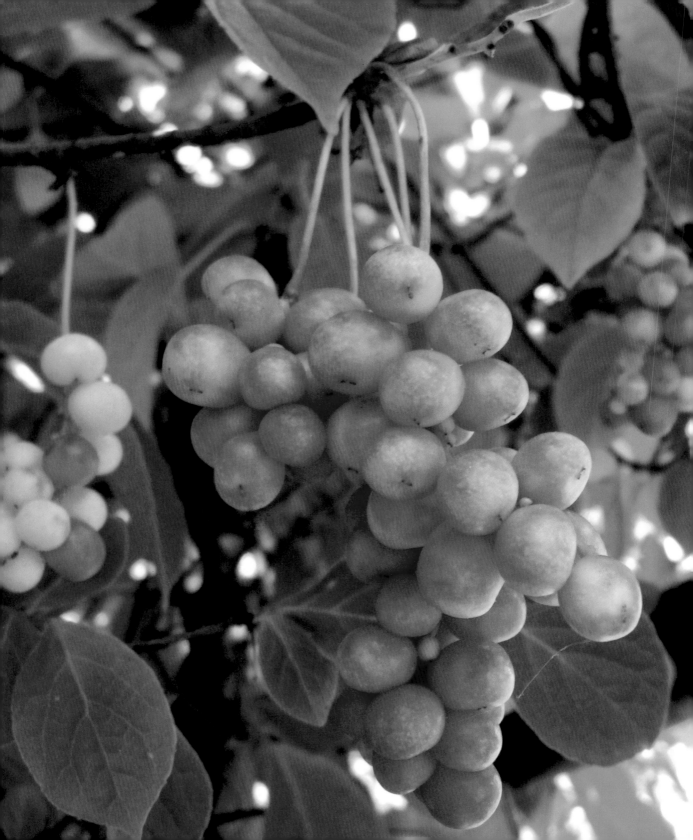

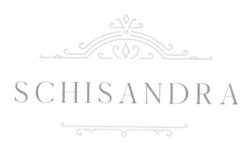

SCHISANDRA

Schisandra chinensis

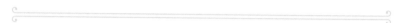

Each bite of schisandra berry is a taste sensation that brings us awake and alive to the present moment. The Chinese name, *wu wei zi*, means "five-flavored fruit." Schisandra has sweet and sour flavors in the peel and pulp, along with acrid, bitter, and salty flavors in the seeds, so each bite of berry has all five tastes! Schisandra strengthens, enlivens, and energizes us, so that we are ready to relate in powerful ways.

How Does Schisandra Work in Our Bodies?

Schisandra is a whole-body tonic that strengthens and tones our organs, is restorative, and energizing. According to a review conducted by Nowak et al.,[1] schisandra has some very unique bioactive compounds known as schisandra lignans. These compounds were shown to improve mitochondrial function, which is important for overall health because the mitochondria produce energy for the body and regulate the metabolism. Schisandrin A, one of the schisandra lignans, was shown to have powerful effects on DNA repair and other important antioxidant properties. These antioxidative properties protect cells against fatigue-induced stress. Gomisin A, another bioactive compound in schisandra, was also shown to protect cells against stress.[2]

These berries are great for our hearts, helping to regulate the cardiovascular system and protect the heart, lungs, and liver while also purifying the blood and helping to normalize blood pressure.[3]

Schisandra also has positive influences on our central and sympathetic nervous systems. Its antioxidant qualities contribute to the way it can enhance cognitive function, and improve mental clarity, concentration, coordination, and sensory perception. Schisandra can also ease depression, quiet the spirit, and calm the heart, reducing irritability and helping with insomnia, especially when combined with ashwagandha.[4]

As an adaptogen schisandra can help us withstand stress and resist disease. It helps strengthen our adrenals, fortify our immune system, and is great for endurance and stamina.[5]

It is also known as a reproductive system tonic for both women and men.[6] It helps nourish our sexual fluids and increases sexual stamina.[7] It also increases sexual desire.[8] Brigitte Mars says that schisandra can help support people in overcoming the trauma associated with sexual abuse.[9]

For women in menopause, this herb can be useful in helping control hot flashes and night sweats by helping dry up excess fluids.[10] One trial shows a significant beneficial effect of schisandra on sleep disorders in peri- and postmenopausal women.[11]

In ancient China, schisandra was known as a youth preserver and beautifier.[12] Some of the lignans in schisandra have now been shown to protect and even prevent skin aging from UV radiation and oxidation.[13]

A Bit about Schisandra Plants

Schisandra is a climbing deciduous vine with pointed oval leaves. It blooms in late spring with solitary cream to pink fragrant flowers, which are then followed by clusters of shiny red berries. It is native to northern and northeast China and the adjacent regions of Russia and Korea. It prefers rich, well-drained but moisture-retentive soil. It is a shade-loving plant.

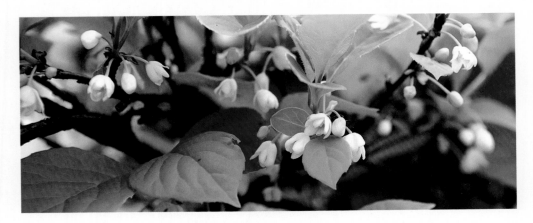

Herbal Shorthand

APHRODISIAC ACTIONS: *adaptogen, cardiotonic, cardioprotective, brain tonic, emotionally uplifting, endocrine system tonic, energy building, energizing, ergogenic, nervine, neuroprotective, reproductive system tonic, restorative, soothing and healing for skin*

OTHER ACTIONS: *antioxidant, astringent, hepatoprotective (protects liver), immune tonic*

ENERGETICS: *warming, drying*　　**TASTES:** *sweet, sour, salty, pungent, bitter*

NOTABLE APHRODISIAC CONSTITUENTS: *Lignans such as Schisandrin A and Gomisin A, vitamin C*

DOSAGE SUGGESTIONS: *Schisandra is a tonic herb and should be taken regularly in medium dosages for a specific period of time. A medium dose might look like ½ cup of tea or a dropperful of tincture three times daily.*

SPECIAL CONSIDERATIONS: *Avoid schisandra during pregnancy as it may stimulate uterine contractions.*

Large doses may cause appetite loss.

Some people experience GERD or heartburn when taking schisandra; if this happens, reduce the dose, or stop taking it altogether.

Schisandra is metabolized by the liver and may interact with certain pharmaceutical drugs including tacrolimus (immunosuppressant), talinolol (beta blocker), and warfarin (blood thinner).

How to Use Schisandra

PARTS USED: *Berry*

For an energy boost or to awaken senses, eat the berries fresh or dried.

Brew schisandra tea, warm or iced. Play with steeping or decocting time to find the flavor intensity you like best. **(Five Springs Tea, page 89)**

Make schisandra-infused honey.

Make pastilles using powdered berries.

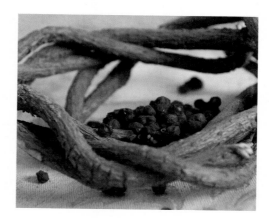

Participant Experiences

Overall, Aphrodisiac Circle participants reported feelings of increased vitality, strength, and courage when engaging with schisandra. When we took it regularly (either as a tincture, tea, or just eating dried berries daily) we noticed feeling a consistent flow of energy that increased our endurance and resilience and helped us feel more connected to our personal power.

Eating schisandra berries also served to bring us fully into the present moment and awaken our senses. We noticed a nourishing and cleansing feeling associated with the zing of ingesting these berries. This sense awakening quality was a wonderful precursor to sexual expression, and two participants noticed a marked increase in their sexual desire from taking schisandra regularly. Angela says this herb had the most pronounced positive effect on her libido of any of the herbs we experimented with.

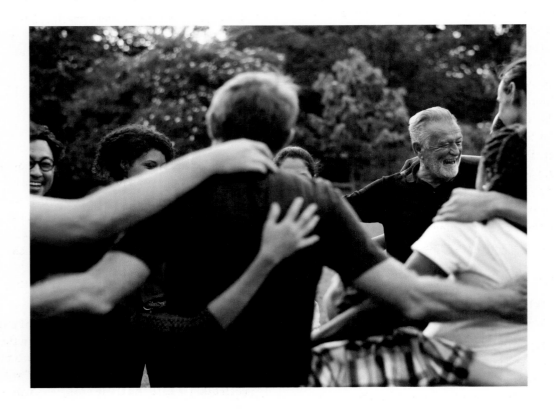

CREATING YOUR OWN APHRODISIAC CIRCLE

When we took time to reflect on what we got out of our year of exploration together, the Aphrodisiac Circle participants agreed that having others to talk with about issues involving sensuality and sexuality was one of the most profound gifts of our time together. I have spoken over and over again about what a bold act it is to prioritize these aspects of our lives. To harvest the gifts of healthy sexuality—gifts like increased confidence and creativity—we must overcome decades of sexual repression. To do so, we must connect with one another and encourage each other. We are social animals. We need each other to grow and learn and find new ways of being, and new levels of connection to ourselves and each other. In these times we are truly being called to meet ourselves and each other with both courage and vulnerability.

So how do we form the kind of circle that will allow for and open up this deep level of interaction? Well, I can tell you what we did for the Aphrodisiac Circle. I created an invitation to participate and sent it out to those I thought might be interested. Those who took me up on it gathered together and we created some group agreements. These are the agreements we made:

CONFIDENTIALITY:

1 What is shared in the group stays in the group.

2 If you are sharing something about your experience beyond the group please be very conscious to speak from your experience and not use the names of others in the group.

3 Be conscious about talking with other members of the group in public spaces about what they have shared in the group. (They likely will not want to discuss their deep share at the grocery store.) Ask permission of each other if you want to talk with them about what they shared.

SOVEREIGNTY:

1 You choose how you participate in this group. We are trusting each other to say yes or no to requests for discussion or participation. When we know we can trust each other to set clear personal boundaries, we feel more free to make requests. We all agree that we want everyone to be participating from a clear yes.

2 That said, few of us are very practiced at being clear, and we may make mistakes. We agree to help each other be clear with our boundaries.

RESPECT:

1 We respect and honor each other's yes's and no's.

2 We see conflict as an opportunity for growth and we deal with it directly. If we find we are having a conflict with someone else in the group, we bring up our issue with them directly in order to resolve it in the best way possible. If we are struggling to reach resolution, we can reach out to Kimberly (or another group member) for help with mediation.

3 We agree to leave "pickup" energy out of our interactions. We are not participating in the group to meet romantic partners and will be very conscious about how "hooking up" with each other might affect the group as a whole.

COMMITMENT:

1 Our commitment to the group is that we will attend the circle and actively participate as often as possible.

2 We want our participation to be from a place of excited yes energy. If you find that is waning for you, we request your communication about that truth. Please do not simply stop attending meetings, but communicate with us about what is coming up for you so that we have an opportunity to adjust the circle if we feel it is appropriate or that we have an opportunity to problem solve together.

3 If you do need to leave the group, please communicate that to the group as a whole.

Your agreements may be similar or different, but it is important to get clear with those that gather about what you are expecting of one another in order for everyone to feel safe. Once the agreements have been made, it is also important to follow through with them. If someone is not living up to the commitments you have made to one another, it is appropriate and important to take action. You may give them an opportunity to adjust their behavior or ask them to leave the group. This is intimate and delicate work you are doing together, and following the group commitments is how you show your respect and care for one another.

Beyond that, you need to decide some logistical things. How will leadership work in your group? Is the person who sent out the invitation going to lead the group, or are you going to share leadership among the participants? Will you take turns hosting and facilitating? How often will you

OPPORTUNITY FOR CULTIVATING EROTIC ENERGY FLOW

Considering Your Next Step

1 Look back at your journal or the art you created as you worked your way through this book.

2 Do a sensory meditation or other practice to bring yourself into a sensually embodied state.

3 Ask yourself if there are pieces of what you learned that you would like to integrate further? Do you see a next step you want to take on your personal journey of sexual empowerment? (Perhaps there is a book you want to read, a workshop you want to take, a recipe you want to try, or a friend you want to reach out to in order to begin building your own Aphrodisiac Circle.)

4 Commit to taking action on this next step!

meet? Where and when? How will you structure your meetings? Are you going to make aphrodisiac preparations together, try them out and come back and discuss your findings? Are you going to read a book together (this one or another) or listen to a podcast and have discussions about what you are learning? It is important to be as clear as possible about your intention and the expectations for each participant in order to set yourselves up for success. You may find that the intention, the expectations, or the agreements need to change over time. That is healthy and to be expected. Taking time to consciously communicate about the changes will help everyone move forward in the best way possible.

I would also encourage lots of grace. Assume the best of each other, and set yourselves up with conflict resolution practices and recovery strategies. As humans, even with the best of intentions, we will make mistakes. Mistakes are part of stretching into new realms. If we can hold each other through them and work through conflicts that arise, we will find our relationships grow stronger and more resilient over time. Those of us who participated in the Aphrodisiac Circle gained a deep respect and appreciation for one another, and when the project was complete, there was definitely a sentiment of not wanting it to end.

discern what new information resonates for you and connect it to your personal experience. Let's pause once more before completing the book to consider your next step.

I feel honored that you chose to take this journey with me. My vision for this book was that the experience of reading it would be a sensual delight, that it would add to the flow of erotic energy in your life. I envisioned readers falling in love with the plants, savoring the sensual experience of creating aphrodisiac delights, and finding new depths of connection and new levels of rapture and ecstasy within their relationships. I imagined each of you finding your unique ways of bringing more erotic energy to your life and in so doing, gaining the confidence, creativity, and resilience to bring your gifts more fully to the world and create the lives you most want to live.

I hope you will return to this book again and again to try out a new recipe, reread a section that touched you, or to just delight in its visual beauty. There is no hurry. Choose one thing, one step forward for yourself. Step by sustainable step, you can build the erotic flow until it becomes a strong current of source energy that carries you to previously unimagined realms of satisfaction and creativity.

Many blessings on your journey.

With love,

Kimberly

CREATING A FLOW OF EROTIC ENERGY IN YOUR OWN LIFE

Throughout the book, I have encouraged you to pause and reflect on the information I have presented. I hope these pauses have helped you

We have come to be danced
Not the pretty dance
Not the pretty pretty, pick me, pick me dance
But the claw our way back into the belly
Of the sacred, sensual animal dance
The unhinged, unplugged, cat is out of its box dance
The holding the precious moment in the palms
Of our hands and feet dance.

We have come to be danced
Not the jiffy booby, shake your booty for him dance
But the wring the sadness from our skin dance
The blow the chip off our shoulder dance.
The slap the apology from our posture dance.

We have come to be danced
Not the monkey see, monkey do dance
One two dance like you
One two three, dance like me dance
but the grave robber, tomb stalker
Tearing scabs and scars open dance
The rub the rhythm raw against our soul dance.

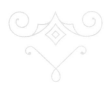

We have come to be danced
Not the nice, invisible, self-conscious shuffle
But the matted hair flying, voodoo mama
Shaman shakin' ancient bones dance
The strip us from our casings, return our wings
Sharpen our claws and tongues dance
The shed dead cells and slip into
The luminous skin of love dance.

We have come to be danced
Not the hold our breath and wallow in the shallow end of the floor dance
But the meeting of the trinity, the body breath and beat dance
The shout hallelujah from the top of our thighs dance
The mother may I?
Yes you may take 10 giant leaps dance
The olly olly oxen free free free dance
The everyone can come to our heaven dance.

We have come to be danced
Where the kingdoms collide
In the cathedral of flesh
To burn back into the light
To unravel, to play, to fly, to pray
To root in skin sanctuary
We have come to be danced

WE HAVE COME
— Jewel Mathieson

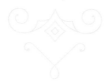

APHRODISIAC CIRCLE PARTICIPANT INTRODUCTIONS

Rebecca: She is a mother to an elementary school daughter and is in the midst of her transition through menopause. She and her husband, Simon, run a home business together complete with a small-scale farm. Rebecca is interested to see how herbs can support her in finding more time for intimacy and reinvigorating her libido.

Simon: At 40, Simon is working with Rebecca to keep their business up and running. He is dealing with high stress and overwork as a block to the kind of intimacy and sexuality he would like in his life.

James: He is a 30-year-old married, polyamorous, bisexual man. He is a healer in the process of becoming a couple and family therapist. Having "encountered a great deal of shame and fear when diving into deeper pleasure states," he is actively engaged in his personal erotic healing work. He enjoys being embodied through contact improv and fusion dance. James is interested in learning how aphrodisiacs will expand the eroticism in his life and affect his life and relationships.

Gabrielle: She has not had an intimate partner in many years. Since her husband passed away, her relationship energy has gone toward her children, two daughters now college age. She is involved in political activism, particularly around the health of our planet, and she loves to travel. She participated in the project to reengage the sensual, sexual aspects of herself.

Sarah: At age 34, Sarah is deepening into her own sensuality and sexuality and engaging in a process with her husband around the possibility of opening their marriage. She is a body worker with a young son.

Cassie: She is a priestess to the goddess. She is 43 years old and has been married to Joe for almost 14 years. She has only been in monogamous heterosexual relationships, but she has also been attracted to women. She is working through the blocks and sexual shame that formed through her upbringing in a strict Roman Catholic household. Her intention for the year is to cultivate her sexual power. She is exploring tantra and erotic dance and developing a jade egg practice as well as exploring how herbs can support her journey.

Joe: He is a 42-year-old leadership workshop facilitator. He is a ceremonialist, professional life coach, and soul guide. Joe is a survivor of childhood sexual abuse, and through his own personal growth work, has come to deeply love sensual and sexual exploration. He is seeking to rekindle the fire in his relationship with Cassie.

Lisa: She is a 50-year-old, married, polyamorous woman in the early stages of menopause who has been taking a deep dive into exploring her sexuality. She has two teenage children and loves being a mother.

Michelle: She is menopausal and a healthy, active bisexual in a relationship with a partner who is excited to explore sensuality and sexuality with her. Michelle also nourishes her own sensuality through dance and her connection to nature. She is outside and engaged in physical activities as much as possible. She is also exploring sexuality, feminine ecophilosophy, and tantric and Taoist practices.

Robert: Robert, 65, is Michelle's partner. He is recently retired from a career in accounting and plans to dedicate some of his retired time to writing erotic adventure stories. He and Michelle love to travel and adventure together and are greatly enjoying their sensual and sexual explorations.

Rachel: She identifies as bisexual and has recently ended an eight-year intimate relationship with a woman. She is participating in the project to engage with her own relationship to her sensuality and sexuality and to move herself toward the frame of mind that would eventually allow her to enter romantic and physical relationship with others again.

Angela: She is 41 and recently married, and she and her husband are raising two children together. While she is "madly in love with and attracted to her husband," she finds her libido does not match her desire.

Artemis: She is a 45-year-old single mother of four smallish boys. She left her marriage of 20 years because she did not have the kind of deep connection she desired with her husband. Since leaving she found tantra and contact improvisation dance and began singing and writing again. She has experienced beautiful spiritual and very sexually sacred relationships and has deepened her love and commitment to herself.

Christina: She is a 47-year-old soul purpose guide, dancer (and dance instructor), and theater manager. She is unpartnered and has no children. She is also a survivor of sexual abuse and is recovering from having been in an abusive long-term relationship that she ended in 2013. Christina is healing and seeking ways to make her life juicier.

APHRODISIAC ACTIONS

adaptogen: works in wide-ranging ways to support overall body functioning, leading to an increased ability to navigate and withstand stress

antidepressant: alleviates depression

aromatic: has a pleasant and distinctive smell

brain tonic: supports brain health

circulatory stimulant: increases circulation

cardioprotective: protects the heart and arteries

cardiotonic: strengthens and tones heart muscle and arteries

demulcent: soothes and protects mucous membranes, often mucilaginous

eases menstrual pain

emotionally uplifting

endocrine system tonic: supports endocrine system health

energizing: brings vitality and energy in the moment

energy building: increases overall energy available

ergogenic: enhances physical performance and stamina

euphoric: contributes to feelings of happiness and excitement

hormone balancing

improves fertility

muscle relaxant

nervine: supports the nervous system; calms nerves

neuroprotective: protects nerve cells from damage

nutritive: provides nourishment

reproductive system tonic: supports health of reproductive system

restorative: helps to bring back energy, vitality, and health

soothing and healing for skin

vasodilator: dilates blood vessels

SAFETY CONSIDERATIONS FOR HERBS NOT FEATURED IN MONOGRAPHS

PERFUME HERBS

(These considerations were all taken into account in the Evoke Perfume formulation.)

Bergamot (*Citrus bergamia*) essential oil: Phytotoxic if used in a dilution of more than 0.4 percent of a blend.

Vetiver (*Vetiveria zizanioides*) essential oil: Nontoxic, nonirritating. Has isoeugenol, so under 15 percent dilution is advised.

Ylang-ylang (*Cananga odorata*) essential oil: Nontoxic, though it may cause skin irritation or be sensitizing, especially on inflamed or damaged skin. Use in low (0.8% or less) dilution when applying to skin. If overused, it may irritate skin or cause headaches or nausea.

HOT LIPS LIP BALM

Sweet orange (*Citrus sinensis*) essential oil: Nontoxic. It may cause skin irritation in dilution over one percent. Older, oxidized oils increase potential for skin irritation. It's best to buy citrus oils from organically grown fruit, as citrus trees are heavily sprayed. The citrus oils are cold pressed, and the pesticides come through the process and are found in the oils.

CHAI HERBS

(those with safety issues)

Nutmeg (*Myristica fragrans*): Avoid during pregnancy.

Whole cloves (*Syzygium aromaticum*): Can be irritating in large doses.

Black peppercorns (*Piper nigrum*): Large doses may cause nausea and may increase the effects of pharmaceutical drugs in unexpected ways.

Fennel (*Foeniculum vulgare*): Not recommended in pregnancy for medicinal use. Caution is recommended in women with a history or risk of estrogen receptor–positive cancer.

Astragalus (*Astragalus membranaceus*): Make sure you buy *Astragalus membranaceous*. Avoid during acute illness. Do not use with immunosuppressive drugs.

Burdock root (*Arctium lappa*): Not for use in first trimester of pregnancy.

OTHER HERBS

Calendula (*Calendula officinalis*): Not recommended during pregnancy.

Gingko (*Ginkgo biloba*): Use caution when taking blood thinners. Not for use in pregnancy or lactation.

Lavender (*Lavandula angustifolia*): Not recommended in large doses during pregnancy.

Nettle (*Urtica dioica*): Not recommended to be eaten after plant has gone to flower/seed. Use with caution if you have a dry constitution.

Rosemary (*Rosmarinus officinalis*): Not recommended in large doses during pregnancy. May lower blood glucose.

CHAPTER 1: SLOWING DOWN TO ENJOY THE EROTIC ENERGY OF LIFE

1. K. Baser, A. Altintas, and M. Kürkçüoglu, "Turkish Rose: A Review of the History, Ethnobotany, and Modern Uses of Rose Petals, Rose Oil, Rose Water, and Other Rose Products," *Herbal-Gram* 96 (2012): 40–53, http://cms.herbalgram.org/herbalgram/issue96/hg96-feat-rose.html.

2. M. Mahboubi, "*Rosa damascena* as Holy Ancient Herb with Novel Applications." *Journal of Traditional and Complementary Medicine* 6, no. 1 (January 2016): 10–16, doi: 10.1016/j.jtcme.2015.09.005.

3. Mahboubi, "*Rosa damascena* as Holy Ancient Herb with Novel Applications."

4. P. Pattanittum et al., "Dietary Supplements for Dysmenorrhoea," *Cochrane Database of Systematic Reviews*, March 22, 2016, doi: 10.1002/14651858.cd002124.pub2.

5. B. Mars, *The Sexual Herbal: Prescriptions for Enhancing Love and Passion* (Rochester, VT: Healing Arts Press, 2002); G. F. Edwards, *Opening Our Wild Hearts to the Healing Herbs* (Woodstock, NY: Ash Tree Publishing, 2000).

6. Z. Ayati et al., "Phytochemistry, Traditional Uses and Pharmacological Profile of Rose Hip: A Review," *Current Pharmaceutical Design* 24, no. 35 (2019): 4101–4124, doi: 10.2174/1381612824666181010151849; Baser, "Turkish Rose"; U. Andersson et al., "Effects of Rose Hip Intake on Risk Markers of Type 2 Diabetes and Cardiovascular Disease: A Randomized, Double-Blind, Cross-Over Investigation in Obese Persons," *European Journal Of Clinical Nutrition* 66, no. 5 (2011): 585–590, doi: 10.1038/ejcn.2011.203.

7. A. Leahu et al., "Influence of Processing on Vitamin C Content of Rosehip Fruits," *Scientific Papers: Animal Science and Biotechnologies* 47, no. 1 (2014): 116–120.

8. L. Phetcharat, K. Wongsuphasawat, and K. Winther, "The Effectiveness of a Standardized Rose Hip Powder, Containing Seeds and Shells of *Rosa canina* on Cell Longevity, Skin Wrinkles, Moisture, and Elasticity," *Clinical Interventions in Aging* 2015, no. 10 (November 2015): 1849–1856, doi: 10.2147/cia.s90092.

9. Baser, "Turkish Rose."

CHAPTER 2: CREATING ENVIRONMENTS WHERE LOVE AND EROS FLOURISH

1. D. Winston and S. Maimes, *Adaptogens: Herbs for Strength, Stamina, and Stress Relief* (Rochester, VT: Healing Arts Press, 2007); G. F. Edwards, *Opening Our Wild Hearts to the Healing Herbs* (Woodstock, NY: Ash Tree Publishing, 2000); S. Mills and K. Bone, *Principle and Practices of Phytotherapy* (London, UK: Churchill Livingstone, 2000).

2. V. P. Saka, S. R. Challa, and A. B. Raju, "Effect of *Avena sativa* (Oats) on Spermatogenesis and Reproductive Health," *Journal of Endocrinology and Reproduction* 20, no. 2 (2016): 83–92, doi: 10.18311/jer/2016/15471.

3. R. Gladstar, *Rosemary Gladstar's Family Herbal: A Guide to Living Life with Energy, Health, and Vitality* (North Adams, MA: Storey Publishing, 2001).

4. D. Hoffmann, *Medical Herbalism: The Science and Practice of Herbal Medicine* (Rochester, VT: Healing Arts Press, 2003); Gladstar, *Rosemary Gladstar's Family Herbal.*

5. G. Nemecz, "Hawthorn," *Pharmacists Manitoba Communication Journal*, February 2001: 10–13, https://www.pharmacistsmb.ca/files/2001/Jan-Feb/Hawthorn.pdf.

6. Hoffmann, *Medical Herbalism*; Gladstar, *Rosemary Gladstar's Family Herbal.*

7. jim mcdonald, personal communication with author.

8. Y. Luo, P. Shang, and D. Li, "Luteolin: A Flavonoid That has Multiple Cardio-Protective Effects and Its Molecular Mechanisms," *Frontiers in Pharmacology* 8 (2017): 692, doi: 10.3389/fphar.2017.00692.

9. X. Che et al., "Vitexin Exerts Cardioprotective Effect on Chronic Myocardial Ischemia/Reperfusion Injury in Rats via Inhibiting Myocardial Apoptosis and Lipid Peroxidation," *American Journal of Translational Research* 8, no. 8 (August 15, 2016): 3319–3328.

10. B. Mars, *The Sexual Herbal: Prescriptions for Enhancing Love and Passion* (Rochester, VT: Healing Arts Press, 2002).

CHAPTER 3: FALLING IN LOVE WITH YOUR BODY

1. G. F. Gonzales et al., "Maca (*Lepidium meyenii Walp*), a Review of Its Biological Properties" [Article in Spanish], *Revista Peruana de Medicina Experimental y Salud Publica* 31, no. 1 (2014): 100–110.

2. H.O. Meissner et al., "Hormone-Balancing Effect of Pre-gelatinized Organic Maca (*Lepidium peruvianum Chacon*): (III) Clinical Responses of Early-Postmenopausal Women to Maca in Double Blind, Randomized, Placebo-Controlled, Crossover Configuration, Outpatient Study" *International Journal of Biomedical Science* 2, no. 4 (2006): 375–394; B. Mars, *The Sexual Herbal: Prescriptions for Enhancing Love and Passion* (Rochester, VT: Healing Arts Press, 2002).

3. S. Wang and F. Zhu, "Chemical Composition and Health Effects of Maca (*Lepidium meyenii*)" *Food Chem* 288 (2019): 422–443, doi: 10.1016/j.foodchem.2019.02.071; Mars, *The Sexual Herbal.*

4. M. S. Lee et al., "Maca (*Lepidium meyenii*) for Treatment of Menopausal Symptoms: A Systematic Review," *Maturitas* 70, no. 3 (2011): 227–233, doi: 10.1016/j.maturitas.2011.07.017; Meissner et al., "Hormone-Balancing Effect of Pre-gelatinized Organic Maca"; Mars, *The Sexual Herbal.*

5. Mars, *The Sexual Herbal.*

6. Y. Zhang, F. Zhou, and F. Ge, "Effects of Combined Extracts of *Lepidium meyenii* and *Allium tuberosum Rottl.* on Erectile Dysfunction," *BMC Complementary and Alternative Medicine* 19, no. 1 (December 2019): 135, doi: 10.1186/s12906-019-2542-4.

7. M. S. Lee et al., "The Use of Maca (*Lepidium meyenii*) to Improve Semen Quality: A Systematic Review, *Maturitas* 92 (2016): 64–69, doi: 10.1016/j.maturitas.2016.07.013.

8. T. Zenico et al., "Subjective Effects of *Lepidium meyenii* (Maca) Extract on Well-Being and Sexual Performances in Patients with Mild Erectile Dysfunction: A Randomised, Double-Blind Clinical Trial," *Andrologia* 4, no. 2 (2009): 95–99, doi: 10.1111/j.1439-0272.2008.00892.x.

9. G. F. Gonzales, "Ethnobiology and Ethnopharmacology of *Lepidium meyenii* (Maca), a Plant from the Peruvian Highlands," *Evidence-Based Complementary and Alternative Medicine* 2012 (2012): 1–10, doi: 10.1155/2012/193496.

10. J. J. Chen et al., "Macamides Present in the Commercial Maca (*Lepidium meyenii*) Products and the Macamide Biosynthesis Affected by Postharvest Conditions," *International Journal of Food Properties* 20, no. 12 (2017): 3112–3123, doi: 10.1080/10942912.2016.1274905; D. Winston and S. Maimes, *Adaptogens: Herbs for Strength, Stamina, and Stress Relief* (Rochester, VT: Healing Arts Press, 2007).

11. K. Jeager, "Some Foods, Activities Can Stimulate Your Endocannabinoid System," *Integr8 Health/Healer.com*, January 24, 2019, accessed April 8, 2020, https://healer.com/some-foods-activities-can-stimulate-your-endocannabinoid-system.

12. Gonzales, "Ethnobiology and Ethnopharmacology of *Lepidium meyenii* (Maca)."

13. Mars, *The Sexual Herbal.*

CHAPTER 4: THE JOY OF PAMPERING

1. R. Gladstar, *Rosemary Gladstar's Family Herbal: A Guide to Living Life with Energy, Health, and Vitality* (North Adams, MA: Storey Publishing, 2001).

2. Harvard SPH, "Oats," *The Nutrition Source, Harvard T.H. Chan School of Public Health*, accessed April 8, 2020, https://www.hsph.harvard.edu/nutritionsource/food-features/oats.

3. R. Singh, S. De, and A. Belkheir, "*Avena sativa* (Oat), a Potential Neutraceutical and Therapeutic Agent: An Overview," *Critical Reviews in Food Science and Nutrition* 53 (2013): 126–144, doi: 10.1080/10408398.2010.526725; G. F. Edwards, *Opening Our Wild Hearts to the Healing Herbs* (Woodstock, NY: Ash Tree Publishing, 2000).

4. B. Mars, *The Sexual Herbal: Prescriptions for Enhancing Love and Passion* (Rochester, VT: Healing Arts Press, 2002).

5. P. Rasane et al., "Nutritional Advantages of Oats and Opportunities for Its Processing as Value Added Foods—A Review," *Journal*

of Food Science and Technology 52, no. 2 (2013): 662–675, doi: 10.1007/s13197-013-1072-1.

6. Edwards, *Opening Our Wild Hearts to the Healing Herbs*; jim mcdonald, "Nettles, Oats, and You," *jim mcdonald Herbalist*, https://herbcraft.org/nettles%20oats%20and%20you.pdf.

7. S. Weed, *Down There: Sexual and Reproductive Health the Wise Woman Way* (Woodstock, NY: Ash Tree Publishing, 2011).

8. Mars, *The Sexual Herbal.*

9. D. Winston and S. Maimes, *Adaptogens: Herbs for Strength, Stamina, and Stress Relief* (Rochester, VT: Healing Arts Press, 2007); Edwards, *Opening Our Wild Hearts to the Healing Herbs*; S. Mills and K. Bone, *Principle and Practices of Phytotherapy* (London, UK: Churchill Livingstone, 2000).

10. Weed, *Down There.*

11. V. P. Saka, S. R. Challa, and A. B. Raju, "Effect of *Avena sativa* (Oats) on Spermatogenesis and Reproductive Health," *Journal of Endocrinology and Reproduction* 20, no. 2 (2016): 83–92, doi: 10.18311/jer/2016/15471.

CHAPTER 5: THE DANCE OF RELATIONSHIP

1. M. Orr, "Damiana," *The Essential Herbal* issue 99, May-June 2018, 10–12.

2. R. Gladstar, *Rosemary Gladstar's Family Herbal: A Guide to Living Life with Energy, Health, and Vitality* (North Adams, MA: Storey Publishing, 2001).

3. S. Palacios et al., "Effect of a Multi-Ingredient-Based Food Supplement on Sexual Function in Women with Low Sexual Desire," *BMC Women's Health* 19, no. 1 (2019): 58, doi: 10.1186/s12905-019-0755-9; B. Mars, *The Sexual Herbal: Prescriptions for Enhancing Love and Passion* (Rochester, VT: Healing Arts Press, 2002).

4. Orr, "Damiana"; Gladstar, *Rosemary Gladstar's Family Herbal.*

5. Mars, *The Sexual Herbal*; Gladstar, *Rosemary Gladstar's Family Herbal.*

6. Palacios et al., "Effect of a Multi-Ingredient-Based Food Supplement on Sexual Function"; K. Szewczyk and C. Zidorn, "Ethnobotany, Phytochemistry, and Bioactivity of the Genus *Turnera* (*Passifloraceae*) with a Focus on Damiana—*Turnera diffusa*," *Journal of Ethnopharmacology* 152, no. 3 (2014): 424–443, doi: 10.1016/j.jep.2014.01.019.

7. S. Weed, *Down There: Sexual and Reproductive Health the Wise Woman Way* (Woodstock, NY: Ash Tree Publishing, 2011).

8. Gladstar, *Rosemary Gladstar's Family Herbal.*

9. D. B. Ana María et al., "Neurobehavioral and Toxicological Effects of an Aqueous Extract of *Turnera diffusa Willd* (*Turneraceae*) in Mice," *Journal of Ethnopharmacology* 236 (2019): 50–62, doi: 10.1016/j.jep.2019.02.036.

10. D. Winston and S. Maimes, *Adaptogens: Herbs for Strength, Stamina, and Stress Relief* (Rochester, VT: Healing Arts Press, 2007).

11. Mars, *The Sexual Herbal.*

12. N. Chaurasiya et al., "Selective Inhibition of Human Monoamine Oxidase B by Acacetin 7-Methyl Ether Isolated from *Turnera dif-*

fusa (*Damiana*)," *Molecules* 24, no. 4 (2019): 810, doi: 10.3390/molecules24040810.

13. S. Kumar, R. Madaan, and A. Sharma, "Pharmacological Evaluation of Bioactive Principle of *Turnera aphrodisiaca*," *Indian Journal of Pharmaceutical Sciences* 70, no. 6 (2008): 740, doi: 10.4103/0250-474x.49095.

CHAPTER 6: STOKING YOUR FIRE FOR SEXUAL FULFILLMENT

1. S. Mills and K. Bone, *Principle and Practices of Phytotherapy* (London, UK: Churchill Livingstone, 2000).

2. Q. Q. Mao et al., "Bioactive Compounds and Bioactivities of Ginger (*Zingiber officinale Roscoe*)," *Foods* 8, no. 6 (2019): 185, doi: 10.3390/foods8060185.

3. M. Sahardi, N. F. Nabilah, and S. Makpol, "Ginger (*Zingiber officinale Roscoe*) in the Prevention of Ageing and Degenerative Diseases: Review of Current Evidence," *Evidence-Based Complementary and Alternative Medicine* 2019 (August 20, 2019): 1–13, doi: 10.1155/2019/5054395; Mills and Bone, *Principle and Practices of Phytotherapy*.

4. R. Gladstar, *Rosemary Gladstar's Family Herbal: A Guide to Living Life with Energy, Health, and Vitality* (North Adams, MA: Storey Publishing, 2001).

5. S. A. Banihani, "Effect of Ginger (*Zingiber officinale*) on Semen Quality," *Andrologia* 51, no. 6 (July 2019): e13296, doi: 10.1111/and.13296; B. Mars, *The Sexual Herbal: Prescriptions for Enhancing Love and Passion* (Rochester, VT: Healing Arts Press, 2002).

6. N. Yilmaz et al., "Ginger (*Zingiber officinale*) Might Improve Female Fertility: A Rat Model," *Journal of the Chinese Medical Association* 81, no. 10 (2018): 905–911, doi: 10.1016/j.jcma.2017.12.009.

7. P. Pattanittum et al., "Dietary Supplements for Dysmenorrhoea," *Cochrane Database of Systematic Reviews*, March 22, 2016, doi: 10.1002/14651858.cd002124.pub2; C. X. Chen, B. Barrett, and K. L. Kwekkeboom, "Efficacy of Oral Ginger (*Zingiber officinale*) for Dysmenorrhea: A Systematic Review and Meta-Analysis," *Evidence-Based Complementary and Alternative Medicine* 2016 (2016): 1–10, doi: 10.1155/2016/6295737; E. Jenabi, "The Effect of Ginger for Relieving of Primary Dysmenorrhea," *Journal of Pakistan Medical Association* 63, no. 1 (2019): 8–10.

8. F. Kashefi et al., "Effect of Ginger (*Zingiber officinale*) on Heavy Menstrual Bleeding: A Placebo-Controlled, Randomized Clinical Trial," *Phytotherapy Research* 29, no. 1 (January 2015): 114–119, doi: 10.1002/ptr.5235.

9. M. Nikkah Bodagh, I. Maleki, and A. Hekmatdoost, "Ginger in Gastrointestinal Disorders: A Systematic Review of Clinical Trials," *Food Science & Nutrition* 7, no. 1 (January 2019): 96–108, doi: 10.1002/fsn3.807; R. de la Forêt, *Alchemy of Herbs: Transform Everyday Ingredients into Foods and Remedies That Heal* (Carlsbad, CA: Hay House, 2017); Mills and Bone, *Principle and Practices of Phytotherapy*.

10. Sahardi, Nabilah, and Makpol, "Ginger (*Zingiber officinale Roscoe*) in the Prevention of Ageing and Degenerative Diseases."

11. Mao et al., "Bioactive Compounds and Bioactivities of Ginger (*Zingiber officinale Roscoe*)."

CHAPTER 7: CHANNELING EROTIC ENERGY INTO VITALITY AND CREATIVITY

1. R. de la Forêt, *Alchemy of Herbs: Transform Everyday Ingredients into Foods and Remedies That Heal* (Carlsbad, CA: Hay House, 2017); K. P. S. Khalsa and M. Tierra, *The Way of Ayurvedic Herbs* (Twin Lakes, WI: Lotus Press, 2008); D. Winston and S. Maimes, *Adaptogens: Herbs for Strength, Stamina, and Stress Relief* (Rochester, VT: Healing Arts Press, 2007).

2. R. Gladstar, *Rosemary Gladstar's Family Herbal: A Guide to Living Life with Energy, Health, and Vitality* (North Adams, MA: Storey Publishing, 2001).

3. de la Forêt, *Alchemy of Herbs*.

4. de la Forêt, *Alchemy of Herbs*.

5. Khalsa and Tierra, *The Way of Ayurvedic Herbs*.

6. Winston and Maimes, *Adaptogens*.

7. M. K. Kaushik et al., "Triethylene Glycol, an Active Component of Ashwagandha (*Withania somnifera*) Leaves, Is Responsible for Sleep Induction," *PLOS One* 12 no. 2 (February 16, 2017): e0172508, doi: 10.1371/journal.pone.0172508.

8. Kaushik et al., "Triethylene Glycol, an Active Component of Ashwagandha."

9. Khalsa and Tierra, *The Way of Ayurvedic Herbs*.

10. J. Prakash et al., "*Withania somnifera* Alleviates Parkinsonian Phenotypes by Inhibiting Apoptotic Pathways in Dopaminergic Neurons," *Neurochemical Research* 39, no. 12 (December 2014): 2527–2536, doi: 10.1007/s11064-014-1443-7; B. Mars, *The Sexual Herbal: Prescriptions for Enhancing Love and Passion* (Rochester, VT: Healing Arts Press, 2002).

11. K. Narinderpa, N. Junaid, and B. Raman, "A Review on Pharmacological Profile of *Withania somnifera* (Ashwagandha)" *Journal of Botanical Sciences* 2, no. 4 (2013): 6–14, http://www.rroij.com/open-access/a-review-on-pharmacological-profile-of-withania-somnifera-ashwagandha.php?aid=33844.

12. D. S. Mandlik (Ingawale) and A. G. Namdeo, "Pharmacological Evaluation of Ashwagandha Highlighting Its Healthcare Claims, Safety, and Toxicity Aspects," *Journal of Dietary Supplements*, April 3, 2020 (2020): 1–4, doi: 10.1080/19390211.2020.1741484; Khalsa and Tierra, *The Way of Ayurvedic Herbs*.

13. G. Kaur et al., "*Withania somnifera* Shows a Protective Effect in Monocrotaline-Induced Pulmonary Hypertension," *Pharmaceutical Biology* 53, no. 1 (January 2, 2015): 147–157, doi: 10.3109/13880209.2014.912240; Mars, *The Sexual Herbal*.

CHAPTER 8: RELAXING INTO YOUR BODY

1. H. C. Chua et al., "Kavain, the Major Constituent of the Anxiolytic Kava Extract, Potentiates GABA$_A$ Receptors: Functional Characteristics and Molecular Mechanism," *PLOS ONE* 11, no. 6 (June 22, 2016): e0157700, doi: 10.1371/journal.pone.0157700.

2. F. Schifano et al., "Novel Psychoactive Substances of Interest for Psychiatry," *World Psychiatry* 14, no. 1 (February 2015): 15–26, doi: 10.1002/wps.20174.

3. H. Butler and M. Korbonits, "Cannabinoids for Clinicians: The Rise and Fall of the Cannabinoid Antagonists," *European Journal of Endocrinology* 161, no. 5 (November 2009): 655–662, doi: 10.1530/eje-09-0511.

4. jim mcdonald, "Kava Kava," *jim mcdonald Herbalist,* https: // herbcraft.org/kava.html.

5. mcdonald, "Kava Kava"; B. Mars, *The Sexual Herbal: Prescriptions for Enhancing Love and Passion* (Rochester, VT: Healing Arts Press, 2002); R. Gladstar, *Rosemary Gladstar's Family Herbal: A Guide to Living Life with Energy, Health, and Vitality* (North Adams, MA: Storey Publishing, 2001); D. D. Jamieson et al., "Comparison of the Central Nervous System Activity of the Aqueous and Lipid Extract of Kava (*Piper methysticum*)," *Archives Internationales de Pharmacodynamie et de Therapie* 301 (Sep–Oct 1989): 66–80.

6. mcdonald, "Kava Kava."

7. S. L. Ooi, P. Henderson, and S. C. Pak, "Kava for Generalized Anxiety Disorder: A Review of Current Evidence," *Journal of Alternative and Complementary Medicine* 24, no. 8 (2017): 770–780, doi: 10.1089/acm.2018.0001.

8. R. Trickey, *Women, Hormones, and the Menstrual Cycle: Herbal and Medical Solutions from Adolescence to Menopause,* 2nd ed. (Crows Nest NSW, Australia: Allen & Unwin, 2003).

9. mcdonald, "Kava Kava."

10. Gladstar, *Rosemary Gladstar's Family Herbal.*

CHAPTER 9: DEEP NOURISHMENT

1. J. M. Jung et al., "The Effects of a Standardized *Acanthopanax koreanum* Extract on Stress-Induced Behavioral Alterations in Mice," *Journal of Ethnopharmacology* 148, no. 3 (July 2013): 826–834, doi: 10.1016/j.jep.2013.05.019; D. Winston and S. Maimes, *Adaptogens: Herbs for Strength, Stamina, and Stress Relief* (Rochester, VT: Healing Arts Press, 2007).

2. T. Saito et al., "The Fruit of *Acanthopanax senticosus (Rupr. et Maxim.)* Harms Improves Insulin Resistance and Hepatic Lipid Accumulation by Modulation of Liver Adenosine Monophosphate-Activated Protein Kinase Activity and Lipogenic Gene Expression in High-Fat Diet-Fed Obese Mice," *Nutrition Research* 36, no. 10 (October 2016): 1090–1097, doi: 10.1016/j.nutres.2016.09.004; K. Y. Liu et al., "Release of Acetylcholine by Syringin, an Active Principle of *Eleutherococcus senticosus*, to Raise Insulin Secretion in Wistar Rats," *Neuroscience Letters* 434, no. 2 (March 2008): 195–199, doi: 10.1016/j.neulet.2008.01.054.

3. L. Jin et. al., "A Comparative Study on Root and Bark Extracts of *Eleutherococcus senticosus* and Their Effects on Human Macrophages," *Phytomedicine* 68 (March 2020): article 153181, doi: 10.1016/j.phymed.2020.153181; R. Trickey, *Women, Hormones, and the Menstrual Cycle: Herbal and Medical Solutions from Adolescence to Menopause,* 2nd ed. (Crows Nest NSW, Australia: Allen & Unwin, 2003); B. Mars, *The Sexual Herbal: Prescriptions for Enhancing Love and Passion* (Rochester, VT: Healing Arts Press, 2002).

4. A. Panossian and G. Wikman, "Evidence-Based Efficacy of Adaptogens in Fatigue, and Molecular Mechanisms Related to Their Stress-Protective Activity," *Current Clinical Pharmacology* 4, no. 3 (September 2009): 198–219, doi: 10.2174/157488409789375311; Trickey, *Women, Hormones, and the Menstrual Cycle.*

5. Trickey, *Women, Hormones, and the Menstrual Cycle.*

6. Winston and Maimes, *Adaptogens.*

7. F. Li et al., "Syringin Prevents Cardiac Hypertrophy Induced by Pressure Overload through the Attenuation of Autophagy," *International Journal of Molecular Medicine* 39, no. 1 (2016): 199–207, doi: 10.3892/ijm.2016.2824; Winston and Maimes, *Adaptogens.*

8. Li et al., "Syringin Prevents Cardiac Hypertrophy."

CHAPTER 10: NAVIGATING TIMES OF CHALLENGE AND STRESS

1. R. de la Forêt, *Alchemy of Herbs: Transform Everyday Ingredients into Foods and Remedies That Heal* (Carlsbad, CA: Hay House, 2017); P. Pattanayak et al., "*Ocimum sanctum Linn.* A Reservoir Plant for Therapeutic Applications: An Overview," *Pharmacognosy Reviews* 4, no. 7 (2010): 95, doi: 10.4103/0973-7847.65323; K. P. S. Khalsa and M. Tierra, *The Way of Ayurvedic Herbs* (Twin Lakes, WI: Lotus Press, 2008); D. Winston and S. Maimes, *Adaptogens: Herbs for Strength, Stamina, and Stress Relief* (Rochester, VT: Healing Arts Press, 2007).

2. Winston and Maimes, *Adaptogens.*

3. Winston and Maimes, *Adaptogens.*

4. Khalsa and Tierra, *The Way of Ayurvedic Herbs.*

5. de la Forêt, *Alchemy of Herbs.*

6. de la Forêt, *Alchemy of Herbs;* Pattanayak et al., "*Ocimum sanctum Linn.*"

7. F. Forouzanfar and H. Hosseinzadeh, "Medicinal Herbs in the Treatment of Neuropathic Pain: A Review," *Iranian Journal of Basic Medical Sciences* 21, no. 4 (April 2018): 347–358, doi: 10.22038/IJBMS.2018.24026.6021.

8. de la Forêt, *Alchemy of Herbs;* Khalsa and Tierra, *The Way of Ayurvedic Herbs.*

9. Pattanayak et al., "*Ocimum sanctum Linn.*"; Khalsa and Tierra, *The Way of Ayurvedic Herbs.*

10. Pattanayak et al., "*Ocimum sanctum Linn.*"

11. de la Forêt, *Alchemy of Herbs;* Khalsa and Tierra, *The Way of Ayurvedic Herbs.*

12. A. A. Kamyab and A. Eshraghian, "Anti-inflammatory, Gastrointestinal and Hepatoprotective Effects of *Ocimum sanctum Linn*: An Ancient Remedy with New Application," *Inflammation & Allergy: Drug Targets* 12, no. 6 (2013): 378–384, doi: 10.2174/187 1528112666131125110017.

13. S. P. Gautami and R. P. Sudha, "Efficacy of *Ocimum sanctum,* Aloe Vera and Chlorhexidine Mouthwash on Gingivitis: A Randomized Controlled Comparative Clinical Study," *AYU*

(An International Quarterly Journal of Research in Ayurveda) 40, no. 1 (2019): 23–26, doi: 10.4103/ayu.AYU_212_18.

14. Pattanayak et al., "*Ocimum sanctum Linn.*"

15. Z. Krajcovicová and V. Melus, "Bioactivity and Potential Health Benefits of Rosmarinic Acid," *University Review* 7, no. 2 (August 2013): 8–14.

16. Khalsa and Tierra, *The Way of Ayurvedic Herbs.*

17. Khalsa and Tierra, *The Way of Ayurvedic Herbs.*

CHAPTER 11: HEALING

1. B. Mars, *The Sexual Herbal: Prescriptions for Enhancing Love and Passion* (Rochester, VT: Healing Arts Press, 2002); G. F. Edwards, *Opening Our Wild Hearts to the Healing Herbs* (Woodstock, NY: Ash Tree Publishing, 2000).

2. A. M. Jazani et al., "Herbal Medicine for Oligomenorrhea and Amenorrhea: A Systematic Review of Ancient and Conventional Medicine," *BioMed Research International* 2018 (2018): 1–22, doi: 10.1155/2018/3052768; D. Koupý, H. Kotolová, and J. R. Kuˇserová, "Effectiveness of Phytotherapy in Supportive Treatment of Type 2 Diabetes Mellitus II. Fenugreek (*Trigonella foenum-graecum*)" [Article in Czech], *Ceska a Slovenska Frmacie* 64, no. 3 (June 2015): 67–71; Mars, *The Sexual Herbal*; G. F. Edwards, *Opening Our Wild Hearts to the Healing Herbs* (Woodstock, NY: Ash Tree Publishing, 2000).

3. K. P. S. Khalsa and M. Tierra, *The Way of Ayurvedic Herbs* (Twin Lakes, WI: Lotus Press, 2008).

4. Khalsa and Tierra, *The Way of Ayurvedic Herbs*; R. Trickey, *Women, Hormones, and the Menstrual Cycle: Herbal and Medical Solutions from Adolescence to Menopause*, 2nd ed. (Crows Nest NSW, Australia: Allen & Unwin, 2003); R. Gladstar, *Rosemary Gladstar's Family Herbal: A Guide to Living Life with Energy, Health, and Vitality* (North Adams, MA: Storey Publishing, 2001); Edwards, *Opening Our Wild Hearts to the Healing Herbs.*

5. S. Zameer et al., "A Review on Therapeutic Potentials of *Trigonella foenum graecum* (Fenugreek) and Its Chemical Constituents in Neurological Disorders: Complementary Roles to Its Hypolipidemic, Hypoglycemic, and Antioxidant Potential," *Nutritional Neuroscience* 21, no. 8 (2018): 539–545, doi: 10.1080/1028415X.2017.1327200; Edwards, *Opening Our Wild Hearts to the Healing Herbs.*

6. X. Che et al., "Vitexin Exerts Cardioprotective Effect on Chronic Myocardial Ischemia/Reperfusion Injury in Rats via Inhibiting Myocardial Apoptosis and Lipid Peroxidation," *American Journal of Translational Research* 8, no. 8 (August 15, 2016): 3319–3328.

7. A. M. Jazani et al., "A Comprehensive Review of Clinical Studies with Herbal Medicine on Polycystic Ovary Syndrome (PCOS)" *DARU Journal of Pharmaceutical Sciences* 27, no. 2 (December 2019): 863–877, doi: 10.1007/s40199-019-00312-0; S. Weed, *Down There: Sexual and Reproductive Health the Wise Woman Way* (Woodstock, NY: Ash Tree Publishing, 2011); Mars, *The Sexual Herbal*; Edwards, *Opening Our Wild Hearts to the Healing Herbs.*

8. M. N. Najafi and M. Ghazanfarpour, "Effect of Phytoestrogens on Sexual Function in Menopausal Women: A Systematic Review and Meta-Analysis," *Climacteric* 21, no. 5 (September 3, 2018): 437–445, doi: 10.1080/13697137.2018.1472566; Koupý, Kotolová, and Kuˇserová, "Effectiveness of Phytotherapy in Supportive Treatment of Type 2 Diabetes Mellitus II"; Khalsa and Tierra, *The Way of Ayurvedic Herbs*; Trickey, *Women, Hormones, and the Menstrual Cycle*; Mars, *The Sexual Herbal*; Edwards, *Opening Our Wild Hearts to the Healing Herbs.*

9. R. Kargozar, H. Azizi, and R. Salari, "A Review of Effective Herbal Medicines in Controlling Menopausal Symptoms," *Electronic Physician* 9, no. 11 (November 2017): 5826–5833, doi: 10.19082/5826; Mars, *The Sexual Herbal*; Edwards, *Opening Our Wild Hearts to the Healing Herbs.*

10. Edwards, *Opening Our Wild Hearts to the Healing Herbs.*

11. Weed, *Down There.*

12. Khalsa and Tierra, *The Way of Ayurvedic Herbs.*

13. Khalsa and Tierra, *The Way of Ayurvedic Herbs*; Gladstar, *Rosemary Gladstar's Family Herbal*; Edwards, *Opening Our Wild Hearts to the Healing Herbs.*

14. Khalsa and Tierra, *The Way of Ayurvedic Herbs.*

15. A. Maheshwari et al., "Efficacy of Furosap™, a Novel *Trigonella foenum-graecum* Seed Extract, in Enhancing Testosterone Level and Improving Sperm Profile in Male Volunteers," *International Journal of Medical Sciences* 14, no. 1 (2017): 58–66, doi: 10.7150/ijms.17256; Weed, *Down There*; Mars, *The Sexual Herbal*; Edwards, *Opening Our Wild Hearts to the Healing Herbs.*

16. S. A. Wani and P. Kumar, "Fenugreek: A Review on Its Nutraceutical Properties and Utilization in Various Food Products," *Journal of the Saudi Society of Agricultural Sciences* 17, no. 2 (2018): 97–106, doi: 10.1016/j.jssas.2016.01.007.

17. Koupý, Kotolová, and Kuˇserová, "Effectiveness of Phytotherapy in Supportive Treatment of Type 2 Diabetes Mellitus II."

CHAPTER 12: SHARING DELICIOUS DELICACIES

1. M. J. Baggott et al., "Psychopharmacology of Theobromine in Healthy Volunteers," *Psychopharmacology* 228, no. 1 (July 2013): 109–118, doi: 10.1007/s00213-013-3021-0.

2. E. O. Afoakwa et al., "Chemical Composition and Physical Quality Characteristics of Ghanaian Cocoa Beans as Affected by Pulp Pre-conditioning and Fermentation," *Journal of Food Science and Technology* 50, no. 6 (2013): 1097–1105, doi: 10.1007/s13197-011-0446-5.

3. F. Bianchi-Demicheli, L. Sekoranja, and A. Pechère-Bertschi, "Sexuality, Heart and Chocolate" [Article in French], *Revue Médicale Suisse* 9, no. 378 (2013): 624–629.

4. B. Mars, *The Sexual Herbal: Prescriptions for Enhancing Love and Passion* (Rochester, VT: Healing Arts Press, 2002).

5. J. P. Garcia et al., "The Cardiovascular Effects of Chocolate," *Reviews in Cardiovascular Medicine* 19, no. 4 (December 30, 2018): 123–127, doi: 10.31083/j.rcm.2018.04.3187; R. Franco, A. Oñatibia-Astibia, and E. Martínez-Pinilla, "Health Benefits of Methylxanthines in Cacao and Chocolate," *Nutrients* 5, no. 10 (2013): 4159–4173, doi: 10.3390/nu5104159.

6. R. de la Forêt, *Alchemy of Herbs: Transform Everyday Ingredients into Foods and Remedies That Heal* (Carlsbad, CA: Hay House, 2017); Mars, *The Sexual Herbal*.

7. Q. R. de Araujo et al., "Cocoa and Human Health: From Head to Foot—a Review," *Critical Reviews in Food Science and Nutrition* 56, no. 1 (January 2, 2016): 1–12, doi: 10.1080/10408398.2012.657921.

8. Franco, "Health Benefits of Methylxanthines in Cacao and Chocolate."

CHAPTER 13: WELCOME TO VITAL LIVING!

1. A. Nowak et al., "Potential of *Schisandra chinensis (Turcz.) Baill.* in Human Health and Nutrition: A Review of Current Knowledge and Therapeutic Perspectives," *Nutrients* 11, no. 2 (2019): 333, doi: 10.3390/nu11020333.

2. Nowak et al., "Potential of *Schisandra chinensis (Turcz.) Baill.*"

3. D. Winston and S. Maimes, *Adaptogens: Herbs for Strength, Stamina, and Stress Relief* (Rochester, VT: Healing Arts Press, 2007); B. Mars, *The Sexual Herbal: Prescriptions for Enhancing Love and Passion* (Rochester, VT: Healing Arts Press, 2002).

4. Winston and Maimes, *Adaptogens*; R. Trickey, *Women, Hormones, and the Menstrual Cycle: Herbal and Medical Solutions from Adolescence to Menopause*, 2nd ed. (Crows Nest NSW, Australia: Allen & Unwin, 2003); Mars, *The Sexual Herbal*.

5. S. Weed, *Down There: Sexual and Reproductive Health the Wise Woman Way* (Woodstock, NY: Ash Tree Publishing, 2011); A. Panossian and G. Wikman, "Pharmacology of *Schisandra chinensis Bail.*: An Overview of Russian Research and Uses in Medicine" *Journal of Ethnopharmacology* 118, no. 2 (2008): 183–212, doi: 10.1016/j.jep.2008.04.020; Winston and Maimes, *Adaptogens*; R. Gladstar, *Rosemary Gladstar's Family Herbal: A Guide to Living Life with Energy, Health, and Vitality* (North Adams, MA: Storey Publishing, 2001).

6. Trickey, *Women, Hormones, and the Menstrual Cycle*.

7. Mars, *The Sexual Herbal*.

8. Weed, *Down There*.

9. Mars, *The Sexual Herbal*.

10. Winston and Maimes, *Adaptogens*.

11. T. Khadivzadeh et al., "A Systematic Review and Meta-Analysis on the Effect of Herbal Medicine to Manage Sleep Dysfunction in Peri- and Postmenopause," *Journal of Menopausal Medicine* 24, no. 2 (2018): 92–99, doi: 10.6118/jmm.2018.24.2.92.

12. Mars, *The Sexual Herbal*.

13. Nowak et al., "Potential of *Schisandra chinensis (Turcz.) Baill.*"

Alchemy of Herbs: Transform Everyday Ingredients into Foods and Remedies that Heal, by Rosalee de la Forêt. New York: Hay House, 2017.

Ecosexuality: When Nature Inspires the Arts of Love, by Serenagaia Anderlini-D'Onofrio and Lindsay Hagamen. Puerto Rico: 3WayKiss via CreateSpace, 2015.

Extended Massive Orgasm: How You Can Give and Receive Intense Sexual Pleasure, by Steve Bodansky, Ph.D., and Vera Bodansky, Ph.D. Alameda, CA: Hunter House, 2000.

Female Ejaculation and the G-Spot: Not Your Mother's Orgasm Book, by Deborah Sundahl. Alameda, CA: Hunter House, 2003.

Herbal Healing for Men: Remedies and Recipes, by Rosemary Gladstar. North Adams, MA: Storey Publishing, 2017.

Herbal Healing for Women: Simple Home Remedies for Women of All Ages, by Rosemary Gladstar. New York: Fireside, 1993.

Non-Violent Communication: A Language of Compassion, by Marshall B. Rosenberg. Del Mar, CA: Puddle Dancer Press, 1999.

Pussy: A Reclamation, by Regena Thomashauer. New York: Hay House, 2016.

Vagina, by Naomi Wolf. New York: Ecco, 2012.

Self Compassion: Stop Beating Yourself Up and Leave Insecurity Behind, by Kristin Neff. New York: William Morrow, 2011.

Slow Sex: The Path to Fulfilling and Sustainable Sexuality, by Diana Richardson. Rochester, VT: Destiny Books, 2011.

Taoist Secrets of Love: Cultivating Male Sexual Energy, by Mantak Chai and Michael Winn. Santa Fe: Aurora Press, 1984.

The Artist's Way: A Spiritual Path to Higher Creativity, by Julia Cameron. New York: Tarcher/Putnam, 1992.

Undefended Love, by Jett Psaris, Ph.D., and Marlena S. Lyons, Ph.D. Oakland, CA: New Harbinger, 2000.

Wild Remedies: How to Forage Healing Foods and Craft Your Own Herbal Medicine, by Rosalee de la Forêt and Emily Han. New York: Hay House, 2020.

Women's Anatomy of Arousal: Secret Maps to Buried Pleasure, by Sheri Winston. New York: Mango Garden Press, 2010.

RECOMMENDED RESOURCES

It is always best to source your herbs and supplies locally if you can. You may be able to gather herbs locally right from nature, or you can look for local herbalists, herb shops, co-ops, or organic farms. Local herbs will likely be the freshest, and buying from local folks helps support them and reduces the environmental impacts involved with shipping.

Sometimes you won't be able to find things locally, so I'll suggest some online resources as well.

Mountain Rose Herbs:
mountainroseherbs.com

Pacific Botanicals:
pacificbotanicals.com

Dandelion Botanical Company:
dandelionbotanical.com

Banyan Botanicals:
banyanbotanicals.com

Frontier Co-op:
frontiercoop.com

For quality essential oils:

Appalachian Valley Natural Products:
av-at.com

Snow Lotus:
snowlotus.org

CONTRIBUTORS

Hanna Nicole, healing foods chef, consultant, and caterer

Hanna contributed in many ways to this project. She created and helped develop many unique and wonderful recipes especially for this book. She is also the creative brain behind many of the recipe names.

Hanna also brought her budding skills as an artistic director to this project. She spent countless hours with Peter and me developing photo ideas and then worked with Jen and the models to make those photos come to life.

In her time as my assistant, Hanna fully devoted herself to the success of this project, and she and I shared tears and triumphs throughout the writing and production process. This book would not be what it is without her contributions.

PHOTOGRAPHY

Jen Lee Light, jenleelight.com

Most of the chapter opener photos and many of the recipe photos in *Aphrodisiac* are the work of Jen Lee Light.

Peter Rubens, peterpaulrubens.com

You'll find Peter's photographic work on the cover of *Aphrodisiac*, the Chapter 9 opener photo, and some select recipe photos.

7Song, 7song.com, for his beautiful photos of damiana on pages 148 and 150.

Jenny Barandich for her photo on page 123.

RECIPES

Rebecca Altman, wonderbotanica.comabout-rebecca

Rosalee de la Forêt, *Alchemy of Herbs: Transform Everyday Ingredients into Foods and Remedies that Heal* (New York: Hay House, 2017).

Diana De Luca, *Botanica Erotica: Arousing Body, Mind, and Spirit.* (Rochester, VT: Healing Arts Press, 1988).

Emily Han, *Wild Drinks and Cocktails* (Beverly, MA: Fair Winds Press, 2016).

Rosemary Gladstar, *The Family Herbal: A Guide to Living Life with Energy, Health, and Vitality* (North Adams, MA: Storey Publishing, 2001).

Karin Rose

POETRY

Dona Nieto, www.LaTigresa.net. Excerpt from "Biosexual" from *Naked Sacred Earth Poems,* by Dona Nieto (La Tigresa) (Berkeley: Regent Press, 2010), copyright Donna Nieto 2010, used by permission of the author.

Meredith Heller, www.BonesofSynchronicity.com.

Lorin Roche, *The Radiance Sutras: 112 Gateways to the Yoga of Wonder and Delight* (Boulder, CO: Sounds True, 2014).

Wahkeena Sitka, www.wahkeenasitka.com

Danna Faulds, *Prayers to the Infinite: New Yoga Poems* (Kearney, NE: Morris Publishing, 2004).

Artemis Mandala

Rachel Naomi Remen, M.D., *Kitchen Table Wisdom: Stories That Heal* (New York: Berkley, 1996).

Jewel Matheison, jewel@vom.com

Courtney Walsh, soul-lit.com/poems/v4/Walsh/index.html

CONTENT

Betty Martin, bettymartin.org

Kushad Watson and **Wendy Jarvis,** for sharing their Relating Meditation.

Jon Young and **Wilderness Awareness School**, for the inspiration for the Sensory Meditation.

METRIC CONVERSION CHART

Standard Cup	Fine Powder (e.g., flour)	Grain (e.g., rice)	Granular (e.g., sugar)	Liquid Solids (e.g., butter)	Liquid (e.g., milk)
1	140 g	150 g	190 g	200 g	240 ml
³/₄	105 g	113 g	143 g	150 g	180 ml
²/₃	93 g	100 g	125 g	133 g	160 ml
½	70 g	75 g	95 g	100 g	120 ml
⅓	47 g	50 g	63 g	67 g	80 ml
¼	35 g	38 g	48 g	50 g	60 ml
⅛	18 g	19 g	24 g	25 g	30 ml

Useful Equivalents for Cooking/Oven Temperatures

Process	Fahrenheit	Celsius	Gas Mark
Freeze Water	32° F	0° C	
Room Temperature	68° F	20° C	
Boil Water	212° F	100° C	
Bake	325° F	160° C	3
	350° F	180° C	4
	375° F	190° C	5
	400° F	200° C	6
	425° F	220° C	7
	450° F	230° C	8
Broil			Grill

Useful Equivalents for Liquid Ingredients by Volume

¼ tsp			1 ml
½ tsp			2 ml
1 tsp			5 ml
3 tsp	1 tbsp	½ fl oz	15 ml
	2 tbsp	⅛ cup	1 fl oz	30 ml
	4 tbsp	¼ cup	2 fl oz	60 ml
	5⅓ tbsp	⅓ cup	3 fl oz	80 ml
	8 tbsp	½ cup	4 fl oz	120 ml
	10²/₃ tbsp	²/₃ cup	5 fl oz	160 ml
	12 tbsp	¾ cup	6 fl oz	180 ml
	16 tbsp	1 cup	8 fl oz	240 ml
	1 pt	2 cups	16 fl oz	480 ml
	1 qt	4 cups	32 fl oz	960 ml
			33 fl oz	1000 ml	1 L

Useful Equivalents for Dry Ingredients by Weight

(To convert ounces to grams, multiply the number of ounces by 30.)

1 oz	¹/₁₆ lb	30 g
4 oz	¼ lb	120 g
8 oz	½ lb	240 g
12 oz	¾ lb	360 g
16 oz	1 lb	480 g

Useful Equivalents for Length

(To convert inches to centimeters, multiply the number of inches by 2.5.)

1 in			2.5 cm	
6 in	½ ft		15 cm	
12 in	1 ft		30 cm	
36 in	3 ft	1 yd	90 cm	
40 in			100 cm	1 m

INDEX

ACKNOWLEDGMENTS

Oh my goodness! There are so many people to thank for their help with this book project. I had no idea when I set out on this endeavor how many people would devote time and energy to helping me make this book a reality.

First, I must thank my devoted husband, John, whose unflagging love and support has seen me through all of the intense ups and downs of the research, writing, and book production process. John's belief in me and my work is what led to the book contract with Hay House, and his willingness to apply his marketing genius to getting this book out into the world may very well be what led to it being in your hands right now.

I must thank my son and daughter as well, as they have continually encouraged me to follow my passions and do my work in the world, even though it has meant I've had less time with my "mom hat" on as I've made my way through this book-writing process.

I also want to thank each of the Aphrodisiac Circle participants who stepped into this project with me when I wrote to them on my 50th birthday. They dedicated time and energy to this project over the course of a whole year and shared deeply and vulnerably with me and with each other so that we could gift you with substantive stories of real people and the effects of the herbs on their lives. Several of these participants were also early readers for the book, offering feedback and suggestions.

I must also thank my editor at Hay House, Anne Barthel, who has been a delight to work with, has improved this manuscript many times over with her excellent suggestions, and whose human connection with me through the trials and tribulations of my production process helped me to continue on.

I am grateful to the whole production team at Hay House for all of their work to make *Aphrodisiac* what it is. Thank you to Reid Tracy for giving me this opportunity to become a Hay House author, and to Tricia Breidenthal and Karla Baker and the rest of the layout team for taking on the complex task of making this book beautiful!

Thank you also to George Rezendes of Toolshed Soundlab, who was my sound engineer and producer for the audio version of *Aphrodisiac*. This was a vulnerable book to read aloud and George made the experience a complete delight. I am thankful for his professionalism, expertise, and genuine interest in my project.

I want to thank all of my models for volunteering their time and vulnerably sharing their beautiful bodies and spirits with all of us.

I am grateful to Susan Marynowski and Emma Jaqueth for their help with monograph researching and to Emma for playing with Hanna and me in the kitchen as we developed and tested recipes for the book. I want to thank all of the LearningHerbs community members who volunteered time, energy, and ingredients to test the recipes in the book.

I also want to thank Rosalee de la Forêt, who consulted with me regularly over the time that I was writing and always encourages me to share my voice with the world. I want to thank Karin Rose from LearningHerbs, who graciously helped with some of my herbal research as well.

I must thank all of my many friends who provided moral support along the way, and a special thank you to friends who dove in and read my manuscript and offered helpful suggestions and encouragement. Most especially, I want to thank my circle of women friends, the Pussy Posse, for their ongoing unconditional love and support.

Thank you to all of the herbalists whose experiences and research added richness to this work. Thank you to Sally King, and EagleSong Gardner, my herbal mentors at RavenCroft Garden, who got me started on this herbal path.

I want to especially thank my *Aphrodisiac* production team. Thank you to Tanya Brakeman for her project management time, energy, and effort. She organized the recipe testing process and helped me gain permission to include some of my favorite poetry in this book. Tanya put in *many* volunteer hours during our photo shoot and worked above and beyond the call of duty in countless ways throughout the production process.

Peter Rubens was a core part of that team as well. Peter embarked on this project with me thinking he would be the main photographer for the book. He devoted countless hours to the project, offering editing suggestions and developing ideas for photographic illustration of the material. He spent hours in the rain photographing plants for me, and generated the amazing cover photo for this book. More than that, though, he was a pillar of enthusiastic support for both me and the book, bringing his full self to this work. I will be forever grateful for his contributions.

And thank you, thank you to Hanna Nicole, who also jumped into the project with her whole being. Hanna contributed in all the ways detailed on the Contributors page and was devoted to me and to the success of *Aphrodisiac* throughout the process of its creation.

Finally, I want to thank Jen Lee Light, who stepped in as photographer late in the game and created incredible beauty for us all to enjoy!

ABOUT THE AUTHOR

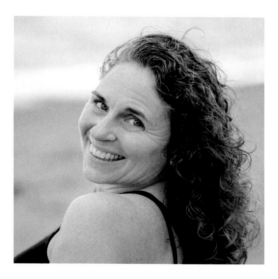

Kimberly Gallagher is an herbalist who has been working with healing plants for over 20 years. She is co-founder with her husband, John Gallagher, of LearningHerbs, one of the most respected online herbal education websites. She is the creator of the *Wildcraft!* board game, which has sold more than 100,000 copies worldwide, and author of the *Herb Fairies* children's books. Kimberly and John have two grown-up children and are into their third decade of marriage. For many years, Kimberly has been actively exploring healthy sexuality, which involves the power of sexuality for healing and erotic energy as source energy for creative, vital living. Kimberly is an ordained minister at her Trail of Beauty ministry, where sacred sensuality is at the heart of her work.
Website: learningherbs.com

How to make sure your lotion comes out perfect every time.

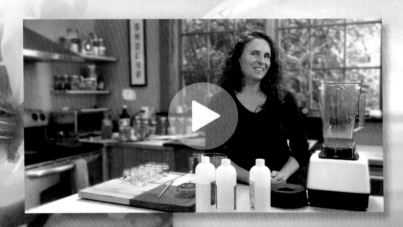

Kimberly invites you into her kitchen to show you the subtle secrets to making one of her most popular recipes in this book. You'll learn, step by step, how to make your first luscious batch of "Love Your Body Lotion."

Watch the video FREE at

www.Aphrodisiac.recipes

We hope you enjoyed this Hay House book. If you'd like to receive our online catalog featuring additional information on Hay House books and products, or if you'd like to find out more about the Hay Foundation, please contact:

Hay House, Inc., P.O. Box 5100, Carlsbad, CA 92018-5100
(760) 431-7695 or (800) 654-5126
(760) 431-6948 (fax) or (800) 650-5115 (fax)
www.hayhouse.com® • www.hayfoundation.org

———

Published in Australia by: Hay House Australia Pty. Ltd.,
18/36 Ralph St., Alexandria NSW 2015
Phone: 612-9669-4299 • *Fax:* 612-9669-4144
www.hayhouse.com.au

Published in the United Kingdom by: Hay House UK, Ltd.,
The Sixth Floor, Watson House, 54 Baker Street, London W1U 7BU
Phone: +44 (0)20 3927 7290 • *Fax:* +44 (0)20 3927 7291
www.hayhouse.co.uk

Published in India by: Hay House Publishers India,
Muskaan Complex, Plot No. 3, B-2, Vasant Kunj, New Delhi 110 070
Phone: 91-11-4176-1620 • *Fax:* 91-11-4176-1630
www.hayhouse.co.in

———

Access New Knowledge.
Anytime. Anywhere.

Learn and evolve at your own pace
with the world's leading experts.

www.hayhouseU.com

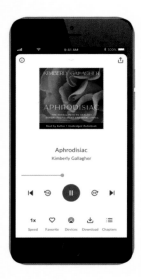